ICSU Short Reports 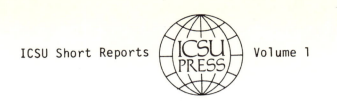 Volume 1

Advances in Gene Technology: Human Genetic Disorders

Proceedings of the Sixteenth
Miami Winter Symposium
Miami, Florida, U.S.A.
January 16-20, 1984

Edited by

Walter A. Scott, Fazal Ahmad, Sandra Black,
Julius Schultz and William J. Whelan

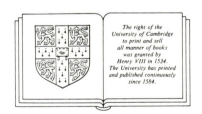

The right of the
University of Cambridge
to print and sell
all manner of books
was granted by
Henry VIII in 1534.
The University has printed
and published continuously
since 1584.

CAMBRIDGE UNIVERSITY PRESS
Cambridge
London New York New Rochelle
Melbourne Sydney

Published by the Press Syndicate of the University of Cambridge
The Pitt Building, Trumpington Street, Cambridge CB2 1RP
32 East 57th Street, New York, NY 10022, USA
296 Beaconsfield Parade, Middle Park, Melbourne 3206, Australia

© The ICSU Press 1984

First published 1984

Printed in Great Britain at the University Press, Cambridge

Library of Congress catalogue card number: 84-550

British Library Cataloguing in Publication Data

Miami Winter Symposium (16th: 1984)
    Advances in gene technology. –
    (ICSU short reports; v. 1)
    1. Medical genetics
    I. Title   II. Scott, W. A.
    616'.042   RB155

    ISBN 0 521 26749 8

Contents

SYMPOSIUM PRESENTATIONS

ONCOGENES

TRANSLOCATIONS AND GENE ACTIVATION

MECHANISMS OF GENE ACTIVATION

THE MAJOR HISTOCOMPATIBILITY LOCI

HUMAN GENETIC ORGANIZATION

HYBRIDIZATION, IMMUNOLOGICAL AND ENZYMIC TECHNIQUES

POSTER SESSION REPORTS

PREFACE

This is the record of the 16th Miami Winter Symposium, the joint venture of the Department of Biochemistry of the University of Miami School of Medicine and the University-affiliated Papanicoloau Cancer Research Institute, both located in Miami, Florida, U.S.A. with the Symposium being held at the Konover Hotel, Miami Beach, during January 16-20, 1984.

The proceedings are published in the form of "Short Reports", presented to the registrants and, after revision, available simultaneously for open sale. The first part of the reports (Symposium Presentations) represents the contributions from the invited speakers, the second part (Poster Session Reports), constitutes the free communications that were presented in three sessions on January 16, 17 and 19.

The aforementioned revision of the Short Reports has consisted in deleting five poster reports that, while originally submitted, were not presented at the Symposium. Three late-entry posters have been added. The topicality of this state-of-the-art compilation is shown by its going to press less than 3 weeks after the Symposium ended.

Not included here is the keynote address at the Symposium, the Lynen Lecture, delivered by Philip Leder on January 16, 1984, under the title: "A New Genesis for Genetics and Medicine". This will appear in Vol. 1, no. 1 (July 1984) of BioEssays, a new current-awareness journal to be published for the ICSU Press by Cambridge University Press.

INTRODUCTION

We are happy to collaborate with the ICSU Press in this new-style format for the proceedings of the Miami Winter Symposia. We have enjoyed working these many years first with the North-Holland Publishing Company and then since 1972 with Academic Press, Inc. in publishing the proceedings of the Miami Winter Symposia in the form of extended presentations by the invited speakers together with the abstracts of the poster sessions.

We feel now, however, that the times call for a new style of reporting symposia. The ICSU Short Reports represent this new style and offer the opportunity to disseminate research results and conclusions as rapidly as possible.

This is an experiment. We would like to hope that it will succeed and we have the confidence to believe that we have made the right decision in changing the reporting route. We welcome your comments and suggestions for the future.

William J. Whelan
Professor and Chairman
University of Miami
School of Medicine

Julius Schultz
President, Papanicolaou
Cancer Research Institute

ICSU SHORT REPORTS

A MESSAGE FROM THE ICSU PRESS

This is the first volume of what will be a continuing series of meeting reports arising from the ICSU Press. What, it may be asked, is ICSU? It is the International Council of Scientific Unions, an international, non-governmental, scientific organization made up of 20 international scientific unions together with more than 80 national members, scientific and national associates. Many of you will be familiar with individual members such as the International Union of Biochemistry or the U.S. National Academy of Sciences but probably not with ICSU itself. ICSU is the "United Nations" umbrella organization that allows these different unions and national members to come together to confront problems of common interest and take advantage of opportunities for collaboration that are only possible on an international, interdisciplinary scale.

ICSU and its member unions and committees are active through most parts of the world in arranging conferences, congresses, symposia, training schools, meetings of experts, as well as meetings to decide policies and programs. Interdisciplinary committees function in multi- or transdisciplinary fields such as genetic experimentation, problems of the environment, space and oceanic research. Close relations are maintained with UNESCO, particularly in helping scientists in developing areas in such matters as teaching and the development of science and technology. Programs of global scope are mounted such as the World Climate Research Program, the International Geological Correlation Project, International Biosciences Network, etc.

The individual family members produce a wide range of publications including monographs, symposia, congress proceedings, scientific journals for original research or reviews, data compilations, standards, etc. The decision was taken in January 1983 that, in parallel with the organized publication activities of individual ICSU members, ICSU itself would create its own publishing house, the ICSU Press.

Now one year old, the Press already has a number of projects in hand of which these ICSU Short Reports is one. Others include semi-popular expositions of the scientific activities of the ICSU family, symposia proceedings, a news and review journal, BioEssays, to cover the new biology, as well as service publications.

The ICSU Press may be contacted via its Chairman, Dr. W.J. Whelan, P.O. Box 016129, Miami, Florida 33101, U.S.A. or its Secretary/Treasurer, Dr. D.P. Den Os, Bureau van de Rijksuniversiteit te Leiden, Postbus 9500, Stationsweg 46, NL-2300 RA Leiden, Netherlands.

The ICSU Short Reports are based on a style which is becoming increasingly popular and which addresses a problem associated with the widespread use of posters to present short communications at scientific meetings. These posters are extremely informative. Their presenters go to a great deal of pains to put their message across in a compact, easily understandable fashion, but the poster is displayed for no more than half a day and in a large meeting often is not seen even by participants in whose area of research it falls. All that remains for posterity is the abstract that was prepared many months before the meeting, is out of date at the time of the meeting and contains but a fraction of the information imparted by the poster.

The reporting format used here is an attempt to allow the presenter to commit the poster to paper. The two-page spread can be used to convey a great deal of information by way of introduction, methodology, results, conclusions, bibliography, diagrams, figures and tables. Produced to a very tight deadline, only two months before the meeting, the short report acts as an up-to-date, permanent record of the poster, and the immediate availability of the volume of short reports to libraries and persons who could not attend the meeting makes this a very timely and we hope effective method of publication. To our invited speakers we have allotted more space, hopefully enough to convey the essence of their message and, at the same time, to remove the burden that afflicts the active scientist who attracts a host of symposia speaking engagments. None of us wish to burden the literature with repetitive publications of the same material. The summary presented here allows the speaker to present a digest of his findings and, through the bibliography, to direct the person who wishes to explore the subject in more depth to the original seminal papers on which the speaker's contribution is based.

It is a pleasure to acknowledge that this reporting concept was brought to the ICSU Press by a prominent member of the Board of Management, Professor Lars Ernster, who at the same time is the Secretary General of ICSU.

We thank all the contributors to this first volume of the ICSU Short Reports, the beginner of what will be a continuing and important series. When referring to any paper from this volume you should use the citation:

ICSU Short Reports, 1 (1984) first page-last page.

Oncogenes

ACTIVATION OF CELLULAR TRANSFORMING GENES

IN NEOPLASMS

Geoffrey M. Cooper

Laboratory of Molecular Carcinogenesis,
Dana-Farber Cancer Institute,
and Department of Pathology,
Harvard Medical School
Boston, MA 02115

Many neoplasms contain transforming genes which efficiently induce transformation of NIH 3T3 mouse cells upon transfection (see 1 for review). Since DNAs of normal cells lack efficient transforming activity, these results indicate that the development of neoplasms can involve dominant genetic alterations resulting in the activation of cellular transforming genes which are then detectable by their biological activity in transfection assays. Activated transforming genes have been identified in a wide variety of neoplasms including carcinomas, sarcomas, neuroblastomas, lymphomas and leukemias of human, rodent and chicken origin. These neoplasms include spontaneously-occurring tumors, chemically-induced tumors and virally-induced tumors. In addition, transforming genes have been detected by transfection of DNAs from primary neoplasms as well as tumor-derived cell lines.

At present several distinct cellular transforming genes have been identified in different types of neoplasms. The biochemical properties and distribution of these genes in tumors is discussed below.

ras genes:

Blot-hybridization analysis initially identified the transforming genes activated in a human bladder and lung carcinoma cell line as cellular homologs of the transforming genes of Harvey (ras^H) and Kirsten (ras^K) sarcoma viruses, respectively (2-4). Activation of ras^H has been reported in only one additional human tumor, so it is not a commonly occurring transforming gene in human neoplasms. However, activation of ras^K has been reported in a variety of different human tumors, including carcinomas of the bladder, colon, lung, gall bladder and pancreas, a rhabdomyosarcoma, and a T cell leukemia. Another member of the ras gene family, ras^N, has also been detected as an activated transforming gene in several human neoplasms including a neuroblastoma, a colon carcinoma, fibrosarcomas, a Burkitt's lymphoma, and myeloid and T cell leukemias.

These three different members of the ras gene family are thus activated in a variety of neoplasms without apparent specificity in relation to cell type. However, they are activated in a relatively small fraction (10-20%) of human neoplasms. It is possible that ras genes can contribute to development of neoplasia in a wide variety of different cells but are not essential for development of any particular type of neoplasm. Alternatively, further studies may reveal a common underlying biological property of neoplasms specifically correlated with ras gene activation.

The ras genes encode proteins of approximately 21,000 daltons (designated p21) which are localized in the plasma membrane and bind guanine nucleotides. Comparisons of ras gene expression in normal and malignant human cells have indicated that the level of p21 expression in neoplasms which contain activated ras genes is elevated only about 5-fold compared to normal bladder epithelial cells and is not different from the level of p21 in human carcinoma cell lines which do not contain activated ras genes detectable by transfection (5). In several cases, it has now been found that activation of transforming activity of ras[H] (6,7) and ras[K] (5,8,9) genes is a consequence of mutations which affect the structure of ras gene expression. In addition, different mutations can activate the same ras gene in different individual neoplasms. How these alterations affect the biochemical activities of ras gene products remains to be elucidated.

Blym-1

The Blym-1 transforming gene was initially identified by transfection of DNAs of chicken B cell lymphomas (10). Activation of Blym-1 was detected in DNAs of six out of six chicken lymphomas analyzed, but not in DNAs of normal tissues of the same individual birds, indicating that in contrast to ras genes, activation of this gene is a highly reproducible event in lymphomagenesis.

The isolated chicken Blym-1 transforming gene is unusually small (approximately 0.6 kb) and its nucleotide sequence indicated that it encodes a predicted protein product of 65 amino acids (7,800 daltons) (11). Comparison of the amino acid sequence of the predicted chicken Blym-1 gene product with amino acid sequences of known cellular proteins revealed partial homology (36%) between the chicken Blym-1 transforming protein and the amino-terminal region of transferrin family proteins. This homology is concentrated in regions which are conserved between legitimate members of the transferrin family, suggesting a common ancestry for the chicken Blym-1 transforming protein and the amino terminal sequences of transferrins. Since transferrin has been implicated as a lymphocyte growth factor, it is intriguing to speculate that this homology may also suggest a functional relationship.

Blot hybridization analysis indicated that the chicken Blym-1 transforming gene was a member of a family of 6-8 related genes in both chicken and human DNAs. The detection of human genes homologous to Blym-1 suggested the possibility that the transforming genes detected by transfection of some human lymphocyte neoplasm DNAs might be members of this Blym gene family. This was initially approached by analysis of a transforming gene detected by transfection of DNAs of Burkitt's lymphomas, which are human B-cell lymphomas representing the same stage of B cell differentiation (surface immunoglobulin-positive) as the chicken B-cell lymphomas from which chicken Blym-1 was isolated. These experiments (12) indicated that a human homolog of chicken Blym-1 was activated in DNAs of six out of six Burkitt's lymphomas investigated. Characterization of the isolated human Blym-1 transforming gene indicates that, like chicken Blym-1, it is less than 1 kb and is not homologous to retroviral transforming genes.

Blot hybridization analysis indicated that Blym-1 is not re-arranged in either chicken or human lymphomas. In addition, activation of Blym-1 in Burkitt's lymphomas is not associated with an increased level of gene expression. It therefore appears likely that activation of Blym-1, like ras genes, is a consequence of structural mutations.

Transforming Genes of Other Lymphoid Neoplasms

Distinct transforming genes have been identified by transfection of DNAs of human and mouse neoplasms representing other stages of B- and T- lymphocyte differentiation (13). Like Blym-1, these genes are activated in a high fraction (80-100%) of the neoplasms which have been investigated. Analysis of the susceptibility of these transforming genes to cleavage with a series of restriction endonucleases indicates that they include a gene common to human and mouse pre B cell neoplasms, a different gene common to human myelomas and mouse plasmacytomas, a third gene common to human and mouse neoplasms of intermediate T lymphocytes and a fourth gene common to human and mouse neoplasms of mature T lymphocytes.

The transforming genes activated in lymphocyte neoplasms thus appear to be specifically related to the stage of normal cell differentiation exhibited by those neoplasms. This suggests the possibility that transformation may result from alterations in genes that are normally involved in differentiation-specific control of cell proliferation. In addition, the specificity of the transforming genes activated in these neoplasms further supports the role of these genes in the disease process.

Transforming Genes and Pathogenesis of Neoplasms

The development of neoplastic disease is classically considered a multi-step process involving a series of progressive changes, rather than a single-step conversion of a normal cell to a neoplastic cell. Thus, most neoplasms develop with long latent periods and through a series of progressive pre-neoplastic and neoplastic pathological stages. It is therefore expected that oncogenesis will involve more than simply the activation of a single transforming gene.

Candidates for such events have been identified in both chicken and human B cell lymphomas. Induction of chicken B cell lymphomas by retroviruses involves transcriptional activation of c-myc as a consequence of adjacent integration of viral regulatory sequences (14). Burkitt's lymphomas are closely associated with chromosomal translocations which have recently been found to occur in the region of c-myc (15,16). Since c-myc is not homologous to Blym-1, these observations suggest that at least two distinct transforming genes are involved in pathogenesis of B cell lymphomas of both chicken and man.

Activation of multiple transforming genes has also been observed in neoplasms other than B-cell lymphomas, including mouse mammary carcinomas, Abelson virus-induced mouse pre-B-cell lymphomas, and mouse plasmacytomas. It is an attractive hypothesis that activation of multiple transforming genes in neoplasms identifies genes which function at different stages of tumor development.

REFERENCES

1. Cooper, G.M. (1982) Science 217, 801.
2. Der, C.J., Krontiris, T.G. and Cooper, G.M. (1982) Proc. Natl. Acad. Sci. USA 79, 3637.
3. Parada, L.F., Tabin, C.J., Shih, C., and Weinberg, R.A. (1982) Nature 297, 474.
4. Santos, E., Tronick, S.R., Aaronson, S.A., Pulciani, S., and Barbacid, M. (1982) Nature 298, 343.
5. Der, C.J. and Cooper, G.M. (1983) Cell 32, 201.
6. Tabin, C.J., Bradley, S.M., Bargmann, C.I., Weinberg, R.A., Papageorge, A.G., Scolnick, E.M., Dhar, R., Lowy, D.R., and Chang, E.H. (1982) Nature 300, 143.
7. Reddy, E.P., Reynolds, R.K., Santos, E., and Barbacid, M. (1982) Nature 300, 149.
8. Shimizu, K., Birnbaum, D., Ruley, M.A., Fasano, O., Suard, Y., Edlund, L., Taparowsky, E., Goldfarb, M., and Wigler, M. (1983) Nature 304, 497.
9. Capon, D.J., Seeburg, P.H., McGrath, J.P., Hayflick, J.S., Edman, U., Levinson, A.D., and Goeddel, D.V. (1983) Nature 304, 507.
10. Cooper, G.M. and Neiman, P.E. (1980) Nature 287, 656.
11. Goubin, G., Goldman, D.S., Luce, J., Neiman, P.E. and Cooper, G.M. (1983) Nature 302, 114.
12. Diamond, A., Cooper, G.M., Ritz, J., and Lane, M.-A. (1983) Nature 305, 112.
13. Lane, M.-A., Sainten, A., and Cooper, G.M. (1982) Cell 28, 873.
14. Hayward, W.S., Neel, B.G. and Astrin, S.M. (1981) Nature 290, 475.
15. Dalla-Favera, R., Gregni, M., Erikson, J., Patterson, D., Gallo, R.C., and Croce, C.M. (1982) Proc. Natl. Acad. Sci. USA 79, 7824.
16. Taub, R., Kirsch, I., Morton, C., Lenoir, G., Swarz, D., Tronick, G., Aaronson, S., and Leder, P. (1982) Proc. Natl. Acad. Sci. USA 79, 7837.

HUMAN ONC GENES, T-CELL GROWTH FACTORS (IL-2) AND THE FAMILY OF
HUMAN RETROVIRUSES CALLED HTLV

R. C. Gallo, P. S. Sarin, W. C. Saxinger, M. Robert-Guroff, and
F. Wong-Staal, Laboratory of Tumor Cell Biology, National Cancer
Institute, Bethesda, Maryland 20205

Retroviruses are a major cause of naturally occurring leukemias
and lymphomas in several animal species, including chickens, mice,
cows, cats and subhuman primates. These viruses are useful tools
for the study of the genes involved in abnormal growth (cellular onc
or c-onc genes) and the DNA nucleotide sequences which regulate the
c-onc sequences.
Retroviruses can be classified as endogenous or exogenous.
Endogenous retroviruses are transmitted genetically, are not generally associated with the production of malignancy, and do not carry
onc genes. Exogenous retroviruses, on the other hand, have a replication cycle which requires integration of viral genetic material
into the host cellular DNA. The exogenous retroviruses are subdivided into (a) the chronic leukemia viruses and (b) the acute leukemia viruses. The chronic leukemia viruses induce a wide spectrum
of disease in animals after a long latency period and are usually
believed to be unable to transform cells in culture because they do
not contain a viral transforming or onc gene (v-onc). The acute
leukemia viruses have been isolated from both laboratory induced and
naturally occurring tumors. Their genomes contain onc genes which
code for a transforming protein. These onc genes are derived from
normal cellular genes of the host and are highly conserved. Some
c-onc genes are activated in tumors caused by avian chronic leukemia
viruses, e.g., the avian leukosis virus-induced B-cell lymphoma.
The v-onc genes, identified and subsequently molecularly cloned from
the acutely transforming retroviruses, have been used to identify,
isolate and characterize various c-onc genes from humans.
HUMAN C-ONC GENES. We have been interested in the role of c-onc
genes in growth, differentiation and neoplastic transformation of
human blood cells. Molecular cloning of human DNA sequences homologous to several v-onc genes has been carried out in our laboratory
and include sis, fes, myb, and myc. We have examined a number of
human cells for the expression of (abl), myc, myb, (ras^H), sis, and
fes. The abl and ras^H genes are expressed at low levels (1-5 copies
per cell) in all hematopoietic cells examined and may be important
for some basic cellular functions. Myc is transcribed in all hematopoietic cells examined, including normal peripheral blood lymphocytes
before or after stimulation with PHA. The only exception is term-
inally differentiated HL60 cells where myc and myb transcription is
turned off. The myb gene is expressed in the early precursor cells
of lymphoid, myeloid, and erythroid lineages, but there is little or
no expression relatively early in B-cell differentiation, or late
in T-cell or myeloid cell differentiation. The sis and fes genes
are not commonly transcribed in hematopoietic cells. An exception
is the human T-cell transformed by HTLV which frequently express
c-sis (see below). We found the c-myc gene amplified in a human

promyelocytic leukemia (HL-60) and in collaboration with C. Croce we and others (see P. Leder's paper) found c-myc translocated in human Burkitt's lymphoma. In this report we will summarize our findings on a human chronic leukemia virus and its role in T-cell malignancies.

HUMAN T-CELL LEUKEMIA VIRUS (HTLV): BACKGROUND AND ISOLATION. Consideration of an etiological role of retroviruses in human cancers was frequently met with skepticism until the recent isolation of HTLV because of the difficulty of detection of low levels of retroviruses in human cells, while the animal models, especially murine and feline leukemias, were associated with abundant virus production and viraemia. In addition, all mammalian retroviruses shared some common antigenic determinants so that immunological reagents for one virus could be used to detect the presence of other viruses. One animal system, bovine leukosis, however, offered several interesting parallels for the subsequent isolation of a human retrovirus. Although the involvement of bovine leukemia virus (BLV) in the enzootic form of bovine leukosis is well established, the fresh tumor tissues are always virus negative and BLV expression occurs only after prolonged culture of the tumor cells in vitro. These studies point to the importance of long term in vitro culture of appropriate human target cells for the isolation of a human retrovirus.

The discovery of T-cell growth factor (TCGF) or interleukin 2 (Il-2) in 1976 in our laboratory made it possible for the first time to grow both normal and neoplastic mature human T-cells in long term suspension culture. T-cells from normal donors can be grown only after lectin or antigen stimulation. In contrast, certain neoplastic mature T-cells responds to TCGF without prior lectin or antigen activation in vitro. These cells already contain TCGF receptors, now routinely detected by a monoclonal antibody called anti-TAC. It was from some of these cultured T-cell lines established from sporadic cases in the United States with a certain subtype of adult T-cell leukemia-lymphoma (HTLV) that the first unambiguous human retrovirus, HTLV, was isolated.

The first isolate of HTLV was obtained from a lymph node derived T-cell line from a patient (CR) with an aggressive variant of cutaneous T-cell lymphoma; the second isolate, HTLV$_{MB}$ was obtained from a patient with Sezary leukemia. There are now about 35 isolates of HTLV. Isolates have been obtained from cell lines established from patients with mature T-cell malignancies from different parts of the world. These patients include individuals born in the United States, Israel, Japan, the Caribbean, Africa, and South America. Our laboratory in collaborative studies with Y. Ito, T. Nakao, and T. Aoki have isolated HTLV from T-lymphocytes of adult T-cell leukemia-lymphoma (ATLL) patients from Japan and have demonstrated serum antibodies directed against determinants on cells producing these particles in almost all Japanese ATLL patients as well as in 5 to 20% of normal individuals from the endemic areas of Japan. Independent work of other Japanese investigators led to similar findings. All virus isolates from Japan are indistinguishable from the prototype U.S. HTLV isolates. Multiple isolates have been obtained from ATLL patients from blacks originating from the Caribbean. Most of the isolates belong to a particular strain we call HTLV-I. In 1982 we isolated another T-lymphotropic human retrovirus which is distantly related to HTLV-I. This isolate, which we call HTLV-II, was obtained from the cell line MO, derived from a young white male with hairy cell leukemia of a T-cell subtype. Since then HTLV-II has been isolated once from a black IV drug user with AIDS. Very recently we identified possibly a third subgroup (HTLV-III) from a black Caribbean man with ATLL. Old World monkeys are also infected with viruses related to but distinguishable from HTLV-I.

SEROEPIDEMIOLOGY. Most ATLL patients have specific antibodies to HTLV, and there is a high incidence of infection of their normal family members, but sera of the vast majority normal healthy donors and patients with a wide variety of other malignancies in the U.S. were negative for antibody. It has become apparent that most HTLV positive lymphomas and leukemias fall into a clinical syndrome consisting of adult onset, usually with a rapid disease course, often associated with lymphadenopathy and hepatosplenomegaly, circulating large and usually pleomorphic lymphocytes with lobulated nuclei, T-cell surface phenotypic markers (usually OKT4$^+$), and frequent hypercalcemia and skin manifestations.

A seroepidemiological survey of patients with ATLL and normal people from endemic and non-endemic regions of Japan shows that almost all patients with a clinical diagnosis of ATLL have HTLV specific antibodies and that a number of normal individuals from this region are also antibody positive. In collaborative studies with W. Blattner at N.C.I. and N. Gibbs in Jamaica we found an unusually high incidence of antibody to HTLV in patients with lymphoid malignancies from the Caribbean and in a small percentage of normal individuals in this area. Finally, more recent related findings have been made in blacks from southeastern U.S.A., Africa, and South America.

MOLECULAR EPIDEMIOLOGY. The genomes of HTLV-I and HTLV-II have been cloned and the complete nucleotide sequence of an HTLV-I prototype has been determined. Like other retroviruses, HTLV-I contains a long terminal repeat sequence (LTR) as well as sequences coding for the gag, pol, and env proteins. In addition, a region (called pX) between the env gene and 3' LTR can potentially code for four small peptides. We have used the cloned genomes of both HTLV-I and HTLV-II to survey various human hematopoietic malignancies for the presence of viral DNA sequences. This allowed detection of HTLV infection even in the absence of virus expression or antiviral antibodies. In seropositive cases where the patients' diseases are not ATLL, this analysis would also tell us if HTLV played a direct role in these diseases. Our results are as follows:

All of the typical ATLL samples as well as a few cases of more benign cutaneous T-cell lymphoma were positive. All other malignancies including acute and chronic myeloid leukemias, acute lymphocytic leukemias and hairy cell leukemia were negative. Thus, HTLV-I is tightly associated with mature T-cell malignancies, and HTLV-II is an extremely rare variant of HTLV, obviously not the agent associated with hairy cell leukemia in general. With one exception, all fresh tumor cells appear to be clonally infected. One patient (HSt) with

ATLL who migrated to London from the Caribbean was unique in that his cells were polyclonally infected. More detailed analysis of this case is underway. The other leukemic cells contained 1 to 3 copies of proviruses that are either complete or defective. The DNA from leukemic cells of a patient (JM) whose sera was negative for HTLV antigens, contained a single defective provirus.

Leukemic cells of two patients who were seropositive for HTLV but whose diseases were not ATLL were examined. Both samples, a child-hood acute leukemia and a B-CLL did not contain detectable HTLV sequences, although cultured T-cells of the latter did contain HTLV. This result indicates that HTLV does not have a direct role in these patients disease. However, since it has been observed that in HTLV endemic regions, a higher percentage of HTLV positivity was found in patients with lymphoid malignancies in general than normal, it is possible that HTLV-infected T-cells may stimulate the abnormal pro-liferation of B-cells or immature T-cells secondarily. Alterna-tively, HTLV infected individuals may be immune compromized and more prone to develop other malignancies.

IN VITRO TRANSFORMATION. HTLV was transmitted into fresh new-born human or adult bone marrow T-cells and most of the newly infected cells produce virus cord blood cells as observed by the expression of p24, p19 and reverse transcriptase activity. The infected cells resemble neoplastic T-cells in many aspects: (a) they develop lobulated nuclei and some grow as multinucleated giant cells; (b) they have potential for indefinite growth. In contrast, mitogen stimulated cord blood T-cells from the same patients consistently exhibited growth crises after one month in culture, even in the con-tinued presence of TCGF. (c) They have decreased or no requirement for TCGF for growth; and (d) they express high levels of TCGF recep-tors.

Mechanisms of Initiation and Maintenance of Transformation. The normal T-cells infected and transformed in vitro by HTLV and the fresh leukemic cells provide excellent models for studying the mech-anisms of initiation and maintenance of transformation, respectively. We have investigated the role of viral and some cellular genes of possible relevance in these two separate stages. In all of the in vitro infected cells, multiple species of viral mRNA were transcribed at high levels, including a 9.0 Kb genomic size mRNA probably coding for gag, pol, a 4 Kb species that hybridized preferentially to env sequences and was probably the env mRNA and a 2.0 Kb RNA containing only pX and LTR sequences. These results suggest that expression of viral proteins, including the pX region, may be necessary for initia-tion of transformation. However, when fresh leukemic cells were examined, some expressed low levels of viral mRNA while others not at all, suggesting that viral expression is not necessary for mainte-nance of transformation.

We also examined gene activation as a possible mechanism of leukemogensis by HTLV. The obvious candidates are growth factor genes and c-onc genes. All HTLV-infected cells express a high den-sity of T-cell growth factor (TCGF) receptor. A gene we call HT-3, which may be the gene for the receptor, is also expressed at high levels in all HTLV-infected cells. Therefore an attractive model would be expression of TCGF in these same cells resulting in auto-stimulation. Using a cloned TCGF gene as a probe, we detected only an extremely low level of transcripts in a few HTLV-positive cell lines and not in most. Neither is TCGF expressed in the fresh leukemic cells. Therefore, a simple autostimulation mechanism cannot be operative either in initiation or maintenance of the leukemic state. However, it is possible that the TCGF receptor expressed on these cells has been altered so that it now recognizes another growth factor or that in its altered state, it is activated without binding to any factor. There is some evidence that the TCGF receptor expressed in HTLV-infected T-cells may be qualitatively different from that of normal cells (W. Greene, personal communication). Therefore, the receptor for TCGF is a natural focus for future efforts to understand the mechanism of transformation by HTLV. We have also examined the possibility of onc gene activation after HTLV infection. Using cloned probes of sis, myc, myb, fes, abl, src, H-ras, Ki-ras, we failed to find consistent activation of any onc gene in either the in vitro infected cells or fresh leukemic cells, thus negating a requisite role of the onc genes tested in either initiation or maintenance of transformation. However, it is of interest to note that a significant number of in vitro HTLV infected cells and some cell lines established from HTLV positive tumors express c-sis, a gene not normally expressed in hematopoietic cells. Since c-sis is now known to code for a growth factor (PDGF), which normally acts on fibroblasts, smooth muscle cells and glial cells, it would be of interest to see if the sis product produced in these cells can stimulate their own proliferation.

In summary, HTLV consist of a family of related human exogenous retroviruses which are highly T-cell tropic. They are very likely causes of certain human leukemias and lymphomas. Despite the fact that they do not carry an onc gene they transform fresh human bone marrow or blood derived T-cells. The molecular mechanism of this phenomenon is not understood, but current results lead us to focus on three areas: (1) the TCGF (Il-2) receptor; (2) the c-sis gene and its product; and (3) certain viral proteins, the latter two, however, only in initiation of transformation.

References. Bishop, J. M. (1978) Ann Rev Biochem 47:35-88; Dalla Favera, R., et al. (1981) Nature 292:31-35; Gallo, R. C., et al. (1982) Proc Natl Acad Sci USA 79:4680-4683; Gallo, R. C., et al. (1983) Cancer Res 43:3892-3899; Gallo, R. C., Wong-Staal, F. (1982) Blood 60:545-557; Gallo, R. C., Wong-Staal, F., Sarin, P. S. (1983) In Leukemia Today - Mechanisms of Viral Leukemogenesis (Dacie, J. V., Goldman, J. M., Jarrett, J. O., eds), in press; Haynes, B. F., et al. (1983) Proc Natl Acad Sci USA 80:2054-2058; Hayward, W. S., Neel, B. G., Astrin, S. M. (1981) Nature 209: 475-480; Kalyanaraman, V. S., et al. (1982) Science 218:571-573; Manzari, V., et al. (1983) Proc Natl Acad Sci USA 80:11-15; Manzari, V., et al. (1983) Proc Natl Acad Sci USA 80:1574-1578; Miyoshi, I., et al. (1981) Nature 294:770-771; Morgan, D. A., Ruscetti, F. W., Gallo, R. C. (1976) Science 193:1007-1008; Poiesz, B. J., et al. (1980) Proc Natl Acad Sci USA 77:7415-7419; Popovic, M., et al. (1983) Science 219:856-859;

Robert-Guroff, M., et al. (1982) Science 215:975-978; Sarin, P. S., et al. (1983) Proc Natl Acad Sci USA 80:2370-2374; Seiki, M. et al. (1983) Proc Natl Acad Sci USA 80:3618-3622; Takatsuki, K., Uchiyama, T., Ueshima, Y., Kattori, T. (1979) Jpn J Cl Oncol 9:317-324; Wong-Staal, F., et al. (1983) Nature 302:626-628; Yoshida, M., Miyoshi, Himuma, Y. (1982) Proc Natl Acad Sci USA 79:2031-2035.

MECHANISMS OF c-myc ACTIVATION IN AVIAN AND HUMAN B-CELL LYMPHOMAS

W. Hayward[1], C.-K. Shih[1], M. Goodenow[1], K. Wiman[1], A. Hayday[2], H. Saito[2], and S. Tonegawa[2]. [1]Sloan-Kettering Institute for Cancer Research, New York, NY 10021; [2]Massachusetts Institute for Technology, Cambridge, MA 02139

The c-myc gene has been implicated in a wide variety of neoplasms, including B-cell lymphomas, myeloid leukemias, and carcinomas. The oncogenic potential of this gene can be activated by many different types of mutational events, including proviral insertion, gene amplification, and translocation (1-7). In each case the c-myc gene is altered in some way that perturbs the normal expression of the gene.

Sequence organization of the c-myc gene--The coding sequences of the c-myc gene are located within two exons, interrupted by an intron of about 1 kb (8-10). An additional exon has been localized approximately 1.5 kb upstream of the coding exons of mouse and human c-myc (11-13). Although this exon is apparently non-coding, the nucleotide sequence is highly conserved in mouse and human, suggesting a strong selective pressure to maintain the sequence of this region. This sequence is not, however, conserved in the avian c-myc gene (14).

We have tentatively localized the first exon of the avian c-myc gene to a position approximately 700 bases upstream of the coding exons (Fig. 1) (14). Nucleotide sequence analysis suggests that the first exon in the avian gene, like that in mammals, is non-coding. No detectable homology exists between the first exons of the avian and mammalian genes.

ALV-induced B-cell lymphomas--Induction of B-cell lymphomas by avian leukosis virus (ALV) results from insertion of proviral sequences adjacent to, and transcriptional activation of, the host c-myc gene (15). This conclusion is based on the following lines of evidence: (i) In more than 80% of ALV-induced lymphomas proviral sequences are integrated adjacent to the c-myc gene. (ii) Levels of c-myc mRNA are elevated 30-100 fold in the lymphomas, compared to equivalent normal tissues. (iii) In most tumors, the myc-specific mRNA contains viral sequences derived from the long terminal repeat (LTR) of the integrated provirus. Thus, transcription initiates within the viral LTR, and reads into the adjacent c-myc gene, causing transcriptional activation of the gene.

Integration of proviral sequences occurs at a number of sites adjacent to c-myc (14-19). In the vast majority of lymphomas, the provirus is integrated within the first intron; most of the integrations are clustered within the first 300 bases upstream of the coding exon (see Fig. 1). Thus, insertion of the provirus results in displacement of the cellular promoter and regulatory sequences, and placement of the c-myc gene under the transcriptional control of viral regulatory sequences. Integration at these sites also results in synthesis of a truncated message

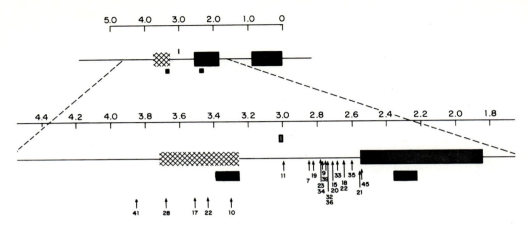

FIG. 1: Chicken c-myc locus and sites of proviral integrations in avian B-cell lymphomas. The two c-myc coding exons are designated by dark hatched boxes. Localization of the first c-myc exon (light hatched box) is tentative. Regions that share significant sequence complementarity are designated by black bars beneath the exons. Integration sites in different tumors are designated by arrows.

that lacks the first exon (14). Because the deleted sequences are non-coding, the protein product of the truncated mRNA would presumably be unaltered. However, loss of these sequences may alter the translational efficiency of the mRNA. In both the avian and human c-myc genes, complementarity exists between sequences in the first and second exons (20,21). It has been postulated that this complementarity plays a role in translational control of the normal c-myc gene (20).

   In a minority of lymphomas, the provirus is integrated at more distal sites, or in the opposite transcriptional orientation (17). Presumably, enhancer sequences located within the viral LTR influence transcription from a cellular promoter in these tumors.

Human Burkitt lymphomas--In approximately 90% of Burkitt lymphomas, the c-myc gene is translocated from its normal position on chromosome 8(q24) (24), and joined to the IgH locus on chromosome 14 (6,7). A similar translocation event has been observed in murine plasmacytomas (5).

   Efforts to deduce the mechanism by which translocation causes activation of c-myc have been complicated by the fact that the juxtaposition of sequences from the two loci is variable from one tumor to another (5-7,11,13,20,21,25,26). In a high proportion of murine plasmacytomas and in many Burkitt lymphomas the breakpoint in c-myc is located within the first intron, but breakpoints within, or considerably upstream of, the first exon are also common. Breakpoints in the Ig locus often occur within the switch region, but sites have also been observed both upstream and downstream of this region.

   Two examples of c-myc rearrangements are shown in Fig. 2. In

15

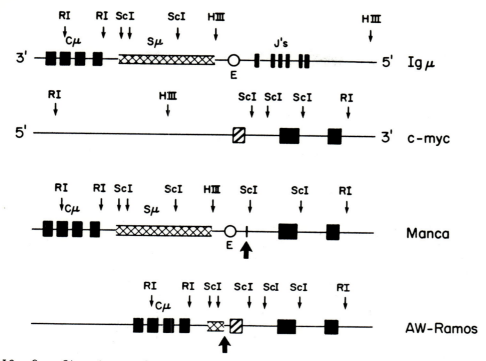

FIG. 2: Structure of rearranged c-myc genes in two human lymphoma
lines. The structural organization of normal and rearranged human
genes, shown schematically as follows (top to bottom): (a) A
portion of the normal IgH locus; (b) the normal c-myc gene; (c)
rearranged c-myc gene from the Manca cell line (a DHL carrying the
8:14 translocation); (d) rearranged c-myc gene from the AW-Ramos
cell line (Burkitt lymphoma). (From Ref. 21).

the Manca cell line, the breakpoints are within the first intron of
c-myc, and within the intron upstream of Sμ in the IgH locus
(20,21,25). The resulting rearranged c-myc thus lacks the first
exon and carries an IgH enhancer sequence just upstream of the
c-myc gene. The enhancer sequences were shown by transfection to
be required for efficient transcription of the c-myc gene from the
Manca cell line (25). In the AW-Ramos cell line the breakpoints
are located approximately 150 bases upstream of the first exon of
c-myc, and within the Sμ region of the IgH locus (21). Thus, c-myc
is not joined to the known enhancer sequences of the IgH locus, and
the first exon of c-myc is not deleted. A point mutation upstream
of the normal c-myc promoter has been identified by nucleotide
sequencing. This single base change might alter a critical control
region of c-myc. Alternatively, changes in the control of c-myc
expression might result from the loss of regulatory sequences
located upstream of the breakpoint in c-myc, or from juxtaposition
of c-myc to an as yet unidentified enhancer in the IgH locus.
    Although no single model has emerged to explain all of the

16

observed rearrangements in different Burkitt lymphomas, in each case the rearrangement appears to influence c-myc expression. In this respect, and in other details, the rearrangements in Burkitt lymphoma and murine plasmacytomas are remarkably similar to those induced by proviral insertion in ALV-induced B-cell lymphoma.

References--(1) HAYWARD, W. S., B. G. Neel, and S. M. Astrin. 1982. In George Klein (ed): "Advances in Viral Oncology", Vol. 1, Raven Press, NY, p207; (2) DALLA-FAVERA, R., F. Wong-Staal, and R. C. Gallo. 1982. Nature 299:61; (3) COLLINS, S. and M. Groudine. 1982. Nature 298:679; (4) ALITALO, K., M. Schwab, C. C. Lin, H. E. Varmus, and J. M. Bishop. 1983. Proc. Natl. Acad. Sci. USA 80:1707; (5) SHEN-ONG, G. L. C., E. J. Keath, S. P. Piccoli, and M. D. Cole. 1982. Cell 31:443; (6) TAUB, R., I. Kirsch, C. Morton, G. Lenoir, D. Swan, S. Tronick, S. Aaronson, and P. Leder. 1982. Proc. Natl. Acad. Sci. 79:7837; (7) DALLA-FAVERA, R., M. Bregni, J. Erikson, D. Patterson, R. C. Gallo, and C. M. Croce. 1982. Proc Nat Acad Sci USA 79:7824; (8) ROBINS, T., K. Bister, C. Garon, T. Papas, and P. Duesberg. 1982. J Virol 41:635; (9) VENNSTROM, B., D. Sheiness, J. Zabielski, and J. M. Bishop. 1982. J. Virol. 42:773; (10) NEEL, B. G., G. P. Gasic, C. E. Rogler, A. M. Skalka, G. Ju, F. Hishinuma, T. Papas, S. M. Astrin, and W. S. Hayward. 1982. J. Virol. 44:158; (11) MARCU, K. B., L. J. Harris, L. W. Stanton, J. Erikson, R. Watt, and C. M. Croce. 1983. Proc. Natl. Acad. Sci. 80:519; (12) WATT, R., L. W. Stanton, K. B. Marcu, R. C. Gallo, C. M. Croce, and G. Rovera. 1983. Nature 303:725; (13) HAMLYN, P. H. and T. H. Rabbitts. 1983. Nature 304:135; (14) SHIH, C.-K., M. Linial, M. M. Goodenow, and W. S. Hayward. In preparation; (15) HAYWARD, W. S., B. G. Neel, and S. M. Astrin. 1981. Nature 290:475; (16) FUNG, Y.-K. T., L. B. Crittenden and H.-J. Kung 1982. J. Virol. 44:742; (17) PAYNE, G. S., J. M. Bishop, and H. E. Varmus. 1982. Nature 295:209; (18) COOPER, G.M.; and P. E. Nieman. 1981. Nature 292:857-858; (19) GOODENOW, M. M., C.-K. Shih, K. Wiman and W. S. Hayward. 1983. "The Transformed Cell" (CSH, NY). (in press); (20) SAITO, H., A. Hayday, K. Wiman, W. S. Hayward, and S. Tonegawa. 1983. Proc. Natl. Acad. Sci. (in press); (21) WIMAN, K., A. Hayday, H. Saito, S. Tonegawa, and W. S. Hayward. (In preparation.); (22) NEEL, B. G., W. S. Hayward, H. L. Robinson, J. Fang, and S. M. Astrin. 1981. Cell 23:323; (23) PAYNE, G. S., S. A. Courtneidge, L. B. Crittenden, A. M. Fadly, J. M. Bishop, and H. E. Varmus. 1981. Cell 23:311; (24) NEEL, B. G., S. C. Jhanwar, R. S. K. Chaganti and W. S. Hayward. 1982. Proc. Natl. Acad. Sci. USA 79: 7842; (25) HAYDAY, A. C., S. D. Gillies, H. Saito, C. Wood, K. Wiman, W. S. Hayward, and S. Tonegawa. 1983. Manuscript submitted; (26) ADAMS, J. M., S. Gerondakis, E. Webb, L.M. Corcoran, and S. Cory. 1983. Proc. Natl. Acad. Sci. 80:1982.

Acknowledgements--The authors would like to thank Lauren O'Connor for help in preparation of this manuscript. This work was supported by grants CA-34502 (WSH) and CA-14051 (ST) from the National Institutes of Health.

Translocations
and
Gene Activation

THE ROLE OF CHROMOSOMAL TRANSLOCATIONS IN ONCOGENE TRANSPOSITION INTO FUNCTIONALLY ACTIVE GENE REGIONS: A MECHANISM IN CARCINOGENESIS.

George Klein

Department of Tumor Biology, Karolinska Institutet
S-104 01 Stockholm, SWEDEN

Nonrandom chromosomal abnormalities, such as deletions, translocations and trisomies are increasingly observed in human and murine cancer cells particularly of the hematopoetic system. Recent investigations are centered upon what roles these specific abnormalities play in the development of cancer and what genes may be involved. There is evidence from rodent and human hematologic malignancies (mouse T-cell lymphomas, rat and mouse plasmacytoma and human Burkitt lymphoma) to illustrate the significance of specific chromosome abnormalities in the genesis of neoplasm development.

In the mouse, spontaneous as well as virally and non-virally induced T-cell leukemias are often chromosomally abnormal (1-4), and trisomy of chromosome 15 is the dominating and frequently the only change. If there are two trisomies, the second one is usually chromosome 17. In some mouse strains, particularly the SJL, trisomy 15 is cryptic. The distal portions of chromosome 15 are translocated to other chromosomes, and only banding analyses can reveal its trisomic state (5). From studies of these cryptic translocations, it was evident that the genes located in the distal portion of chromosome 15 are important for the development of T-cell leukemia in the mouse.

Further supportive evidence comes from studies involving mouse stocks carrying different Robertsonian chromosome translocations (6). These translocations were derived from the centromeric fusion between chromosome 15 and 1, and 5 and 6. In leukemias induced in the mouse stocks by chemicals or by viruses, the entire translocated chromosome is present in triplicate. This indicates that the trisomy of the attached autosome is by no means lethal for the leukemic cells. It also indicates that the presence of certain gene(s) in chromosome 15 in a trisomic state are so essential for leukemogenesis that the duplication of genes in the translocated chromosome is tolerated.

The next question to ask is whether the duplication of chromosome 15 is a random or nonrandom event in heterozygous mice derived from crosses of mice with cytogenetically distinguishable chromosome 15. In crosses between AKR and AKRt(6;15) (carrier of a translocation between chromosomes 6 and 15) as well as CBA and CBAT6T6 (carrier of a translocation between chromosomes 14 and 15) the F_1 hybrids would carry a normal and a translocated chromosome 15. In leukemic cells of these F_1 hybrid mice, the duplication of chromosome 15 is random. In other combinations of crosses, the duplication is nonrandom (7,8). These observations indicate that if one of the parents is an AKR strain, the AKR-derived chromosome 15 is usually duplicated. This suggests that the genetic background of the strain from which the chromosome 15 is derived, rather than the translocated state, dertermines the duplication pattern.

Further experiments were conducted to determine whether the genetic content of the tumor-derived chromosome 15 is different from that of the normal one. Somatic hybrid cells were obtained by fusing trisomic 15 AKR leukemic cells and normal CBAT6T6 fibroblasts or lymphocytes. Chromosome analysis of high tumorigenic hybrids and high tumorigenic segregants of originally low tumorigenic hybrids shows that the tumor derived chromosome 15 is increased from an expected frequency of 3 to an average of 5.5 ± 0.2 per cell with a concomitant decrease of the normal derived translocated chromosome 15 from 2 to $0.9 \pm 0.2(9)$. In the low tumorigenic hybrids, an opposite pattern is observed: the tumorigenic hybrids, an opposite pattern is observed: the tumor derived chromosome is decreased from 3 to 2.6 ± 0.1 with the maintenance also of two copies of the normal derived ones. These findings indicate the existence of a qualitative difference in the genetic content between the tumor and the normal chromosome 15. In addition, the amplification of tumor-derived chromosome 15 and a decrease in the normal counterpart appear to favor tumorigenicity. This phenomenon indicates that the normal chromosome 15 may be expressing some form of transacting control over the expression of the tumor-derived homolog. One way to counteract such control is by amplification of the tumor-derived chromosome 15.

A working hypothesis was generated from the studies of the mouse T-cell leukemia. It states that an oncogene is present in chromosome 15 and is located distal to band D3. This oncogene is activated in one of the chromosomes either by insertion of retrovirus proviral DNA or by mutation. The expression of such genes is under a trans-acting control by the normal homolog. For the oncogene to be expressed, an extra copy of the gene may be required, and duplication of this chromosome by non-disjunction is the simplest means of achieving this.

The idea that there is an oncogene located in the distal portion of chromosome 15 was further substantiated by the observation in a completely different kind of tumor, the mouse plasmacytoma. In 90% of the plasmacytomas, the specific chromosome abnormality involves the translocation from chromosome 15 to 12. The break-point in chromosome 15 is at the D3 band, the region considered critical for the T-cell leukemia. The terminal region of chromosome 12 is known to carry the heavy-chain immunoglobulin gene. The remaining 10% involve reciprocal translocations between the same region in chromosome 15 and 6. Chromosome 6 is known to carry the Kappa locus although the exact location is still unknown. It appears that in the mouse plasmacytoma, the activation of the oncogene in chromosome 15 is by a mechanism different from that of the T-cell leukemia. We have suggested that the activation in this case is by translocation of the same oncogene to a functionally active region (the immunoglobulin gene region) of another chromosome.

In the rat, translocation of the distal region of chromosome 7 to 6 is consistently observed in the spontaneously derived plasmacytoma. The distal region of chromosome 6 in the rat is similar to chromosome 12 in the mouse with respect to the isozyme marker distribution. Thus, it is likely that the rat chromosome 6 carries genes that activate the oncogene translocated from chromosome 7.

The specific translocation of one of the two homologous chromoso-

mes to another chromosome that carries immunoglobulin genes in the
plasmacytomas suggests that specific gene(s) are expressed when located next (cis) to the immunoglobulin genes. Such cis-acting mechanisms apparently can overcome other controls as well as the trans-acting control by the normal homolog.

In patients with Burkitt lymphomas, Manolov and Manolova (10)
first identified the consistant presence of the 14q+ marker chromosome in the cancer cells. Subsequently, it was shown that there are
three consistant and related translocations in Burkitt lymphoma. In
90% of the cases, the translocation is between chromosomes 8 and 14,
5% between 8 and 2 and the remaining 5% between 8 and 22. Interestingly, the three recipient chromosomes (14, 2 and 22) have been
shown to contain immunoglobulin gene loci (the heavy chain genes are
in 14, Kappa light chain genes in 2 and Lambda light chain genes in
22). And, there is significant concordance between the light chains
being produced and the recipient chromosomes involved in the translocation. Thus, the mechanisms involved in the Burkitt lymphomas appeared to be similar to that in plasmacytomas, namely, activation of an
oncogene by translocating to a recipient chromosome with functionally
active genes.

Recently, our hypothesis received strong support from molecular
evidence obtained by other groups (for review see 11), showing that
the distal part of human 8 and of mouse 15 carries the oncogene c-myc.
In both MPC and BL, c-myc is often transposed to the immediate vicinity of, or even inserted into, the appropriated Ig-locus on the recipient chromosome. As a result, a normal or abnormal myc transcript is
produced at a high level, in line with our original hypothesis. Similar transposition of oncogenes into functionally active chromosome
regions may play a role in certain other forms of carcinogenesis as
well. The most recent developments in this area and its potential implications will be discussed.

References. (1) Dofuku, J.L., Biedler, B.A. and Lloyd, L.J. (1975)
Proc.Natl.Acad.Sci.72, 1515; (2) Wiener, F., Ohno, S., Spira, J.,
Haran-Ghera, N. and Klein, G. (1978) J.Natl.CancerInst. 61, 227; (3)
Wiener, F., Spira, J., Ohno, S., Haran-Ghera, N. and Klein, G. (1978)
Int.J.Cancer 22, 447; (4) Chan, F.P.H., Ball, J.K. and Sergovich, F.R.
(1979) J.Natl.CancerInst. 62, 605; (5) Spira, J., Babonits, M., Wie-
ner, F., Ohno, S., Wirschubsky, Z., Haran-Ghera, N. and Klein, G.
(1980) CancerRes. 40, 2609; (6) Spira, J., Wiener, F., Ohno, S. and
Klein G. (1979) Proc.Natl.Acad.Sci. 76, 6619; (7) Wiener, F., Spira,
J., Babonits, M., Haran-Ghera, N. and Klein, G. (1980) Int.J.Cancer
26, 661; (8) Wiener, F., Spira, J., Babonits, M. and Klein, G. (1982)
Int.J.Cancer 30, 479; (9) Spira, J., Wiener, F., Babonits, M., Miller,
J. and Klein, G. (1981) Int.J.Cancer 28, 785; (10) Manolov G. and Manolova, Y. (1972) Nature 237, 33; (11) Klein, G. (1983) Cell 32, 311.

ACTIVATION OF C-MYC ONCOGENE BY CHROMOSOME TRANSLOCATION TO IMMUNOGLOBULIN GENES IN MURINE PLASMACYTOMAS

Kenneth B. Marcu[1], Lawrence W. Stanton[1], Jian-qing Yang[1], Elaine F. Remmers[1], Paul Fahrlander[1], Robert Greenberg[1,2], Laurel Eckhardt[3], Barbara K. Birshtein[3], Linda J. Harris[1,4], and Rosemary Watt[5]

[1]Dept. Biochemistry SUNY at Stony Brook, Stony Brook, NY 11794
[2]Shearing Corp. 86 Orange St. Bloomfield, NJ 07003
[3]Dept. Cell Biology Albert Einstein College of Medicine Bronx, NY 10462;[4]Genetic Systems Corp., 3005 First Avenue Seattle, WA 98121
[5]Smith Kline and French Laboratories, Philadelphia, PA 19101

Specific chromosomal abnormalities have long been associated with various human and murine neoplasias (1-3). Activated cellular oncogenes (generally found to be the cellular homologues of retroviral transforming genes) are now known to be causative agents of cellular transformation. In the past year, a number of oncogenes have been localized to chromosome bands displaying abnormalities in specific neoplasias ((2,3). The mammalian c-myc gene represents the best understood example in molecular terms. C-myc has been localized to 8q24 in man (4-6) and to chromosome 15 in mice (7-9). A t(8;14) (q24;q32) in man has been associated with the majority of Burkitt lymphomas (1-3). Mineral oil induced murine plasmacytomas possess a characteristic t(12;15) involving the distal ends of these chromosomes (10,11). The consequences of the 12;15 chromosome translocation for c-myc gene structure and activation in murine plasmacytomas are discussed in this presentation.

Chromosome translocation breaks the c-myc gene thereby removing its normal regulatory sequences.

The 12;15 chromosome translocation breaks the c-myc gene in an exon on intron juxtaposing the remaining two myc exons with an immunoglobulin heavy chain gene switch (S) region (4,7-9,12-18). The anatomy of the c-myc locus and the myc breakpoints in four plasmacytomas are presented in Figure 1. The locations of myc exons and introns in the J558 rearranged myc gene were determined by comparison to a c-myc cDNA clone prepared from normal BALB/c spleen RNA (18). The unrearranged myc gene expresses a ∿2.4 kb RNA (14-17, 20). Elevated levels of ∿2.0 kb RNAs are produced from the rearranged myc gene (16,20). DNA probes prepared from myc intron and exon sequences have revealed that these truncated myc RNAs are initiated from novel promoters within the first myc intron (see Figure 1) (17,18).

Chromosome translocation does not alter the structure of the c-myc product.

The first c-myc exon is an atypically large noncoding sequence (18,19). Multiple termination codons are found in all three reading frames of exon 1 (Figure 2B) (18,19). The first initiation codon is found at the beginning of exon 2 (see Figure 1) (18). A transcription initiation site for normal sized myc RNAs was identified by S_1 nuclease mapping of the 2.4 kb myc RNA produced by the PC 3741 plasmacytoma (see boxed TATA sequence and downstream RNA cap site in Figure 2a) (19). The lengths of the 5' noncoding exons in mouse and

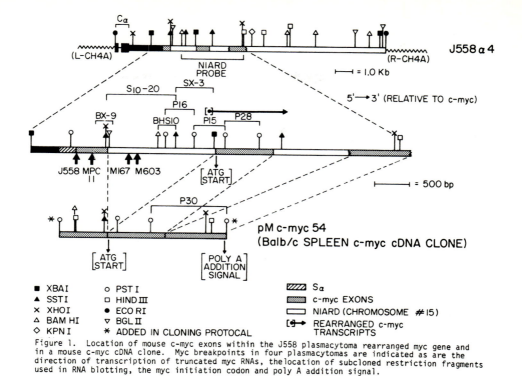

Figure 1. Location of mouse c-myc exons within the J558 plasmacytoma rearranged myc gene and in a mouse c-myc cDNA clone. Myc breakpoints in four plasmacytomas are indicated as are the direction of transcription of truncated myc RNAs, the location of subcloned restriction fragments used in RNA blotting, the myc initiation codon and poly A addition signal.

man are essentially identical (569 bp compared 572 bp respectively) and are ~78% homologous (see Figure 3). Like the murine first exon, the human sequence possesses multiple termination codons and lack an initiation codon (21,22). Two TATA promoter sequences, 155 bp apart, are conserved at the 5' end of exon 1 in the murine and human genes (see Figure 3). The existence of different quantities of two human myc RNAs of 2.2 and 2.4 kb in Burkitt lymphomas and Epstein-Barr-Virus (EBV) transformed human lymphoblastoid cell lines would be consistant with two closely spaced promoters (23). Two promoters in exon 1 would also explain the heterogeneous profiles of the 2.4 kb RNAs present in plasmactyomas without myc rearrangements (16). The conservation of a large 5' non-coding exon may be important for normal c-myc regulation since the expression of the normal, unrearranged myc allele in plasmacytomas (17,18) and Burkitt lymphomas (24) is suppressed. The inappropriate, generally elevated expression of myc RNAs in plasmacytomas may result from either the complete loss or alteration of exon 1 sequences.

C-myc translocation is a fairly precise reciprocal exchange which does not occur by homologous recombination.

C-myc 5' flanking sequences are retained in plasmacytomas in a rearranged context with S region sequences (25). Southern hybridizations and molecular cloning experiments performed with a 5' flanking c-myc probe have demonstrated that the c-myc rearrangement is generated by a reciprocal chromosome translocation (i.e. RcpT(12;15) (19,25). The 5' flanking and exon 1 sequences, which are lost from

A

```
AAAWATACAGAGAGGTGGGGAAGGGAGAAAGAGAGATTCTCTGGCTAAT      50
CCCCGCCCACCCGCCCTTTATATTCCGGGGGTCTGCGCGGCCGAGGACCC    100
CTGGGTGCGCTGCTCTCAGCTGCCGGGTCCGACTCGCCTCACTCAGCTCC   150
CCTCCTGCCTCCTGAAGGGCAGCTTCGCCGACGCTTGGCGGGAAAAAGAA   200
GGGAGGGGGAGGGATCCTGAGTCGCAGTATAAAAGAAGCTTTTCGGGCGTT  250
TTTTTCTGACTCGCTGTAGTAATTCCAGCGAGAGACAGAGGGAGTGAGCG   300
GACGGTTGGAAGAGCCGTGTGTGCAGAGCCGCGCTCCGGGGCGACCTAAG   350
AAGGCAGCTCTGGAGTGAGAGGGGCTTTGCCTCCGAGCCTGCCGCCCACT   400
CTCCCCAACCCTGCGACTGACCCAACATCAGCGGCCGCCAACCCTCGCCGC  450
CGCTGGGAAACTTTGCCCATTGCAGCGGGCAGACACTTCTCACTGGAACT   500
TACAATCTGCGAGCCAGGACAGGACTCCCCAGCCTCCGGGGAGGGAATTT   550
TTGTCTATTTGGGGACAGTGTTCTCTGCCTCTGCCCGCGATCAGCTCTCC   600
TGAAAAGAGCTCCTCGAGCTGTTTGAAGGCTGGATTTCCTTTGGGCGTTG   650
GAAACCCCG   ——— intron 1  ——▶
```

B

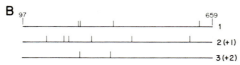

Figure 2. A. Complete nucleotide sequence of murine c-myc exon 1 and 5' flanking region. Sequences were derived from the 5' MPC-11 rearrangement (19) and from a c-myc cDNA clone (18). Promoter like sequences 5' of an S₁ nuclease mapped transcription start site at position 97 are boxed. Arrows indicate Exon-1 breakpoints and double arrows where 5' and 3' reciprocal breakpoints are known. B. Locations of multiple termination codons in each of three reading frames.

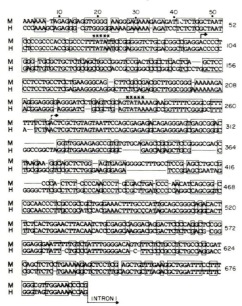

Figure 3. Comparison of c-myc 5' noncoding exons from mouse (M) (19) and man (H) (22). Homologous sequences are boxed. Two conserved TATA sequences are indicated by asterisks. Transcription start sites are denoted with solid and dashed horizontal arrows. Vertical lines represent gaps in either sequence.

the transcribed portion of the rearranged myc gene, have recombined with Sμ or Sα sequences in most BALB/c plasmacytomas (25). In the MPC-11 plasmacytoma, the c-myc gene has recombined directly with the Sγ2a region with both 5' and 3' rearrangement products remaining attached to Sγ2a sequences (19) (Figure 4).

Myc sequences in the vicinity of seven myc breakpoints are presented in Figure 5. Three of these rearrangements occur in the first exon and four in the major c-myc intron. These recombination sites span ~1.0 kb of myc sequences (13, 14,18,19,25). The reciprocal translocations in MPC-11 (19) and P3 (26) are remarkably precise resulting in losses of only 11 and 5 bp of c-myc sequence respectively. Short inverted repeats (4-7 bp in length) are found 2-35 bp apart, 5' and 3' of each myc breakpoint. However, these inverted repeats are not conserved between different recombination sites and the frequency of short palindromic sequences within the c-myc recombination region is no more than expected for a DNA sequence with a high G + C content (~62% in this case). It is interesting to note that S regions consist of large numbers of tandemly repeated GAGCT sequences which contain the palindromic sequence AGCT (27). If a higher order secondary structure somehow facilitates c-myc translocation, S region sequences may provide numerous acceptable targets for this rearrangement (19).

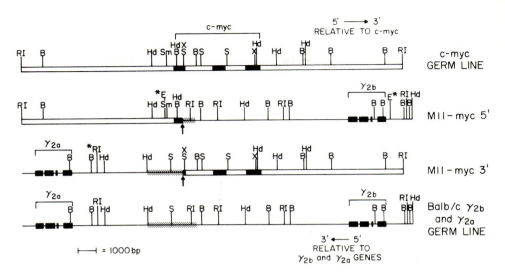

Figure 4. Restriction endonuclease maps of the products of a reciprocal exchange involving the c-myc locus and the $S_{\gamma 2a}$ region in the MPC-11 myeloma. Only relevant restriction sites are shown. * indicates clone boundaries. RI=EcoRI, B=BamHI, Hd=HindIII, S=SstI, X=XhoI, Sm=SmaI and E=EcoRI*.

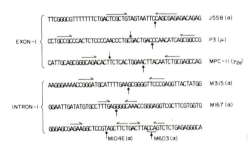

Figure 5. Inspection of nucleotide sequences in the vicinity of seven c-myc breakpoints. Horizontal arrows indicated inverted repeats and vertical arrows signify myc breakpoints (5' breakpoints above and 3' sites below the sequences). Multiple arrows for MOPC 603 indicate ambiguity of the precise breakpoint. Switch region targets are indicated beside each plasmacytoma. J558 (14,18), MPC-11 (19), P3 (26), MOPC 603 and 167 (8), M104E and MOPC 315 (M. Cole, personal communication).

References-(1) Klein, G. (1981) Nature 294, 313; (2) Rowley, J.P. (1982) Science 216, 749; (3) Yunis, J.L. (1983) Science 221, 227; (4) Taub, R., et al., (1982) Proc. Natl. Acad. Sci. USA 79, 7837; (5) Dalla-Favera, et al., (1982) Proc. Natl. Acad. Sci. USA 79, 7824; (6) Neel, B.G., et al., (1962) Proc. Natl. Acad. Sci. USA 79, 7843; (7) Harris, L.J., et al., (1982) Proc. Natl. Acad. Sci. USA 79, 6622; (8) Calame, K., et al., (1982) Proc. Natl. Acad. Sci. USA 79, 6994; (9) Cory, S. et al., (1983) EMBO J. 2, 213; (10) Ohno, S. et al., (1979) Cell 18. 1001; (11) Weiner, F. et al., (1980) Somatic Cell Genet. 6, 731; (12) Kirsch,I.R., et al., (1981) Nature (London) 293, 585; (13) Harris, L.J., et al., (1982) Proc. Natl. Acad. Sci. USA 79, 4175; (14) Adams, J.M., et al., (1982) Proc. Natl. Acad. Sci. USA 79, 6966; (15) Shen-Ong, G.L.C. et al., (1982) Cell 31, 443; (16) Marcu, K.B. et al., (1983) Proc. Natl. Acad. Sci. USA 80, 519; (17) Adams, J. et al., (1983) Proc. Natl. Acad. Sci. USA 80, 1982; (18) Stanton, L.W. et al., (1983) Nature (London) 303, 401; (19) Stanton, L.W. et al., (1983) Proc. Natl. Acad. Sci. USA in press; (20) Mushinski, J.F. et al., (1983) Proc. Natl. Acad. Sci USA 80, 1073; (21) Watt, R. et al., (1983) Nature (London) 303, 725; (22) Watt, R. et al., (1983) Proc. Natl. Acad. Sci. USA in press. (23) Hamlyn, P.H. and Rabbitts, T.H. (1983) Nature (London) 304, 135; (24) Nishikura, K., et al., (1983) Proc. Natl. Acad. Sci. USA 80, 4822; (25) Cory, S., et al., (1983) EMBO J. 2, 697; (26) Dunnick, W., et al., (1983) Proc. Natl. Acad. Sci. USA, in press. (27) Nikaido, T., et al., (1982) J. Biol. Chem. 257, 7322.

Acknowledgements-This research was supported by NIH and ACS grants awarded to KBM and an NIH grant to BKB. KBM is a recepient of an NIAID research career development award. P.F. is a postdoctoral fellow of the American Cancer Society and Elaine Remmers is a Damon-Runyon Walter Winchell Cancer fund fellow.

THE CHROMOSOMAL BASIS OF HUMAN NEOPLASIA

Jorge J. Yunis

Dept. of Laboratory Medicine and Pathology, University of Minnesota Medical School, 420 Delaware Street S.E., Minneapolis, MN 55455

At present, there are 22 specific chromosomal defects associated with over 30 distinct types of human neoplasia (1,2). These abnormalities are mostly represented by either a reciprocal translocation, or a loss of a given band (1). In the non-Hodgkin's lymphomas and acute leukemias we have recently found that two-thirds of all cases have a specific chromosomal lesion, with a reciprocal translocation commonly observed (1,3,4). Such exchange is now visualized as a crucial event that sets a stem cell toward a malignant path (1,5). An example is found in Burkitt's lymphoma where a translocation 8;14, with breakpoints at subbands q24.1 and q32.3 [t(8;14)(q24.1;q32.3)], is often found. In this instance, the oncogene **c-myc** of chromosome 8 becomes activated when rearranged with the heavy chain immunoglobulin genes in chromosome 14 (6).

In leukemias, consistent defects may also be linked to one of 8 other oncogenes, mapped to specific chromosome bands or subbands (7-11). One possibility is the t(8;21)(q22.1;q22.3) in acute myelogenous leukemia with cell maturation (AML-M2), where **c-mos** has been localized to the same band (8q22) involved in the translocation (7). Another is the t(9;22)(q34.1;q11.21) in chronic myelogeneous leukemia (1), where the oncogene **c-abl** from subband 9q34.1 (8) translocates to the abbreviated chromosome 22 known as the Philadelphia (Ph^1) chromosome (9). Similarly, a newly discovered ANLL-M2 subgroup shows a breakpoint at 9q34 [t(6;6;9)(p23;q23-25;q34)] where the 9q34 translocation to 6p23 is the crucial event (3).

Besides oncogenes and chromosome defects, 14 inheritable autosomal chromosomal fragile sites have been recently defined (13). Eight of them (fragile sites 6p23, 8q22, 9p21, 11q13, 11q23, 12q13, 16p12, 16q22) are localized at or near the breakpoint of the one inversion and six of ten specific translocations defined to date in leukemias and non-Hodgkin's lymphomas. Using high resolution chromosome analysis, we observed that in most cases there is a very close correlation between the two, since the fragile site and the breakpoint of the chromosomal rearrangement occur at the same height within a band or subband. In one instance, an oncogene **(c-mos)**, a fragile site and a breakpoint of a chromosome defect coincide in the same band, 8q22. Another fragile site and a "gene" involved in two different types of leukemias with monocytic features [t(4;11) and t(9;11)] have been assigned to the distal end of band 11q23 (1,13,14).

An intriguing observation is our recent finding of a fragile site 16q22 in the normal blood cells of three of three patients with an inversion 16 [inv 16 (p13q22)] in a newly discovered acute myelomonocytic leukemia (1,3); a fragile site 11q13.3 in one of two patients with t(11;14)(q13.3;q32.3) and small lymphocytic cell lymphoma; and a fragile site 12q12.1 in a single patient with t(12;14)(q13.1;q32.3) and diffuse mixed T-cell lymphoma (1.4). Because of these findings, there is now need to correlate the presence of fragile sites in normal blood cells with breakpoints of chromosomal rearrangements in the malignant cells of a large number of lymphohematopoeitic malignancies. Confirmation of our findings would suggest that some individuals could be preordained to develop certain malignancies and may explain why leukemias and lymphomas with a translocation appear to arise "spontaneously".

The molecular mechanism involved in the expression of fragile sites is unknown. Fragile sites appear as either a chromosome gap, stretch or break when cells are deprived of folic acid and thymidine during the last few hours of culture (15). This suggests that a fragile site may have a unique DNA structure and, when a cell is deprived of certain DNA precursor substances, becomes prone to rearrangement.

Most of the known fragile sites have an approximate population frequency of 0.2% each (13) and are inherited in a simple mendelian co-dominant fashion. In the case of the fragile sites 16p12 and 16q22, it has been briefly reported that some of the patients developed lymphohematopoeitic malignancies (16,17). Since cancer is a multi-stage process, and a given chromosome defect can be shared by 2 to 5 related neoplasias (1), a careful study of malignancies among families with fragile sites is indicated. This would help uncover a possible relationship between some of these "curiosities" of nature and a predisposition factor to cancer in man.

Acknowledgement

Supported in part by grants CA-31024 and CA-33314 from the National Cancer Institute.

References

1. Yunis, J.J. (1983) Science, 221:227-240.
2. Yunis, J.J. (1983) Current Hematology III, NY: Wiley and Sons.
3. Yunis, J.J. (1984) Cancer Genet Cytogenet.
4. Yunis, J.J., Oken, M.M. Theologides, A., Howe, R.R., Kaplan, M.E., In press, Cancer Genet Cytogenet.
5. Klein, G. (1981) Nature (London), 294:313-318.
6. Erikson, J., Ar-Rushidi, A., Drwinga, H.L., Nowell, P.C., Croce, C.M. (1983) Science, 219:963-967.
7. Neel, B.G., Jhanwar, S.C., Chaganti, R.S.K., Hayward, W.S. (1982) Proc. Natl. Acad. Sci., 79:7842-7846.

8. Chaganti, R.S.K., Jhanwar, S.C. (1983) 34th Annual Meeting Am. Soc. Hum. Genet. Norfolk, Virginia.
9. de Klein, A., van Kessel, A.G., Grosveld, G., Bartram, C.R., Hagemeijer, A., Bottsma, D., Spurr, N.K. London, Heisterkamp., N., Groffen, J., Stephenson, J.R. (1982) Nature, 300:765-767.
10. Jhanwar, S.C., Neel, B.G., Hayward, W.S., Chaganti, R.S.K. (1983) Proc. Natl. Acad. Sci., 80: 4794-4797.
11. Harper, M.E., Franchini, G., Love, J., Simon, M.I., Gales, R.C., Whang-Staal, F. (1983) Nature (London), 304:169-171.
12. Vermaelen, K., Michaux, J-L., Louwage, A., van den Berghe, H. Cancer Genet Cytogenet. In press.
13. Sutherland, G.R., Jacky, P.B., Baker, E., Manuel, A. (1983) Am. J. Hum. Genet., 35:432-437.
14. Nagasaka, M., Maeda, S., Maeda, H., Chen, H-L., Kita, K., Mabuchi, O., Misu, H., Matsuo, T., Sugiyama, T. (1983) Blood, 61:1174-1181.
15. Sutherland, G.R. (1979) Am. J. Hum. Genet., 31:125-135.
16. Sutherland, G.R. (1979) Am. J. Hum. Genet., 31:136-148.
17. Shabatai, F., Bichacho, S., Halbrecht, I. (1980) Hum. Genet., 55:19-22.

Mechanisms of Gene Activation

DNA METHYLATION, X INACTIVATION, AND CANCER. Arthur D. Riggs, Judith Singer-Sam, Douglas Keith, and Brian I. Carr*. Division of Biology, Beckman Research Institute of the City of Hope, Duarte, CA 91010, and (*) Department of Medical Oncology, City of Hope Medical Center, Duarte, CA 91010.

Although not immediately obvious, the three subjects in the title are interrelated, and in this abstract we will try to explain why they are. In essence, the thinking is as follows. It has become increasingly evident that the postreplicational formation of 5-methylcytosine (MeCyt) in DNA is part of a new mechanism for gene control. Among experimental data supporting such a statement, the data for X-chromosome inactivation is the strongest and, moreover, indicates that methylation is involved in normal cellular differentiation and embryonic development. We will review X inactivation in some detail, including some of our recent data on X-linked PGK, and then present our data indicating that perturbations in DNA methylation also may be involved in an abnormal developmental process--the progression of cells to malignancy.

In 1975 Riggs (1) and Holiday and Pugh (2) proposed that DNA methylation may provide a new mechanism for somatic inheritance. It was proposed that a maintenance methylase exists capable of quickly methylating hemimethylated symmetrical sites in duplex DNA but having little activity on unmethylated sites. With this system, a methylated site becomes a somatically heritable entity capable of influencing sequence-specific, DNA-binding regulatory proteins (1,3). These notions are now supported by a large body of experimental evidence, which, when taken together, suggests that DNA methylation may function as a gene silencing mechanism relevant to vertebrate cell heredity and development: (a) MeCyt affects protein-DNA interactions, (b) MeCyt stabilizes Z-form DNA, (c) Maintenance methylases exist, (d) Methylation patterns exist and are tissue-specific, (e) Methylation patterns are somatically heritable, (f) Gene activity correlates with hypomethylation of critical sites, (g) In vitro methylation reduces in vivo gene activity, (h) DNA methylation is involved in the maintenance of X-chromosome inactivation, (i) Treatment of cells with inhibitors of DNA methylation activates many genes. The evidence supporting the above statements has recently been reviewed by Riggs and Jones (4) and Doerfler (5).

X-chromosome inactivation (reviewed in ref. 6) takes place in the early mammalian embryo at about the time of implantation and results in the incredibly stable (reversion rate 10^{-8} or less) genetic silencing of most genes on the X chromosome. Recent evidence has established that efficient reactivation does occur in the germ line; therefore no irreversible changes are made in the DNA. The types of experiments indicating that DNA methylation is involved in X inactivation are summarized in Table 1. Liskay and Evans (7) first obtained evidence that DNA modification is involved in X inactivation. They found that the hpt gene on an inactive X chromosome is less effective than that on the active chromosome in DNA-mediated cell transformation. This result has been confirmed and extended (7-12). Since DNA methylation is known to decrease the efficiency of DNA-mediated cell transformation, this result suggested that methylation might be involved. The next major discovery was that 5-azacytidine (5-AzaC), a potent inhibitor of DNA methylase, efficiently caused the reactivation of genes on the X chromosome (12-14). For example, Graves (14) found that, in a cell line derived from a hybrid Mus musculus X Mus caroli mouse, 5-AzaC increases the reactivation rate of hpt from 10^{-8} or less to as much as 3×10^{-3}.

****

Table 1. Methylation maintains X inactivation.

Experimental Result	References
1. DNA-mediated cell transformation by an hpt gene on an inactive X is inefficient relative to that on an active X.	7 to 12
2. 5-Azacytidine causes efficient reactivation of X-linked genes.	12 to 14
3. 5-Aza-2'-deoxycytidine is 10 times more effective than 5-azacytidine	15
4. 5-Aza-2'-deoxycytidine is most effective in late S for hpt activation.	15
5. After reactivation by 5-azacytidine, the hpt gene functions normally in DNA-mediated cell transformation.	10, 12

****

Jones, et al. (15) have established that 5-aza-2'-deoxycytidine is ten times more efficient than 5-AzaC in causing reactivation of hpt (up to 8.0%) and is most effective in late S phase when the inactive X chromosome is replicating. Finally, to complete the evidence that DNA methylation silences genes on the inactive X chromosome, the hpt gene on the inactive X chromosome functions normally in gene-mediated cell transformation after reactivation by 5-AzaC (10,12). Thus, DNA methylation is involved in at least one important event in early mammalian gene control. As indicated earlier, there are several other reasons for thinking that DNA methylation may function in mammalian cells as an effective gene silencing mechanism. We wish to stress here that there have been more than 20 reports, in a variety of systems, showing that treatment of cells in culture with 5-AzaC is sufficient to activate previously silent genes (reviewed in Ref. 4). For example, Harris (16) reported that the reversion rate of a Chinese hamster Tk⁻ variant increases from 10^{-6} to 0.1 after treatment with 5-AzaC. These and other results have established that methylation variants can masquerade as mutants. 5-AzaC is not a mutagen in the Ames test strains (17), and Landolph and Jones (18) find that it does not significantly increase the frequency of HPRT⁻ mutants or ouabain-resistant mutants in Chinese hamster cells. There is strong experimental evidence that the primary effect of 5-AzaC is to function as a mechanism-based, irreversible inactivator of DNA methylase after incorporation into DNA (see ref. 19 and 20). 5-AzaC also activates genes in vivo. Ley, et al., found that treating beta-thalassemic patients with 5-AzaC induces production of fetal hemoglobin. Similar results have been obtained with patients with sickle-cell anemia, and in these cases, the induction of the fetal globin gene transcription correlated with hypomethylation of a site in the 5'-flanking region (22,23).

Recent data has established convincingly that methylation of the coding region or introns can be relatively unimportant in controlling transcription. At the same time, the notion that methylation of critical sites can control transcription has become increasingly strong. We have recently cloned human phosphoglycerate kinase, an X-linked gene (24). This gene is activated very efficiently by 5-AzaC but our preliminary results indicate that there are no obvious differences in the methylation of HpaII/MspI (CCGG) sites between males (one active X) and fe-males (one active and one inactive X). However, we have not yet examined the 5'-flanking region. Our current working hypothesis is that hypomethylation of certain critical sites is a necessary condition for the efficient transcription of many genes. Methylation functions as a somatically heritable locking mecha-nism, stabilizing the transcriptionally quiescent state (3). Therefore, we reasoned (4) that inappropriate demethylation might activate oncogenes or other genes relevant to oncogenesis. This hypothesis was tested by asking whether or not the most potent inhibitor of methylation, 5-AzaC, was a carcinogen when given to rats by intraperitoneal injection.

****

Table 2. 5-Azacytidine-induced neoplasms in male F334 rats.

Property examined	Tumors	No. rats/group
1. Hepatic tumor initiation		
(a) Phenobarbitol	2	12
(b) Solt-Farber	0	6
2. Hepatic tumor promotion		
(a) 10 mg/kg AzaC	9	10
(b) 2.5 mg/kg AzaC	10	10
3. Complete carcinogenesis		
(a) 10 mg/kg AzaC	6	8
(b) 2 to 5 mg/kg AzaC	11	12
4. Single dose, 10 mg/kg AzaC	4	12
5. DEN control	0	6
6. Phenobarbitol control	0	6
7. Age control	0	12

Outline of protocols: (1a) 10 mg/kg 5-AzaCyt followed at 18 hr by a partial hepatectomy (PH), then dietary phenobarbitol for 9 months; (1b) 20 mg/kg 5-AzaCyt followed by PH and the Solt-Farber procedure (ref. 31); (2) 50 mg/kg diethylnitrosamine (DEN) followed by PH at 28 hr and 5-AzaCyt twice weekly for 9 months; (3) 5-AzaCyt twice weekly for 9 months.

****

As shown in Table 2, 36 of 40 rats had tumors in the groups tested for hepatic-tumor-promoting activity and complete car-cinogenicity. No tumors were detected in the age-matched controls (0/24). A wide variety of tumors was found: skin, testis, renal, lung, liver, leukemia, mesothelioma, and reticu-loendotheliosis. Histological data and other details of this work have been published elsewhere (25). Two rats in the complete carcinogenesis group had multiple primary tumors. An intriguing result, which needs to be followed with a larger study, is that the group receiving only a single dose of 10 mg/kg of 5-AzaC showed 4 of 12 rats with tumors.

   Ours is the first detailed study of the carcinogenicity of 5-AzaC for a variety of tissues and confirms two earlier studies suggesting that 5-AzaC might be a carcinogen for mice (26,27). 5-AzaC also is known to cause the morphologically-transformed phenotype in tissue culture (28). Finally, it has recently been shown that 5-AzaC efficiently changes immunogenic markers and the metastatic phenotype of certain mouse tumor lines (29,30). For these and other reasons (reviewed in ref. 4), we think that per-turbations in DNA methylation must be considered as a possible new mechanism involved in tumor progression.
****

References. (1) Riggs, A.D. (1975) Cytogenet. Cell Genet. 14: 9-25; (2) Holliday, R. and Pugh, J.E. (1975) SCIENCE 187: 226-232; (3) Razin, A. and Riggs, A.D. (1980) Science 210: 604-610; (4) Riggs, A.D. and Jones, R. (1983) Adv. Cancer Res. 40:1-30; (5) Doerfler, W. (1983) Annu. Rev. Biochem. 52:93-124; (6) Gartler, S.M. and Riggs, A.D. (1983) Annu. Rev. Genet. 17: 153-190; (7) Liskay, R.M. and Evans, R.J. (1980) Proc. Natl. Acad. Sci. USA 77:4895-4898; (8) Chapman, V.M., et al. (1982) Proc. Natl. Acad. Sci. USA 79:5357-5361; (9) Kratzer, P.G., et al., (1983) Cell (in press); (10) Venolia, L., et al. (1982) Proc. Natl. Acad. Sci. USA 79:2352-2354; (11) Venolia, L. and Gartler, S.M. (1983) Nature (London) 302:82-83; (12) Lester, S.C., et al. (1982) Somatic Cell Genet. 8:265-284; (13) Mohandas, T., et al. (1981) Science 211:393-396; (14) Graves, J.A.M. (1982) Exp. Cell Res. 141:99-105; (15) Jones, P.A., et al. (1982) Proc. Natl. Acad. Sci. USA 79:1215-1219; (16) Harris, M. (1982) Cell 29:483-492; (17) Podger, D.M. (1983) Mutat. Res. 121:1-6; (18) Landolph, J.R. and Jones, P.A. Cancer Res. 42:817-823; (19) Taylor, S.M. and Jones, P.A. (1982) J. Mol. Biol. 162:679-692; (20) Santi, D.V., et al. (1983) Cell 33: 9-10; (21) Ley, T.J., et al. (1982) New Eng. J. Med. 307: 1469-1475; Ley, T.J., et al. (1983) Blood 62: 370-380; (23) Carache, S., et al. (1983) Proc. Natl. Acad. Sci USA 80: 4842-4846; (24) Singer-Sam, J., et al. (1983) Proc. Natl. Acad. Sci. USA 80:802-806; (25) Carr, B.I., et al. (1984) New Eng. J. Med. (in press); (26) NCI Carcinogenesis Tech. Rep. Series No. 42, 1978. CAS No. 320-67-2; (27) Stoner, G.D., et al. (1973) Cancer Res. 33:3069-3085; (28) Benedict, W.F., et al. (1977) Cancer Res. 37:2202-2208; (29) Frost, et al. (1984) J. Exp. Med., submitted; (30) Olsson and Forschhammer (1984) submitted; (31) Solt, D. and Farber, E. (1976) NATURE (London) 263:701-703.

STUDIES OF X CHROMOSOME INACTIVATION IN HUMAN CELLS

Stanley F. Wolf and Barbara R. Migeon

Dept. of Pediatrics, Johns Hopkins University, Baltimore, MD 21205

Mechanisms have evolved in many eukaryotes with the XX/XY system of sex determination to compensate for the differences in the dosage of X chromosomes between the sexes. In these organisms, dosage compensation seems to be required in somatic cells to equalize the products of those X-linked genes not involved in sex differentiation. Equalization of X-chromosome gene products in mammals occurs by inactivation of one of the two X chromosomes in each female somatic cell, so that there is effectively a single, active X chromosome in both sexes (1).

It is not clear that there must be multiple events involved in the regulation of the mammalian X chromosome. The X chromosome houses genes of all types: those that are expressed only during early development, those that are tissue-specific, and those that are responsible for differentiated functions as well as for housekeeping enzymes. Therefore, all the mechanisms responsible for regulating any other chromosome are also operating in the regulation of genes on the active X chromosome.

The event that initiates dosage compensation for X-linked genes during early embryogenesis results in inactivation of all but a single X-chromosome in diploid cells. Once inactivated, the X-chromosome remains inactive in somatic cells, implying a mechanism that maintains the inactive state. The molecular basis for all of these functions is unknown. A popular working hypothesis is that DNA modification, specifically methylation, might be responsible for initiation and maintenance of the inactive state (2,3). However, studies of methylation of X-chromosome DNA assayed by Southern blot analysis using cloned X-chromosome-specific probes, indicates that X DNA methylation in normal human cells changes with replication, and preclude ubiquitous methylation differences as the molecular basis for X-chromosome inactivation (4,5).

On the other hand, it is clear that methylation of specific sites is important, at least in the maintenance of the inactivation process. Studies of interspecies cell hybrids have shown that 5-azacytidine (5-azaC) can induce local derepression of the inactive X chromosome, presumably because the cytidine analogue has blocked methylation at relevant sites on the active X (6,7).

Fig. 1. _Model for Studies of X-Methylation_. Hybrids derived from the fusion of female 46 XX fibroblasts and A9 mouse cells lacking HPRT are selected in HAT medium. Most of these hybrids retain the human active X, but some retain both. Back selection in medium containing 6-thioguanine (6TG) eliminates the active X, providing hybrids with no human X or only the inactive X. 5-azaC treatment of the hybrids with the inactive X and subsequent selection in HAT medium provides hybrids in which the previously inactive HPRT locus is expressed.

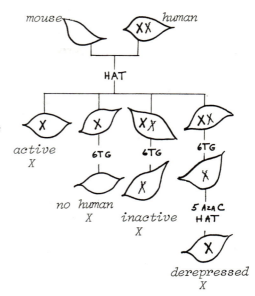

What is not clear is if demethylation is affecting regulation of transcription or regulation of sites specifically related to the inactivation process.

To explore the role of DNA methylation in maintaining dosage compensation of X-linked genes, we analyzed DNA methylation around the locus for hypoxanthine phosphoribosyltransferase (HPRT) on the human X chromosome. Using a genomic DNA probe (8,9) and restriction enzyme analysis, we characterized methylation of active, inactive and derepressed alleles (10). If DNA methylation of active and inactive X chromosomes differs significantly, the restriction fragments generated by digestion with HpaII or Hha I and hybridization with a labeled X-specific probe should differ between DNA of male cells with a single active X and that of female cells that have an inactive X as well. Furthermore, somatic cell hybrids provide the means to isolate the inactive X from its active homologue and enable one to obtain reactivants as well (Figure 1).

Observations of this kind indicate that the methylation of HpaII and Hha I sites in HPRT alleles on the active X was the same in all tissues that were analyzed. The consensus pattern associated with the active locus includes hypomethylation of 5' clustered sites, and extensive methylation of the 3' sequence (Figure 2). The striking feature of methylation of inactive X alleles is nonuniformity and less extensive hypomethylation of 5' clusters. Analysis of inactive alleles which reexpress HPRT activity in response to 5-azaC showed at least partial restoration of the consensus pattern, specifically with respect to 5' demethylation.

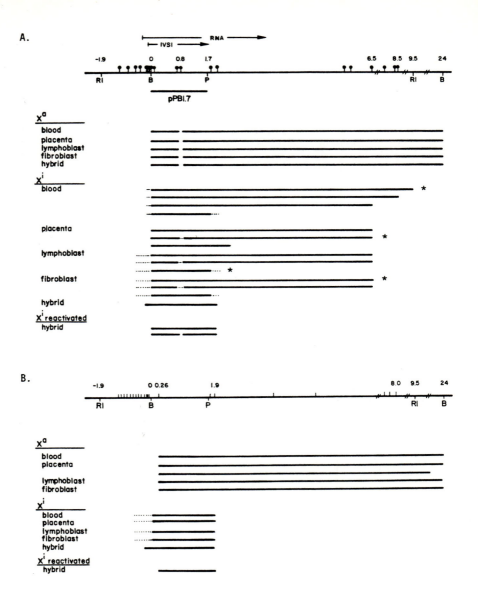

Fig. 2. *Methylation of HPRT at (A) and HpaII and (B) Hha I Sites on Active (X^a) and Inactive X (X^i) X Chromosomes.* Hpa II (⃚), Hha I (|), EcoRI (RI), BamHI (B), and Pst I (P). *The probe used in Southern blot hybridization is indicated by the bar below the map. The lines represent HpaII and Hha I fragments obtained in genomic digests; the predominant X^i fragment in populations studied is indicated (*). The ends of some X^i fragments are represented by dots to indicate that the specific unmethylated site within clusters may not be the same for all chromosomes.*

These observations indicate that methylation of housekeeping genes on the X chromosome is the same as that of autosomal ones and that the overall pattern and the state of methylation of many sites within a cluster may provide a cooperative means to facilitate transcription. Furthermore, the variable methylation of the inactive X, and absence of unique features argues against a specific methylation dependent mechanism for maintaining the silence of the inactive X. The fidelity of methylation of the active allele, and the extensive drift in methylation of the inactive allele suggest that maintenance X-dosage compensation is, in effect, maintenance of the transcriptional _activity_ of genes on the active X.

References.   (1) Lyon, M.F. (1972) Biol Rev 1: 35; (2) Riggs, A.D. (1975) Cytogenet Cell Genet. 14: 9; (3) Razin, A. and Riggs, A.D. (1980) Science 210: 604; (4) Wolf, S.F. and Migeon, B.R. (1982) Nature 295: 667-671; (5) Wolf, S.F. and Migeon, B.R. (1983) in Cold Spring Harbor Symposia on Quantitative Biology 47: 621-630; (6) Mohandas, T., Sparkes, R.S. and Shapiro, L.J. (1981) Science 211: 393-396; (7) Lester, S.C., Korn, N.J. and DeMars, R. (1982) Somatic Cell Genet. 8: 265-284; (8) Jolly, D.J., Okayama, H., Berg, P., Esty, A.C., Filpula, D., Bohlen, P., Johnson, G.G., Shively, J.E., Hunkapillar, T. and Friedmann, T. (1983) Proc. Natl. Acad. Sci. 80: 477-481; (9) Jolly, D.J., Esty, A.C., Bernard, H.U. and Friedmann, T. (1982) Proc. Natl. Acad. Sci. 79: 5038-5041; (10) Wolf, S.F., Jolly, D.J., Lunnen, K.D., Friedmann, T. and Migeon, B.R. (1983) - manuscript submitted.

DROSOPHILA HEAT SHOCK GENES AND THE CONTROL OF THEIR EXPRESSION.

R. Voellmy, R. Lawson, R. Mestril and P. Schiller Dept. of Biochemistry, University of Miami School of Medicine, Miami, Florida and D. Rungger, Dept. of Animal Biology, University of Geneva, Switzerland.

Heat shock proteins (hsp) are made in a wide variety of organisms ranging from bacteria to mammals. As in entire organisms, hsps are either not made at all or only at low levels at the normal growth temperature of cultivated cells but are produced at moderate to high levels at temperatures slightly above normal. In heat-treated Drosophila cells hsps with molecular weights of 84, 70, 68, 27, 26, 23 and 22,000 daltons (hsp 84, 70, etc.) are synthesized. The expression of the corresponding genes is controlled at both the transcriptional and the translational level. Large quantities of hsp mRNAs are present in heat-treated but not in untreated Drosophila cells. In contrast to most other mRNAs, hsp-mRNAs are translated efficiently at elevated temperatures. A subgroup of the hsp genes encoding hsp 27, 26, 23, and 22 are not only heat-induced but are also activated by the insect steroid hormone ecdysterone. All Drosophila hsp genes have been isolated and characterized in detail (5).

Attempts to define the DNA sequences required for the heat-activation of the Drosophila hsp genes have focused on the hsp 70 gene. In the absence of a convenient Drosophila in vivo expression system, the expression of the hsp 70 gene has been studied extensively in mouse cells (6), Xenopus oocytes (7,8) and COS cells (8,9). The Drosophila hsp70 gene was found to be transcribed in a heat-induced fashion in all of these heterologous cell systems. A 66 base pair DNA segment located immediately 5' to the transcription start site is sufficient for the heat-regulated expression of the hsp70 gene in COS cells and Xenopus oocytes (8,9). Sequence comparison suggested that a 15 base pair sequence containing two inverted repeats (consensus sequence) which is present upstream of several of the hsp genes and which is located 10-20 bp 5' to the TATA motif, is responsible for the heat activation of the hsp genes (8). We have been attempting to answer the following questions regarding the regulated expression of Drosophila hsp genes:

1. Are Drosophila genes other than the hsp70 gene expressed in foreign cells?

To be able to follow easily heat-regulated gene expression we prepared fusion genes consisting of hsp gene 5' nontranscribed and nontranslated sequences and short segments of hsp coding sequences (18 base pairs or more) linked in phase to an E. coli B-galactosidase gene. In all constructions the B-galactosidase gene was immediately followed by a 2.2 kilobase pair segment containing hsp 70 gene 3' nontranslated sequences. The fusion genes were inserted into the COS cell vector pSVod (4). The maps of two such constructs, p522 and p523 containing Drosophila hsp 70 and hsp 23 gene sequences respectively are shown in Fig. 1. Both plasmids when introduced into COS cells or Xenopus oocytes direct the heat-induced production of B-galactosidase activity. That α-amanitin blocks the heat-induced B-galactosidase synthesis indicates that control of expression of these genes occurs at the transcriptional level (data not shown).

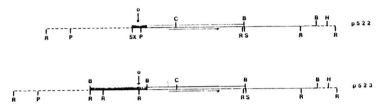

Fig. 1 Maps of plasmids 522 and 523. Black bars represent sequences from the 5' ends of Drosophila hsp genes. p522 contains a 450 base pair XhoI/Sau3A fragment from plasmid 51 (1) including 190 base pairs of 5' nontranscribed sequence and the complete RNA leader region of an hsp70 gene. p523 contains a 1.75 kilobase pair PstI/PvuII segment from plasmid F4 (2) which includes 1.5 kilobase pairs of 5' nontranscribed sequence and the complete RNA leader region of hsp23 gene. Open bars represent the E.coli B-galactosidase gene portion present in pMC 1871 (obtained from M. Casadaban), solid lines a 2.2 kilobase pair SalI/BamHI fragment from p56H8 (3) containing 3' nontranslated sequences of an hsp70 gene and interrupted lines pSVod vector sequences (4). Start and direction of transcription of the fusion genes are indicated by arrows. B: BamHI, C: ClaI, H: Hind III, P: Pst I, R: EcoRI, S: Sal I, SX: SalI/XhoI. The overall length of p522 is 9 kilobase pairs.

2.   How much 5' nontranscribed sequence is required for the heat-induced expression of the hsp 23 fusion gene in p523?

The sequence immediately upstream of the TATA motif in the hsp 23 gene matches the consensus sequence considerably less well (in 8 out of 14 base pairs only) than that of other genes including the hsp 70 gene (in 11 out of 14 base pairs). The main reason for choosing the hsp 23 gene for this study is the existence in this gene of a second sequence element about 90 base pairs 5' to the usual location of the consensus sequence (Fig. 2). This additional element matches the overall consensus sequence equally well as the element at the normal location. The inverted repeat sequences however are conserved better in the more distal element. The question therefore arose as to which element, if any, is recognized by the cells.

```
                    -150                              -120
Hsp23      TTTTCAGCCCGAGAAGTTTCGTGTCCCTTCTCGATGTCGATGTTTGTG

                    -100                    -80
Hsp23      CCCCCTAGCACACAGACACGACGCGCACACACACAGCGCCGACGGGCG                    -60

                                            -30
Hsp23      CCGCACACTTCGACAGCAAGCGGTTGTATAAATA

Hsp70      CTCGAATGTTCGCGAAAAGAGCGCCGGAGTATAAATA

Consensus  CTGGAATNTTCTAGA
Sequence
```

Fig. 2 5' Nontranscribed sequences of the hsp23 and the hsp70 gene (1,2). Sequences resembling the consensus sequence are underlined. Dots indicate identity with the consensus sequence.

A series of mutant fusion genes with 5' nontranscribed sequences of different lengths was prepared (Fig. 3). The heat-induced expression of these mutants was examined in Xenopus oocytes (Fig. 3). All mutants with 5' nontranscribed sequences of 100 base pairs or more were found to be expressed equally well in heat-treated but not in untreated oocytes. A mutant with only 60 base pairs of gene leader sequence was not expressed. We therefore conclude that the second more distal sequence element is not required for heat-regulated gene expression in Xenopus oocytes. The first element and additional sequences of somewhere between 2 and 40 base pairs in length 5' to this element contain all the information necessary for regulated expression.

3. Are the sequence requirements for the regulated expression of the hsp23 gene the same in a homologous as in a heterologous expression system?

To answer this question we have developed a procedure for the transfection of Drosophila melanogaster S3 cells (to be described elsewhere). This procedure allows us to measure the transient expression of heat shock –B-galactosidase fusion genes such as p522 and p523 (see Table 1). The expression of the mutant genes in Fig. 3 was reexamined in Drosophila cells. Surprisingly all mutants with up to 190 base pairs of leader sequence were inactive in Drosophila cells (Fig. 3). Thus the sequences required for hsp23 expression include both of the putative regulatory sequence elements mentioned above and more than 40 base pairs of additional sequence 5' to the most distal element. These results suggest that the consensus sequence elements alone are not sufficient for the expression of at least one of the Drosophila heat-shock genes in homologous cells.

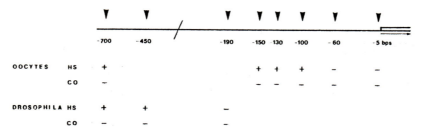

Fig. 3 Expression of hsp 23 fusion gene mutants with 5' nontranscribed segments of different lengths in Xenopus oocytes and Drosophila melanogaster S3 cells. The lengths of the leader segments of the various mutants are indicated by arrows. Details of the experimental procedures will be described elsewhere.

4. Does ecdysterone stimulate the expression of the hsp23 - B-galactosidase fusion gene in Drosophila cells?

Drosophila melanogaster S3 cells are ecdysterone-responsive. The genes encoding hsp27, 26, 23 and 22 have been shown to be activated during larval development and by ecdysterone in hormone-responsive cultivated cells (10, 11). To functionally characterize the DNA sequences responsible for the hormonal activation of these genes, it is necessary to have an expression system that allows the cloned genes to be expressed in a hormone-regulated fashion. We therefore examined the effects of ecdysterone treatment on the activity of the hsp23 fusion gene in p523-containing S3 cells. Ecdysterone was found to stimulate the expression of the hsp23 fusion gene substantially. In contrast, the hsp70 fusion gene in p522 was activated to a much lesser degree (Table 1). Stimulation of p523 gene expression occurs at ecdysterone concentrations between 10^{-7}M and 5×10^{-6}M, thus at concentrations well within the physiological range. Increasing the ecdysterone concentration above 5×10^{-6}M does not lead to any further stimulation of the hsp23 fusion gene activity. The activity of the hsp70 fusion gene, however increases linearly with ecdysterone concentrations from 10^{-7}M to at least 2×10^{-5}M indicating that the observed small degree of stimulation of this gene (Table 1) is not a true hormone effect but rather a response to the general stress imposed upon the cells by the hormone treatment. These results suggest that it will be possible to define the sequences involved in the hormonal regulation of the expression of the hsp23 gene and possibly also of other hormone-activated genes by using transient expression of fusion genes in S3 cells as an assay.

Table 1

Expression of fusion genes in ecdysterone and heat-treated Drosophila S3 cells.

Plasmids	B-Galactosidase Activity (A_{420})		
	No Treatment	Heat Treatment	Ecdysterone Treatment (10^{-6}M)
p 523	0.02	0.76	0.52
p 522	0.00	1.44	0.16

S3 cells were grown to confluency, transfected during 4 hrs and then further cultivated for 24 hrs at 25°C prior to any treatment. Ecdysterone treatment was for 24 hrs at 25°C, heat shock for 2 hrs at 36°C (Lawson et al., manuscript in prep.). B-Galactosidase activity was measured using the standard ONPG assay. All absorbance measurements have been corrected for differences in the protein contents of the cell lysates. Background activity has been determined for each condition using mock-transfected cells and has been subtracted from the experimental activity values shown.

References
(1) Karch, F., Torok, I. and Tissieres, A. (1981) J. Mol. Biol. 148, 219. (2) Southgate, R., Ayme, A. and Voellmy, R. (1983) J. Mol. Biol. 165, 35. (3) Mirault, M.-E., Goldschmidt-Clermont, M., Artavanis-Tsakonas, S. and Schedl, P. (1979) Proc. Natl. Acad. Sci. USA 76, 5254. (4) Mellon, P., Parker, V. Gluzman, Y. and Maniatis, T. (1981) Cell 27, 279. (5) "Heat Shock from Bacteria to Man" (1982) Schlesinger, M., Ashburner, M. and Tissieres, A. eds., Cold Spring Harbor Laboratory. (6) Corces, V., Pellicer, A., Axel. R. and Meselson, M. (1981) Proc. Natl. Acad. Sci. USA 78, 7038. (7) Voellmy, R. and Rungger, D. (1982) Proc. Natl. Acad. Sci. USA 79, 1776. (8) Pelham, H. (1982) Cell 30, 517. (9) Mirault, M.-E., Southgate, R. and Delwart, E. (1982) EMBO J. 1, 1279. (10) Sirotkin, D. and Davidson, N. (1982) Dev. Biol. 89, 196. (11) Ireland, R., Berger, E., Sirotkin, K., Yund, M., Osterbur, D. and Fristrom, J. (1982) Dev. Biol. 93, 498.

REGULATION OF TRANSCRIPTION BY GLUCOCORTICOIDS: IDENTIFICATION OF THE HORMONE REGULATORY ELEMENT AND ANALYSIS OF MECHANISM OF ACTION WITH EPISOMAL FUSIONS CONTAINING THE MMTV PROMOTER

Gordon L. Hager

Lab of Tumor Virus Genetics, Natl. Cancer Inst., Bethesda, MD 20205

INTRODUCTION. The modulation of gene expression by steroid hormones occurs primarily at the level of transcription. The induction of mouse mammary tumor virus (MMTV) transcription by glucocorticoids has emerged as an attractive model for the analysis of this regulatory process (1-4). By utilizing the MMTV promoter for expression of genes with a selectable phenotype in cultured cells, it has been shown that the sequences responsible for hormone regulation are completely encoded within the long terminal repeat (LTR) of the retrovirus (5, 6). It has also been demonstrated that purified glucocorticoid receptor complex has a selective affinity for the MMTV LTR (7-9).

LOCALIZATION OF THE HORMONE REGULATORY ELEMENT WITHIN THE MMTV LTR. Three approaches have been followed for the identification of putative hormone regulatory element(s) in the MMTV LTR. The first two involve the engineering of deletions in fusion chimeras (10) with the MMTV promoter driving expression either of chloramphenicol acetyl transferase (CAT) in a transient expression assay (11), or of the v-ras oncogene in a hormone-dependent transfection assay (12, 13). A third source of information comes from sequencing a variety of endogenous MMTV LTR's, one of which contains a major sequence rearrangement (14). It can be concluded from these studies that the hormone regulatory sequences occur between 100 and 200 base pairs upstream from the cap site for initiation of viral transcription.

A MINICHROMOSOME SYSTEM FOR STUDIES OF HORMONE REGULATION. Activation of gene transcription in mammalian cells is frequently accompanied by alterations in chromatin structure. These changes are most sensitively detected as sites of increased susceptibility to digestion by deoxyribonucleases (15), and are usually referred to as DNase-I hypersensitive sites. These sites can be localized in the vicinity of target genes by the indirect end-labelling technique (16, 17). Although these techniques are quite powerful for locating and mapping hypersensitive sites, the physical characterization of these structural alterations is quite difficult due to the high complexity of mammalian chromatin.

The modulation of target gene activity by glucocorticoids might also involve alterations to the nucleoprotein template. To investigate this question, the MMTV promoter was inserted (with appropriate tester genes) in chimeras with the bovine papilloma virus (BPV) 69% transforming fragment (18). These chimeras have the important property of replicating as free episomes in the nuclei of transformed mouse cells. Furthermore, cell lines harboring these plasmids can be expanded indefinitely with the fusion DNA remaining exclusively

in an unrearranged, episomal state (18). This system therefore
provides an opportunity for investigation of chromatin structure
at a hormone regulated promoter, and potential perturbations of
that structure that would occur during transcription induction.

THE MMTV PROMOTER IS SUBJECT TO REGULATION IN THE EPISOMAL STATE.
Chimeras with the v-ras oncogene driven by the MMTV promoter fused
to the BPV 69% transforming fragment have been used to transform
either NIH 3T3 or C127 mouse cells in culture. Cell lines have been
identified that contain 200-300 episomal copies of these chimeras
per nucleus. No integrated copies of the chimera are present in
these cells, and there is no evidence of sequence rearrangements in
the episomal elements (18). The responsiveness of the MMTV promoter
to induction in the episomal state has been investigated by transcription run-on experiments with minichromosomes prepared from nuclei
of transformed cells. Approximately 50% of the RNA labelled during
transcription extension with the minichromosome fraction is specific
for episomal DNA. The sequence distribution in RNA transcribed with
minichromosomes is analyzed by hybridization with single-stranded
probes that detect specific regions and strands of the plasmid template. The results indicate that approximately 10-25 times as many
RNA polymerase II molecules are initiated at the MMTV promoter with
minichromosomes isolated from hormone-treated cells, compared to
episomes from untreated cells, whereas no effect is observed on the
number of polymerase molecules initiated at the BPV promoter in the
BPV segment of the chimera. The MMTV promoter is therefore respons-
ive to regulation when mobilized in the extrachromosomal state.

GLUCOCORTICOID RECEPTOR ASSOCIATES SPECIFICALLY WITH CHROMATIN
CONTAINING A TARGET PROMOTER. The glucocorticoid receptor-hormone
complex can be specifically tagged by treatment of cells with radio-
labelled hormone. When minichromosomes that contain an MMTV promoter
and associated hormone regulatory element are purified from cells
treated with labelled hormone, an average of 2-4 receptor molecules
per episome are bound to the minichromosome fraction. Receptors
are not found in high affinity association with episomes that do
not include the MMTV LTR. The hormone-receptor complex is therefore
bound specifically to LTR-containing chromatin.

HORMONE EFFECTS ON CHROMATIN STRUCTURE. MMTV-LTR BPV episomal
chromatin has been examined for the presence of sites hypersensitive
to attack by deoxyribonuclease I. A DNase I hypersensitive site has
been localized within the LTR by the indirect end-labelling procedure
(16, 17). This site is only present in episomal chromatin from cells
that have been stimulated with hormone, and maps at current levels
of resolution to the region of the LTR required in gene transfer
experiments to confer hormone responsiveness. These results, coupled
with the finding that activated receptor is specifically associated
with LTR containing chromatin, suggest that the hormone receptor complex binds specifically to a regulatory site within LTR chromatin and
induces a change in the nucleoprotein structure that is detected as
a DNase I hypersensitive site, resulting in increased transcription

at an adjacent promoter. One interpretation of these findings
would be that activation of gene transcription by steroids involves
a local structural alteration to chromatin, creating an "open"
promoter; chromatin would be a necessary template for regulation.
Alternatively, the critical regulatory interactions could occur
between hormone receptor, RNA polymerase II and associated transcription factors and DNA, and the chromatin changes detected as
hypersensitive sites might reflect alterations in the nucleoportein
structure that occur as a result of the primary regulatory events.
The resolution of this question will require reconstitution of
regulation in vitro with DNA and chromatin templates.

(1) Ringold, G.M. (1979) Biochimica et Biophysica Acta 560, 487; (2)
Young, H.A., and Hager, G.L. (1979) In: Steroid Receptors and the
Management of Cancer (E.B. Thompson & M. Lippman, eds.), C.R.C.
Press, Inc., Cleveland, Ohio, p. 45; (3) Hager, G.L. (1983) Progr.
Nucl. Acid Res. Mol. Biol. 28, 193; (4) Hager, G.L., Richard-Foy,
H., Kessel, M., Lichtler, A.C. and Ostrowski, M.C. (1984) Recent
Progress in Hormone Research 40, (in press); (5) Huang, A.L.,
Ostrowski, M.C., Berard, D.S., and Hager, G.L. (1981) Cell 27, 245;
(6) Lee, F., Mulligan, R., Berg, P., and Ringold, G. (1981) Nature
294, 228; (7) Payvar, F., Firestone, G.L., Ross, S.R., Chandler,
V.L., Wrange, O., Carlstedt-Duke, J., Gustafsson, J.-A., and Yamamoto,
K. (1982) J. Cell. Biochem. 19, 241; (8) Govindin, M.V., Spiess, E.
and Majors, J. (1982) Proc. Natl. Acad. Sci. U.S.A. 79, 5157; (9)
Scheidereit, C., Geisse, S., Westphal, H.M., and Beato, M. (1983)
Nature 304, 749; (10) Kessel, M., Khoury, G., Lichtler, A.C., Ostrowski,
M.C., and Hager, G.L. Nuc. Acids Res. (submitted); (11) Gorman,
C.M., Moffat, L.F., and Howard, B.H. (1982) Mol. and Cell. Biology
2, 1044; (12) Ostrowski, M.C., and Hager, G.L. (1983) In: Workshop
on Gene Transfer and Cancer, Raven Press, New York, N.Y. 10036 (in
press); (13) Ostrowski, M.C., Huang, A.L., Kessel, M., Wolford, R.G.,
and Hager, G.L. EMBO Journal (submitted); (14) Johnson, L. and
Hager, G.L. (in preparation) (15) Weintraub, H., and Groudine, M.
(1976) Science 193, 848; (16) Wu, C. (1980) Nature 286, 854; (17)
Nedospasov, A., and Georgiev, S. (1980) Biochem. Biophys. Res. Comm.
92, 532; (18) Ostrowski, M.C., Richard-Foy, H., Wolford, R.G., Berard,
D.S., and Hager, G.L. (1983) J. Cell and Mol. Biol. 11, (in press).

THE SV40 "ENHANCER TRAP"

Frank Weber, Michael Boshart, Jean de Villiers, Julian Banerji, Christoph A. Gehring and Walter Schaffner

Institut für Molekularbiologie II der Universität Zürich, Hönggerberg, CH-8093 Zürich, Switzerland

INTRODUCTION

Transcriptional enhancers are short DNA segments that activate the transcription of linked genes, in either orientation and over distances of many kilobase pairs (kb), which were originally discovered in viral genomes (Banerji et al., 1981; de Villiers and Schaffner, 1981; Moreau et al., 1981; for recent reviews see Khoury and Gruss, 1983, and also Gluzman and Shenk, 1983). Tissue-specific cellular enhancers have recently been found in immunoglobulin genes (Banerji et al., 1983; Gillies et al., 1983; Neuberger, 1983; Queen and Baltimore, 1983; Picard and Schaffner, 1983).

We reasoned that it is possible to generally select for functional enhancers by assaying for the resurrection of enhancerless SV40, after cotransfecting it with short random DNA fragments into monkey cells. In this way we could select for the growth of recombinant viruses which had incorporated DNA with enhancer function. This technique offers clear advantages over the direct and indirect approaches used previously to identify enhancers (Banerji et al., 1981; Lusky et al., 1983; Fried et al., 1983; Folger et al., 1983).

RESULTS

We have transfected monkey CV-1 cells with non-infectious, linear SV40 DNA, lacking the 72 bp repeated enhancer region. Infectious virus was recovered from this "enhancer trap" upon co-transfection with enhancer DNA segments from various viruses such as SV40, polyoma, cytomegalovirus and Rous sarcoma virus. The enhancer DNA segments apparently became integrated into the enhancerless SV40 DNA by intracellular resection/ligation/repair processes. A truncated polyoma "semi-enhancer" (BclI to PvuII fragment; de Villiers and Schaffner, 1981) was incorporated as a dimer and retains the host cell preference (de Villiers et al., 1982) of the complete polyoma enhancer. Co-transfection of the "enhancer trap" with fragmented DNA of mouse, monkey or human origin, yielded no recombinant virus with integrated cellular sequences, with one possible exception. This indicates that there are no more than a few hundred segments per mammalian genome with the strong enhancer activity demanded by our assay. In some transfection experiments without added viral enhancer DNA, SV40 variants were generated which have a segment of their flanking "late" DNA duplicated to substitute for the deleted 72 bp repeat. In one of these variants (SV7.2, see Figure 1) an 88 bp duplication creates a strong enhancer from this previously inactive DNA region. Both the polyoma enhancer fragment and the spontaneously created enhancers lack the physical sequence features which have been associated with enhancer elements, namely the "GTGG(A/T)-box" (Khoury and Gruss, 1983), the "CACA-box" (Lusky et al., 1983) or stretches of alternating purines-pyrimidines (Nordheim and Rich, 1983). It therefore appears that these sequence motifs are not ubiquitously associated with, and may even be redundant for, the function of transcriptional enhancers.

REFERENCES

Banerji, J., Rusconi, S. and Schaffner, W. (1981) Cell 27, 299-308

Banerji, J., Olson, L. and Schaffner, W. (1983) Cell, 729-740

de Villiers, J. and Schaffner, W. (1981) Nucl.Acids Res.9, 6251-6264

50

de Villiers, J., Olson, L., Tyndall, C. and Schaffner, W. (1982) Nucl.Acids Res. 10, 7965-7976
Folger, K.R., Wong, E.A., Wahl, G. and Capecci, M.R. (1982) Mol.Cell.Biol. 2, 1372-1378
Fried, M., Griffiths, M., Davies, B., Bjursell, G., LaMantia, G. and Lania, L. (1983) Proc.Natl.Acad.Sci.80, 2117-2121
Gillies, S.D., Morrison, S.L., Oi, V.T. and Tonegawa, S. (1983) Cell 33, 717-728
Gluzman, Y. and Shenk, T. Editors (1983) Enhancers and eucaryotic gene expression. Cold Spring Harbor Laboratory, Cold Spring Harbor, New York
Khoury, G. and Gruss, P. (1983) Cell 33, 313-314
Lusky, M., Berg, L., Weiher, H. and Botchan, M. (1983) Mol.Cell.Biol. in press
Moreau, P., Hen, R., Wasylyk, B., Everett, R., Gaub, M.P. and Chambon, P. (1981) Nucl.Acids Res. 9, 6047-6068
Neuberger, M.S. (1983) EMBO J. 2, 1373-1378
Nordheim, A. and Rich, A. (1983) Nature 303, 674-679
Picard, D. and Schaffner, W. (1983) Nature, in press
Queen, C. and Baltimore, D. (1983) Cell 33, 741-748
Tooze, J. Ed. (1981) DNA tumor viruses (Cold Spring Harbor, New York: Cold Spring Harbor, New York

LEGEND TO FIGURE 1

SVΔ50: This variant virus has a 54 bp deletion around the KpnI site. It was obtained from a cotransfection of enhancer trap DNA with the enhancer bearing restriction fragment and an excess of sonicated carrier DNA.

SVP2M2: This variant was obtained from an experiment using the mixed-in sonicated plasmid pPySVkl00- where the SV40 enhancer was provided flanked by polyoma virus sequences (de Villiers et al., 1982).

SV15-: This is a virus containing the SV40 enhancer in the opposite orientation, obtained from an experiment with the same transfection protocol as in the case of SVΔ50.

SVFE2 and **SV7.2** grew out of cells transfected with SV40 enhancer trap and carrier DNA without enhancer added. The transfected SV40 DNA was circularized in vivo. 77 bp and 88 bp of the viral "late" region around the HpaII site were duplicated in SVFE2 and SV7.2, respectively, thereby giving rise to variants which grow slowly (SVFE2) or intermediately fast (SV7.2).

FIGURE 1: Maps of SV40-derived enhancers

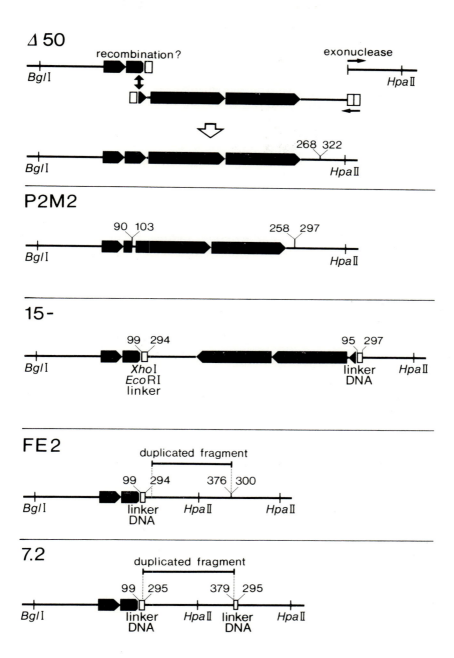

52

THE INTRODUCTION OF METALLOTHIONEIN-GROWTH HORMONE FUSION GENES INTO MICE.

R.E. Hammer[1], R.D. Palmiter[2], and R.L. Brinster[1]
[1]Lab. of Reprod. Phys., Sch. of Vet. Med., University of Pennsylvania, Philadelphia, PA. 19104
[2]Dept. Biochemistry, Howard Hughes Med. Inst., Univ. of Washington, Seattle, WA. 98195

The introduction of foreign DNA into the genome of mice by micro-injecting DNA fragments into the nuclei of early embryos is a unique and powerful approach to studying gene expression. Several foreign genes have been successfully introduced into the mouse genome and in some cases expression of these genes has been demonstrated (1-4). Fusion genes containing the mouse metallothionein I-gene (MT-I) are proving to be particularly useful for studying both gene expression and regulation (5-7).

We chose the MT-I promoter because the endogenous gene is regulated by heavy metals in most tissues (8). Our initial studies demonstrated that this fusion construction could be used to show metal regulation of the herpes virus thymidine kinase gene in transgenic mice (5). The success of these studies raised the possibility of using this promoter to regulate growth hormone (GH) production. Thus, we fused the MT-I promoter to either the rat or human GH structural gene (Fig. 1).

Linear DNA fragments containing these genes were microinjected into male pronuclei of fertilized mouse eggs. Animals that developed from these eggs were analyzed for the presence of the foreign gene by DNA dot hydridization using nucleic acid extracts from tails. Out

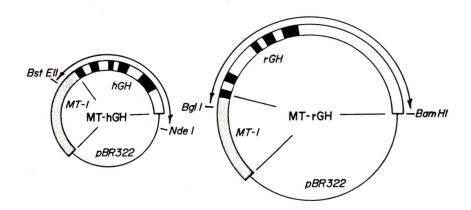

Fig. 1. Plasmids pMT-hGH and pMT-rGH contain the mouse metallothionein-I promoter fused to the human and rat growth hormone structural gene, respectively. The growth hormone exons are shown as solid regions, introns are open and the MT-I region is stippled.

of 122 animals that developed from these eggs, 40 contained the
foreign fusion genes and the majority (29) grew significantly larger
than their littermates.

Transgenic animals exhibiting the accelerated growth rate
expressed the fusion gene in the liver and to a lesser degree in
the intestine and heart. MT-GH transcriptional activity was induced
by metal treatment and in some of the largest mice, about a thousand
rat or human GH mRNA molecules per cell could be detected in the
liver.

Table I Expression of MT-hGH gene in transgenic mice

Animal	Gene Copy number/cell	Serum hGH ng/ml		IGF-I ug/ml	Growth ratio
		-Zn	+Zn		
184-1 ♀	2.0	250	11,900	1.73	2.37
184-5 ♂	10.4	520	18,000	1.21	1.70
186-4 ♀	18.0	8,200	143,000	1.04	2.14
182-3 ♂	45.0	3,700	14,600	1.48	1.67
control			0	0.55	

Copy number was determined by "tail" dot blots (5). Serum
samples were taken either before (-Zn) or during 76mM $ZnSO_4$ water
treatment (17 to 21 weeks of age). Serum GH and IFG-1 were determined by radioimmunoassay (RIA) and radioreceptor assay respectively
(7).

To determine whether high growth rates and high hGH mRNA production were associated with an increased production of human growth
hormone, serum hGH was measured in MT-GH animals (Table I). Transgenic mice produced hGH in large quantities and chronic zinc treatment further increased serum levels.

Growth hormone is thought to mediate growth through stimulation
of insulin-like growth factor (IGF-I) production which increases
growth by acting on bone, muscle and cartilage. Therefore, IGF-I
levels were measured in 4 zinc-treated transgenic mice and were
found to be 2-3 times control levels (Table I).

Although serum GH levels in most MT-GH mice could be increased
by chronic metal treatment, growth rates in treated animals were not
stimulated by metal induction (Table II). Apparently the constitu-
tive level of growth hormone present without metal stimulation is
sufficient to accelerate growth maximally.

If the foreign fusion gene was stably integrated into the host
chromosome and present in the germ line then MT-GH should be transmitted and the phenotype heritable. To determine MT-GH stability,
a transgenic male containing eight copies of MT-rGH was out bred
(Fig. 2). The fusion gene has now been transmitted into the third
generation with continued expression of the foreign gene in every
transgenic offspring. Growth rates remain accelerated with the
average increase in adult size about 2-fold.

54

Table II   Effect of Zn stimulation on serum GH and growth
              in MT-rGH transgenic mice

	Animals	Serum GH (ng/ml)		Weight gain (g)	
MGH mice, -Zn	5	1,250 ±	210*	14.0 ±	2.0
MGH mice, +Zn	5	12,500 ±	4,600	11.6 ±	1.0
Control mice, -Zn	3	410 ±	170	3.3 ±	1.0
Control mice, +Zn	5	330 ±	120	5.0 ±	0.5

*Mean ± SEM. Mice are from two litters of a transgenic male
(MGH 10) containing 8 copies of MT-rGH per cell (6). Animals
drinking water was supplemented with 76mM ZnSO4 from 5 to 11 weeks
of age. Weight gain was for the entire six weeks. Serum GH was
determined by RIA (9).

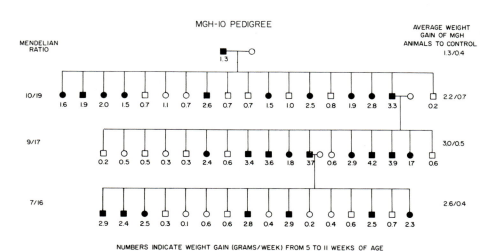

Fig. 2. Pedigree of MGH 10 showing inheritance and expression
of the MT-rGH gene (6). Approximately 50% of the offspring in three
generations of MGH 10 carry the fusion gene (solid symbols). All
of the transgenic offspring grew at an accelerated rate.

These results demonstrate that the mouse MT-I promoter when
fused to the growth hormone structural gene from two different
species regulates GH mRNA production and in turn controls GH synthesis. Many transgenic animals have supraphysiological levels of
serum growth hormone resulting in dramatic growth rates and twice
normal body weights. Although growth hormone levels can be increased
by MT-I induction it is apparent that growth rate is limited by
factors other than circulating GH, possibly IGF-I production.
    Based on these observations we undertook experiments to restore
growth in the dwarf mutant lit/lit mouse which is deficient in

growth hormone, by introducing the fusion gene MT-rGH into mutant eggs. Transgenic <u>little</u> mice grew to approximately 1.5 times the size of normal heterozygote animals. In addition, the fusion gene was stably integrated into the host chromosome and was transmitted into the second generation with continued expression in transgenic mutant offspring. Thus the effects of a single gene defect can be partially overcome by the introduction of a foreign replacement gene.

References: (1) Wagner, T. F., Stewart, T. A. and Mintz, B. (1981) Proc. Nat. Acad. Sci. USA. 78, 5016-5020. (2) Lacy, E., Roberts, S., Evans, E. P., Burtenshaw, M. D. and Constantini, F. D. (1983) Cell 34, 343-358. (3) McKnight, G. S., Hammer, R. E., Kuenzel, E. A. and Brinster, R. L. (1983) Cell 34, 335-341. (4) Brinster, R. L., Ritchie, K. A., Hammer, R. E., O'Brien, R. L., Arp, B. and Storb, U. (1983) Nature, In Press. (5) Brinster, R. L., Chen, H. Y., Trumbauer, M., Senear, A. W., Warren, R. and Palmiter, R. D. (1981) Cell 27, 223-231. (6) Palmiter, R. D., Brinster, R. L., Hammer, R. E., Trumbauer, M., Rosenfeld, M. A., Birnberg, N. C. and Evans, R. M. (1982) Nature 300, 611-614. (7) Palmiter, R. D., Norstedt, G., Gelinas, R. E., Hammer, R. E. and Brinster, R. L. (1983) Science. In Press. (8) Durnam, D. M., and Palmiter, R. D. (1981) J. Biol. Chem. 256, 5712-5716. (9) Doehmer, J., Barinaga, M., Vale, W., Rosenfeld, M. G., Verma, I. M. and Evans, R. M. (1982) Proc. Nat. Acad. Sci. USA 79, 2268-2272.

Acknowledgements: This work was supported by grants from NIH: HD-07155, HD-09172, HD-17321 and AM-31322. NSF: PCM-81-07172 and the American Heart Association: 80-728.

The Major
Histocompatibility Loci

HUMAN HISTOCOMPATIBILITY ANTIGENS: GENES AND PROTEINS

Jack L. Strominger

Department of Biochemistry and Molecular Biology, Harvard
University, Cambridge, MA 02138 (U.S.A.)

The structures of Class I (HLA-A,B,C) and Class II (HLA-DR)
antigens encoded on human chromosome 6 (Fig. 1) will be briefly
reviewed. Despite the differences in function, these molecules have
remarkably similar structures. Each is composed of four
extracellular domains (two of which are conserved Ig-like domains
and one of which is polymorphic) in addition to the transmembrane

Human Chromosome 6

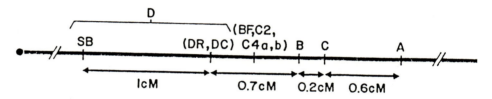

Murine Chromosome 17

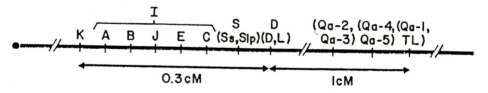

Fig. 1 Structure of the HLA complex on chromosome 6 and its murine
homologue on chromosome 17 based on genetics and serology.
It should be noted that the order within each of the
following groups is unknown: Ss and Slp; L and D; Qa1 and
Qa2; DR and DR; C2, BF, C4A and C4B.

and intracytoplasmic regions (Fig. 2). In homozygous human cell lines <u>at least</u> four subsets of HLA-DR antigens are expressed (SB, DC and two subsets of DR). DR is homologous to murine I-E antigens, and DC is homologous to I-A antigens. All of the light chains and one of the heavy chains are polymorphic. cDNA and/or genomic clones

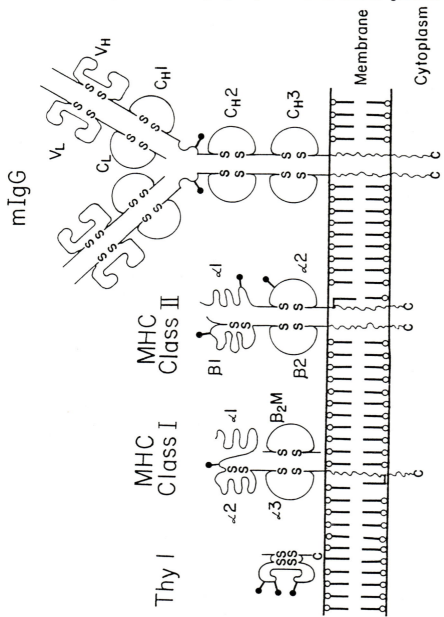

Fig. 2 Models of membrane proteins with homology to immunoglobulin. The Class I and Class II MHC antigens each contain two immunoglobulin-like domains adjacent to the membrane.

have been obtained for five heavy chains (SB, SX, DC, DX and DR plus three additional still unidentified crosshybridizing DNA sequences) and for at least three groups of light chains (Fig. 3). Thus the human HLA-D region appears to be more complex than the corresponding murine Ia region, at least as so far observed, and appears to have been created by a large gene expansion. Sequence comparison of genes has provided some clues to its evolutionary history. In genomic blots one of the heavy chain clones (DCα) reveals an extensive polymorphism which correlates exactly with the polymorphism of the MT alloantisera described by Terasaki. The SB β clone correlates both with SB typing and with SB segregation in a recombinant family. Data on <u>in situ</u> hybridization of clones to metaphase chromosomes of a normal individual and of an individual with apparent duplication of the MHC at 6p21.3 (carried out by Walter Nance, Cynthia Morton and their colleagues) will also be presented.

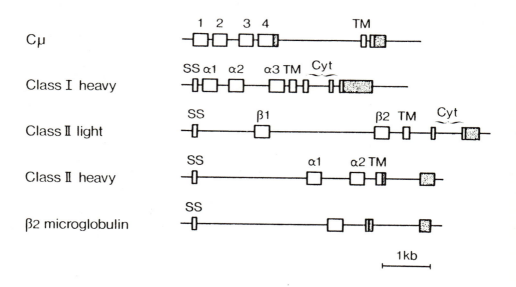

Fig. 3 Genomic structures of six related genes (SS, signal sequence; TM, transmembrane region; cyt, cytoplasmic region; exons representing extracellular domains are so numbered). Shaded boxes denote 3' untranslated regions. Cµ represents the constant region of a Cµ heavy chain gene.

This short account is based mainly on the following recent references from our laboratory and on still unpublished experiments of the authors. References to the work of others can be found in the papers cited.

References - (1) Shackelford, D.A., Kaufman, J.F., Korman, A.J. and Strominger, J.L. (1982) Immunol. Rev. 66, 133; (2) Korman, A.J., Knudsen, P.J., Kaufman, J.F. and Strominger, J.L. (1982) Proc. Natl. Acad. Sci. USA 79, 1844; (3) Korman, A.J., Auffray, C., Schamboeck, A. and Strominger, J.L. (1982) Proc. Natl. Acad. Sci. USA 79, 6013; (4) Auffray, C., Korman, A.J., Roux-Dosseto, M., Bono, R. and Strominger, J.L. (1982) Proc. Natl. Acad. Sci. USA 79, 6337; (5) Auffray, C., Ben-Nun, A., Roux-Dosseto, M., Germain, R.N., Seidman, J.G. and Strominger, J.L. (1983) EMBO J. 2, 121; (6) Auffray, C., Kuo, J., DeMars, R. and Strominger, J.L. (1983) Nature 304, 174; (7) Roux-Dosseto, M., Auffray, C., Lillie, J.W., Korman, A.J. and Strominger, J.L. (1983) in 'Gene Expression' (UCLA Symp. Mol. Cell. Biol.), Vol. 8, eds. D. Hamer and M. Rosenberg. Alan R. Liss, Inc., New York; (8) Roux-Dosseto, Auffray, C., Lillie, J.W., Boss, J., Cohen, D., DeMars, R., Mawas, C., Seidman, J.G. and Strominger, J.L. (1983) Proc. Natl. Acad. Sci. USA 80, 6036; (9) Schamboeck, A., Korman, A.J., Kamb, A. and Strominger, J.L. (1983) Nuc. Acids Res., in press; (10) Kaufman, J.F., Auffray, C., Korman, A.J., Shackelford, D.A. and Strominger, J.L. (1983) Cell, in press; (11) Auffray, C., Lillie, J.W., Arnot, D., Grossberger, D., Kappes, D. and Strominger, J.L. (1983) Nature, submitted; (12) Kirsch, I.R., Morton, C.C., Nance, W.E., Evans, G.A., Korman, A.J. and Strominger, J.L. (1983) Nature, submitted;

With the collaboration of Robert deMars (University of Wisconsin), Daniel Cohen and Jean Dausset (Hopital St. Louis, Paris), Jon Seidman, Avi Ben-Nun and Cynthia Morton (Harvard Medical School), Ronald Germain, Lani Kirsch and Glenn Evans (N.I.H.), Jiri Novotny (Massachusetts General Hospital), Claude Mawas (Centre d'Immunologie, Marseille) and Walter Nance (Medical College of Virginia). Supported by research grants from N.I.H. (AI-10736, AM-13230 and AM-30241) and the Kroc Foundation.

STRUCTURE AND FUNCTION OF I-A MOLECULES

Hugh O. McDevitt

Department of Medical Microbiology, Stanford University Medical School, Stanford, CA 94305

Analysis of cDNA sequences from six A_α cDNA alleles (1), three A_β alleles (2) and two E_β alleles (3,4) reveals several common characteristics in the allelic sequence variation and the gene products of these three I region genes. Almost all of the allelic variability is found in the first domain, while there is very little variation in the second domain or in the transmembrane or cytoplasmic regions. Within the first domain, allelic sequence variation tends to be clustered in three to four "allelic hypervariable" regions which are localized roughly around residues 10 to 15, residues 48 to 60, and residues 75 to 85, with some variation between the three different genes in the exact location of these regions of variability (See Table). The already documented immunoglobulin sequence homology of all three gene products, in combination with the finding of short stretches of allelic hypervariability with, a spacing between these stretches reminiscent of immunoglobulin hypervariable regions in immunoglobulin V region sequences, raises the possibility that the external domains of I region α and β chains are folded in a β sheet conformation in such a way that the allelic hypervariable regions of both the α and β chain come into close contact with one another at one end of the molecule, most probably that end most external with respect to the cell membrane surface. Detailed sequence data will be presented to document these findings.

TABLE I
Regions of Allelic Hypervariablity
in Murine I-A and I-E molecules.+

A. The I-A molecule.

	A_{α_1} (6)[*]	A_{α_2}(6)
10-15	(3/6)[**]	
44-49	(3/6)[++]	--
53-59	(4/7)[++]	--
68-79	(5/9)	--
Total hypervariable residues	15	0
	15	4
Isolated variations	4	4

	A_{β_1} (3)	A_{β_2} (3)
10-18	(5/9)[+++]	--
63-68	(4/6, 2 gaps)	--
85-90	(3/6)	--
Total hypervariable residues	12	0
Isolated Variants	6	4

[+]A region of allelic hypervariability was arbitrarily defined as any stretch of 6 or more amino acid residues in which ar least 50% of the positions exhibited allelic variation.

[*]This number indicates the number of alleles for which complete or nearly complete sequence information is available.

[**]This number gives the number of variant residues/total number of residues in a hypervariable stretch.

[++]Combining these adjacent regions results in a single hypervariable stretch from residues 48-59 in which 5/12 residues vary.

[+++]The first six residues are not yet sequenced.( )

TABLE I
Part 2

B. The I-E molecule.

	$E_{\alpha 1}(2)$	$E_{\alpha 2}(2)$
Hypervariable residues	0	0
Isolated variants		

	$E_{\beta 1}(2)$	$E_{\beta 2}(2)$
	1-13 (7/13)	--
	24-35 (6/12)	--
	68-75 (4/8)	--
Total Hypervariable Residues	17	0
Isolated Variants	5	1

STRUCTURE AND EXPRESSION OF HLA CLASS I GENES

Bertrand R. JORDAN, François A. LEMONNIER, Philippe LE BOUTEILLER,
Marie MALISSEN, Zohair MISHAL, Régis SODOYER, Terry L. DELOVITCH,
Tom STRACHAN, Michèle DAMOTTE, Catherine N'GUYEN, Corine LAYET,
Joëlle DUBREUIL, André J. VAN AGTHOVEN, Jeannine TRUCY and Danielle
CAILLOL.
Centre d'Immunologie INSERM-CNRS de Marseille-Luminy, Case 906,
13288 Marseille Cedex 9, France.

We have screened two libraries of human DNA constructed with
the cosmid expression vector pOPF1 (1) using HLA class I probes
derived from an HLA class I gene obtained and sequenced in our
laboratory (2). The HLA cosmids obtained have been characterized by
restriction mapping (3) and used to transform murine LMTK⁻ cells.
Stable expression of some of these genes has been obtained in this
system (4), and the HLA protein expressed at the surface of the
murine cells has been characterized with monoclonal antibodies and
alloantisera (5). In this way DNA clones encoding particular HLA
allelic products have been identified ; a summary of our results is
presented in Table 1. It is worth noting that in spite of the
relatively small number of clones obtained from the first cosmid
library (DNA from a heterozygous individual is expected to contain
approximately 40 different HLA genes-including pseudogenes) four out
of the six expected HLA specificities are found. Note also that we
have not detected any clone encoding the human equivalents of the TL
and Qa molecules, i.e. that all genes which were positive in the
expression assay turned out to code for HLA-A, -B, -C products.

Individual	HLA specificities	Number of different cosmid clones	Number of different HLA class I genes	Genes identified by expression	
				Cosmid clone	Specificity expressed
JG	A3	15	13	c44+, c64+	A3
	AW24			c27	AW24
	B7			c37	B7
	B27				NOT FOUND
	CW2				NOT FOUND
	CW3			c42	CW3
HHK	A3	35	20	c207*, c220*, c225* c229*, c242*, c277*	A3
	A3				
	B7				
	B7			c276	B7
	CW6				
	CW6				NOT FOUND

+, ★ : OVERLAPPING COSMIDS

TABLE I

68

The availability of A3 and B7 clones obtained from two different unrelated individuals allow comparison of these genes and their surrounding regions to see whether they are identical or different, an important issue with respect to the nature of HLA polymorphism in an outbred population. Such a comparison is particularly instructive in the A3 case since overlapping cosmids allowed us to define a gene cluster covering over 50 kilobases of DNA and containing three class I coding sequences, one of which causes the expression of the A3 protein when assayed in murine cells. This cluster is shown in Fig. 1 and appears identical at the restriction map level in the two individuals studied. A polymorphic restriction fragment characteristic of some HLA-A alleles, in particular A3 and A11 has been identified by Ascanio et al. (6). This 5.8 Kb Bgl I fragment is indeed found in our cloned A3 region but, unexpectedly, does not correspond to the A3 gene itself but to the first gene of the cluster which is not expressed in murine cells and whose restriction map differs markedly from that of the A3 genes (Fig. 1). This indicates extreme conservation of sequences flanking the A3 gene and shows that, although the "blot typing" approach is valid, polymorphic fragments do not necessarily provide a way of isolating the HLA class I gene coding for the corresponding HLA protein.

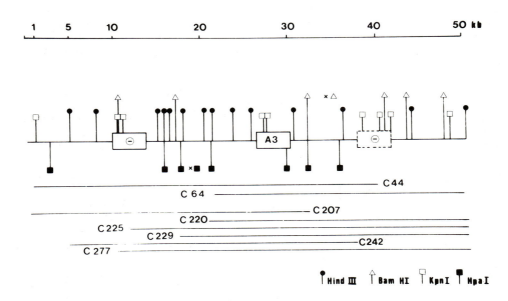

The two HLA-B7 genomic clones which we have obtained appear to have a different restriction map. Further study will indicate whether or not this corresponds to differences in the coding sequences.

Sequencing studies on identified genes allow the determination of new HLA protein sequences ; in addition (since these are performed on genomic clones) they make it possible to examine the extent of divergence of introns and flanking sequences. This data is important to test hypotheses on the mechanism(s) by which polymorphism is generated and maintained. Such studies have been performed on the HLA-CW3 and the HLA-A3 genes and will be reported.

The transformed cells (murine cells expressing a single type of HLA heavy chain at their surface, in association with murine β2-microglobulin) are in themselves useful for a number of studies. For example, they have revealed that a conformational change occurs on murine β2-microglobulin when it is associated with certain HLA heavy chains. This conformational change renders the murine β2-microglobulin molecule reactive with a monoclonal antibody specific for human β2-microglobulin (7). Transformed cells can be used to immunize C3H mice (of the H-2^k haplotype, as L cells) ; anti-HLA sera and monoclonal antibodies are obtained which in some cases distinguish between different HLA allelic products. The action of interferon on these cells has also been studied : the amount of HLA messenger RNA and of HLA protein (both intracellular and at the cell surface) is increased by treatment with murine (and not human) interferon, with kinetics very similar to those observed for the endogenous H-2 products (8).

Exon-shuffling experiments performed with these identified genes show that the HLA allospecificity is essentially determined by the first two external domains of the molecule (9). Further constructions (including genes modified by site-directed mutagenesis) should help to locate the most important regions of the HLA molecule.

References – (1) Grosveld, F.G., Lund, T., Murray, E., Mellor, A., Dahl, A. and Flavell, R.A. (1982) Nucl. Acids Res. 10, 6715; (2) Malissen, M., Malissen, B. and Jordan, B.R. (1982a) Proc. Natl. Acad. Sci. USA 79, 893; (3) Malissen, M., Damotte, M., Birnbaum, D., Trucy, J. and Jordan, B.R. (1982b) Gene 20, 485; (4) Lemonnier, F.A., Malissen, M., Golstein, P., Le Bouteiller, P., Rebai, N., Damotte, M., Birnbaum, D., Caillol, D., Trucy, J. and Jordan, B.R. (1982) Immunogenetics 16, 355; (5) Lemmonier, F.A., Dubreuil, P.C, Layet, C., Malissen, M., Bourel, D., Mercier, P., Jakobsen, B.K., Caillol, D.H., Svejgaard, A., Kourilsky, F.M. and Jordan, B.R. (1983) Immunogenetics 18, 65; (6) Ascanio, L., Paul, P., Marcadet, A., Mahouy, G., Fradelizi, D., Cohen, D. and Dausset, J. (1982) C.R. Acad. Sci. Paris 295, 433; (7) Lemonnier, F.A., Le Bouteiller, P., Malissen, B., Gostein, P., Malissen, M., Mishal, Z., Caillol, D.H., Jordan, B.R. and Kourilsky, F.M. (1983) J. Immunol. 130, 1432; (8) Rosa, F., Le Bouteiller, P., Abadie, A., Mishal, Z., Lemonnier, F.A., Bourrel, D., Damotte, M., Kalil, J., Jordan, B.R. and Fellous, M. (1983) Eur. J. Immunol. 13, 495; (9) Jordan, B.R., Lemonnier, F.A., Caillol, D.H. and Trucy, J. (1983) Immunogenetics 18, 165.

GENES OF THE MAJOR HISTOCOMPATIBILITY COMPLEX

Leroy E. HOOD

Division of Biology, California Institute of Technology
Pasadena, California 91125

The genes of the major histocompatibility complex include two multigene families that are involved in self-nonself recognition phenomena. The class I genes, typified by the transplantation antigens, encode cell-surface molecules about 45,000 daltons in molecular weight and which are associated with β_2-microglobulin, a free immunoglobulin-like domain. The class II genes encode the so-called Ia antigens which are heterodimers made up of α and β chains. The class I genes all appear to have a common structure composed of eight exons which correlate with the various domains and regions of the class I molecule. The same appears to be true of the class II genes. We have employed cosmid libraries to isolate at least 36 different class I genes which map into 13 distinct cosmid clusters. Restriction enzyme site polymorphism mapping has been used to determine the precise location of each of these cosmid clusters in the major histocompatibility complex. All 36 class I genes have been transferred by DNA-mediated gene transfer into mouse L cells and the classically defined serologic products identified. Thus six of the class I genes encode classically defined serologic products and at least 12 other class I genes express class I molecules that have heretofore not been identified. We have used gene transfer techniques to study the basic features of T cell-mediated cytotoxic killing which employ a foreign antigen in conjunction with a particular transplantation antigen. We have manipulated the class I genes by in vitro mutagenesis (exon shuffling) and have used the mutated gene products to delineate the regions that are important in T-cell cytotoxic killing and the specific binding sites of relevant monoclonal antibodies. We have also demonstrated that truncated class I genes can be transferred into mouse L cells and reconstituted presumably by homologous but unequal crossing-over to generate full-length hybrid class I genes whose products can be expressed on the cell surface. This phenomena has obvious importance for specific gene transfer experiments in the future.

Chromosomal walking procedures have been used to isolate 250 kilobases of contiguous DNA in the I region which contains six distinct class II genes. Several of these genes have been sequenced and the region has been mapped extensively by restriction analysis. These studies have demonstrated several striking features including the fact that there are chromosomal domains that are highly polymorphic and other chromosomal domains which are highly conserved, that there is a hot spot for recombination which divides a polymorphic and conservative domain, and that one of the important subregions in the I region (I-J) is missing. The membrane proximal domains of the class I and class II molecules are homologous to one another and to the constant regions of antibody molecules. This suggests that each of these gene families descended from a common ancestral family. One wonders how many additional members of this super gene family will exist and how they might be identified.

References

1. R. S. Goodenow, I. Stroynowski, M. McMillan, M. Nicolson, K. Eakle, B. T. Sher, N. Davidson and L. Hood. Nature **301**: 388-394 (1983).
2. L. Hood, M. Steinmetz and B. Malissen. Ann. Rev. Immunol. 1: 529-568 (1983).
3. M. Steinmetz, K. Minard, S. Horvath, J. McNicholas, J. Frelinger, C. Wake, E. Long, B. Mach and L. Hood. Nature **300**: 35-42 (1982).
4. M. Steinmetz, A. Winoto, K. Minard and L. Hood. Cell **28**: 489-498 (1982).

Human Genetic Organization

INTRODUCTION AND OVERVIEW

William L. NYHAN

Dept. Pediatrics, University of California San Diego
La Jolla, CALIFORNIA

Solution of the structure of DNA and elucidation of the nature of the code provided the promise that technology would be developed directed at the gene itself that would have impact on clinically relevant genetical disorders. The study of human disease and the analysis of pedigree patterns has permitted the mapping of certain portions of the genome, notably on the X chromosome. Techniques of somatic cell hybridization have permitted the development of similar information on the autosomes. The use of cells with translocations and deletions and the advent of new techniques of banding and stretching of the chromosomes have permitted much more precise localization of genes on human chromosomes. A substantial portion of the genome has now been mapped. The development of techniques of recombinant DNA has now permitted direct application to human disease. The isolation and cloning of normal human genes whose altered counterparts code for clinical illness raise the promise that one day a symposium of this type will be devoted to gene therapy. The methodology has already begun to have an impact on diagnosis. New methods are being developed for the detection of heterozygotes and for prenatal diagnosis using restriction fragment polymorphisms. As will be evident as this symposium proceeds, these techniques are providing very precise information on the mechanisms by which genetic disease is caused.

Genetically determined diseases fall generally into three categories. The Mendelian or single gene disorders are the ones that we are beginning to come to grips with on a molecular level that deals not just with the abnormal protein or enzyme molecule but with what has gone wrong with the genetic message in the DNA. Chromosomal abnormalities visible under the microscope were first recognized as causes of major malformation syndromes in which an entire chromosome, such as 18 or 21, was present in an extra copy. Visualization of the elongated chromosomes of the high resolution techniques is permitting the recognition of some much more subtle alterations, such as the abnormality of position q12 on the long arm of chromosome 15 in the Prader-Willi syndrome and the deletion of chromosome 13q14 which appears to remove a suppressor permitting the development of retinoblastomas. Observations like these and techniques of in situ hybridization bring us closer to the anatomy of the abnormal genome and bring the study of chromosomes and single gene defects closer together. The third major category of genetical disease, that of the multifactorial disorders, represents some of the really common diseases of man. The understanding of these disorders at a molecular level appears a bit further off.

The single gene disorders are generally thought of as rare diseases, although this is not always true. Cystic fibrosis is a common disorder in the United States. So is sickle cell anemia and glucose-6-phosphate dehydrogenase deficiency in our black population. The same is true for Tay Sachs disease among the descendents of the original Ashkenazim of central Europe,and thalassemia among those whose ancestors lived around the Mediterranean Sea that gave the disease its name. Furthermore, in the aggregate, Mendelian disorders make up quite a body of diseases. In the most recent 6th Edition of McKusick's catalogs (1) the total number of loci listed was 3368. The rate of growth in knowledge is indicated by the fact that in 1958 the number known was only 412, and the first edition of the McKusick catalogs in 1966 listed 1487.

Among the Mendelian disorders,the inborn errors of metabolism and the other disorders in which the protein product of the altered gene can be tested for chemically have provided our richest current sources of new molecular understandings. In genetic disease in general pleiotropism is the rule; the single abnormal gene produces a wide variety of clinical phenotypic effects. This makes it very difficult in many disorders to see what is the primary problem. When we can identify an abnormal enzyme protein or abnormal hemoglobin molecule, the sequence of events becomes much more clear. It is now (1984) 50 years since Fölling's landmark discovery (2) of the excretion of phenylpyruvic acid in the urine of a series of individuals with mental retardation. The disease he discovered, now known as phenylketonuria or PKU, is understood as an abnormality in the enzyme phenylalanine hydroxylase. A considerable amount is known about the enzyme and its abnormalities, although it is not easy to study since it is confined to the liver. The human gene for phenylalanine hydroxylase has now been cloned (3). Using a cDNA probe, it has been possible to identify a considerable amount of restriction polymorphism.

We described a disorder 20 years ago in which there was a substantial evidence of pleiotropism (4) in which there were effects on the kidneys and the joints, as well as retardation of mental development, prominent neurologic abnormalities and striking alterations in behavior. Its nature as an inherited disorder of metabolism was clear from the markedly elevated concentrations of uric acid in body fluids. This is now understandable on the basis of a fundamental, virtually complete defect in the activity of the enzyme hypoxanthine guanine phosphoribosyl transferase (HPRT) (5). Considerable genetic heterogeneity has been observed in the abnormalities of HPRT and a variety of distinct phenotypes have been observed with a roughly linear correlation between the severity of the clinical phenotypic expression and the degree of abnormality in the enzyme (6). The human gene for HPRT has now been cloned (7-9), and the use of the cDNA probe has identified restriction fragment polymorphisms which have already been useful in heterozygote detection (9) and should be effective in prenatal diagnosis. Kelley and colleagues (10) have determined the amino acid sequence of normal human erythrocyte HPRT and those of some variants including HPRT$_{Toronto}$ in which there is a glycine substitution at position 50. This permitted the prediction that there should be the abolition of a restriction endonuclease site that is recognized by Taq-I. This was confirmed by Southern blot analysis in which a normal 2.0 kb restriction fragment was replaced by a 4.0 kb fragment. This methodology has permitted the identification of heterozygotes not identifiable with other methods.

The field is moving very rapidly forward. We can expect to gain substantially improved understanding of the nature of the genome and the ways in which its alterations produce disease in man. This section of the symposium provides an up to date analysis of the current state of the art.

References. (1) McKusick, V. A., _Mendelian Inheritance in Man, Catalogs of Autosomal Dominant Autosomal Recessive and X-Linked Phenotypes_, 6th Ed., Johns Hopkins Univ. Press, Baltimore-London (1983); (2) Fölling, A. (1934) Z. Physiol. Chem. 277, 169-176; (3) Woo, S.L.C., Lidsky, A., Chandra, T., Stackhouse, R., Guttler, F., and Robson, K.J.H. (1983) Clin. Res. 31, 479A; (4) Lesch, M., and Nyhan, W.L. (1964) Am. J. Med. 36, 561-570; (5) Seegmiller, J.E., Rosenbloom, F. M., and Kelley, W.N. (1967) Science 155, 1682-1684; (6) Page, T., Bakay, B., Nissinen, E., and Nyhan, W. L. (1981) J. Inherit. Metabol. Dis. 4, 203-206; (7) Jolly, D.J., Esty, A.C., Bernard, H.U., and Friedmann, T. (1982) Proc. Natl. Acad. Sci. 79, 5038-5041; (8) Jolly, D. J., Okayama, H., Berg, P., Esty, A.C., Filpula, D., Bohlen, P., Johnson, G.G., Shively, J.E., Hunkepillar, T., and Friedmann, T. (1982) Proc. Natl. Acad. Sci. 80, 477-481; (9) Nussbaum, R.L., Crowder, W.E., Nyhan, W.L., and Caskey, C.T. (1983) Proc. Natl. Acad. Sci. 80, 4035-4039; (10) Wilson, J. M., Young, A.B., and Kelley, W.N. (1983) New Eng. J. Med. 309, 900-910.

GENETIC DIAGNOSIS BY DNA ANALYSIS

Yuet Wai Kan, M.D.
Howard Hughes Medical Institute and Department of Medicine
University of California, San Francisco, California

The availability of recombinant DNA probes has vastly increased the scope of prenatal diagnosis of genetic disorders. Thus it is now possible to diagnose all the inherited conditions of hemoglobin by DNA analysis. As more genes are cloned, other genetic diseases are becoming amenable to this method of detection. Random DNA probes may soon be used to diagnose diseases in which the defective structural gene has not been identified. In addition, the isolation of Y-chromosome-specific probes has provided a rapid method of fetal sex determination, and early diagnosis of genetic disorders in the first trimester is being explored using chorionic villi biopsy.

Hemoglobin Disorders

The most important hemoglobin disorders are sickle cell anemia and the thalassemias. Prenatal diagnosis of these disorders is now accomplished using DNA probes.

Diagnosis of α thalassemia is straightforward since the severe form of the disease is almost invariably due to deletion of all the α-globin structural genes. Hence the condition can be diagnosed by Southern blot analysis of amniotic fluid DNA to demonstrate the presence or absence of the α-globin genes (1).

In sickle cell anemia, the mutation at the β^6 position abolishes a recognition site for the restriction enzyme Mst II which is present at this position in normal DNA. Hence a sickle gene can be distinguished from a normal β-globin gene by the difference in size of the fragments generated by digesting the DNA with Mst II (2-4). An alternate method of diagnosis using synthetic oligomer probes has also been devised (5,6). Two nonadecamers were synthesized, one homologous to normal DNA and the other to sickle DNA in the β^6 region. Under well defined hybridization conditions, the normal probe hybridizes only to normal DNA, and the sickle probe only to sickle DNA.

β thalassemia is caused by a heterogeneous group of mutations that include gene deletion, decreased β-globin gene transcription, abnormal RNA processing, and premature termination of translation (7). Since more than 30 lesions have been described to date, prenatal diagnosis of this disorder is more complicated than either α thalassemia or sickle cell anemia. In the past, linkage analysis with polymorphic restriction sites was used to trace the β-thalassemia gene within a given family (8). Once the precise molecular lesion is defined in the various types of β thalassemia, synthetic oligonucleotide probes can be used for the specific mutation (9). The technique is now being adopted in the Mediterranean area for prenatal diagnosis of β thalassemia.

Other Genetic Disorders in Which the Structural Gene has been Isolated

Recently the defective genes responsible for a number of disorders have been isolated, including factor IX deficiency (10), Lesch-Nyhan syndrome (11,12), α1-antitrypsin deficiency (13), antithrombin III deficiency (14), and phenylketonuria (15). Synthetic oligomer probes or linkage analysis techniques are being explored as methods of prenatal diagnosis. For example several restriction site polymorphisms have been found with the phenylalanine hydroxylase gene, and may potentially be useful for prenatal diagnosis of this disorder. The common form of α1-antitrypsin deficiency is due to a single nucleotide mutation that results in an abnormal enzyme. This condition has been prenatally diagnosed with the aid of synthetic oligonucleotide probes.

Diseases in Which the Genetic Defect is not Known

Prominent among this group are Duchenne's muscular dystrophy, Huntington's chorea and cystic fibrosis. The approach to prenatal diagnosis of these disorders involves isolation of random DNA sequences and a search for polymorphic restriction sites around the sequences. Random DNA fragments on the X chromosome close to the Duchenne's muscular dystrophy locus have been isolated (16), and DNA fragments close to the Huntington's chorea locus have been described. These DNA probes will be useful for prenatal diagnosis and for elucidating the nature of these diseases.

Y-Specific Probes

Prior to prenatal diagnosis of sex-linked disorders, the fetal sex must first be determined. If the fetus is female, further testing is usually unnecessary. A Y-chromosome-specific DNA probe has now been isolated which has over 1000-fold more affinity for male than female DNA. Thus, fetal sex can be determined rapidly by dot blot analysis of amniotic fluid cell DNA (17).

Improvements in Diagnostic Techniques

The method involving the DNA hybridization probe is quite sensitive. DNA from 10-20 ml of amniotic fluid cells is usually sufficient for analysis. At present, diagnosis is routinely performed at the 15th to 16th gestational week. Earlier diagnosis has recently been attempted using chorionic villi biopsy (18). With this technique, DNA can be obtained as early as the 6th week of gestation. The DNA from one chorionic villi is adequate for analysis. The overall safety of this technique must be tested before it becomes generally available.

References — (1) Dozy, A.M., Forman, E.N., Abuelo, D.N., Barsel-Bowers, G., Mahoney, M.J., Forget, B.G. and Kan, Y.W. (1979) JAMA 241, 1610; (2) Wilson, J.T., Milner, P.F., Summer, M.E., Nallaseth, F.S., Fadel, H.E., Reindollar, R.H., McDonough, P.G. and Wilson, L.B. (1982) Proc. Natl. Acad. Sci. U.S.A. 79, 3628; (3) Chang, J.C. and Kan, Y.W. (1982) N. Engl. J. Med. 307, 30; (4) Orkin, S.H., Little, P.F.R., Kazazian, H.H., Jr. and Boehm, C.D. (1982) N. Engl. J. Med. 307, 32; (5) Wallace, R.B., Schold, M., Johnson, M.J., Dembek, P. and Itakura, K. (1981) Nucleic Acids Res. 9, 3647; (6) Conner, B.J., Reyes, A.A., Morin, C., Itakura, K., Teplitz, R.L. and Wallace, R.B. (1983) Proc. Natl. Acad. Sci. U.S.A. 80, 278; (7) Orkin, S.H., Antonarakis, S.E., Kazazian, H.H., Jr. (1983) Progress in Hematology, in press; (8) Boehm, C.D., Antonarakis, S.E., Phillips, J.A., Stetten, G. and Kazazian, H.H., Jr. (1983) N. Engl. J. Med. 308, 1054; (9) Pirastu, M., Kan, Y.W., Cao, A., Conner, B.J., Teplitz, R.L. and Wallace, R.B. (1983) N. Engl. J. Med. 309, 284; (10) Choo, K.H., Gould, K.G., Rees, D.J.G. and Brownlee, G.G. (1982) Nature 299, 178; (11) Jolly, D.J., Esty, A.C., Bernard, H.U. and Friedmann, T. (1982) Proc. Natl. Acad. Sci. U.S.A. 79, 5038; (12) Brennand, J., Chinault, A.C., Konecki, D.S., Melton, D.W. and

Caskey, C.T. (1982) Proc. Natl. Acad. Sci. U.S.A. <u>79</u>, 1950; (13) Kidd, V.J., Wallace, R.B., Tan, Z.-K., Itakura, K. and Woo, S.L.C. (1983) Nature <u>304</u>, 230; (14) Prochownik, E.V., Antonarakis, S.E., Bauer, K., Rosenberg, R., Fearon, E.R., Orkin, S.H. (1983) N. Engl. J. Med. <u>308</u>, 1549; (15) Woo, S.L.C., Lidsky, A., Chandra, T., Guttler, F. and Robson, X. (1983) Nature, in press; (16) Davies, K.E., Pearson, P.L., Harper, P.S. Murray, J.M., O'Brien, T., Sarfarazi, M. and Williamson, R. (1983) Nucleic Acids Res. <u>11</u>, 2303; (17) Lau, Y.-F., unpublished results; (18) Goossens, M., Dumez, Y., Kaplan, L., Lupker, M., Chabret, C., Henrion, R. and Rosa, J. (1983) N. Engl. J. Med. <u>309</u>, 831.

THE MOLECULAR GENETICS OF HUMAN GLOBIN GENE EXPRESSION: IN-VITRO ANALYSIS OF SPLICING MUTATIONS

ADRIAN KRAINER, MICHAEL GREEN, BARBARA RUSKIN AND TOM MANIATIS
Department of Biochemistry and Molecular Biology
Harvard University, Cambridge MA. 02138

Inherited disorders in human globin gene expression (thalassemias) provide a useful model for the study of the molecular basis of human genetic diseases. Thalassemia is well characterized clinically and biochemically, and all of the normal human globin genes have been cloned and sequenced (see 1,2 for reviews). In addition, the structures of the normal nuclear globin mRNA precursors and mature cytoplasmic mRNAs have been determined. Thus, defects in transcription and splicing can be evaluated by comparing the expression of normal and mutant genes. This comparison was made possible by the development of transient expression assays in which cloned globin genes are introduced into mammalian cells in culture in a manner which allows their efficient and accurate transcription, and correct processing of nuclear RNA precursors (see 3 for review). Thus, it is now possible to isolate globin genes from individuals with thalassemia, to identify mutations by comparison of their nucleotide sequences with those of normal globin genes, and to evaluate the consequences of these mutations on transcription and splicing (see 4 for review). Remarkably, most thalassemia genes differ from their normal counterparts by only a single base substitution.

The effect of thalassemia mutations on transcription and splicing has been established for a number of different alleles. In some cases it has been possible to examine RNA from erythroblasts of patients from which the cloned thalassemia genes were isolated. Except for quantitative differences, the data obtained from erythroid cells and from cultured cells transfected with cloned genes are consistent. Thus it has been possible to definitively establish the molecular basis of a number of different types of thalassemia. Defects at virtually every step of globin gene expression have been identified, including transcription, polyadenylation, splicing, and translation. (See 1,2,4 for recent reviews).

SPLICING MUTATIONS

The analysis of thalassemia genes not only provides a molecular description of the disease, it has also provided information regarding the mechanisms of globin RNA splicing (5). For example, examination of a number of β-thalassemia genes has identified four types of splice mutations (4,5). In the first type, single base changes in the conserved GT or AG dinucleotides at the splice junctions prevent normal splicing but lead to the utilization of 'cryptic' splice sites which are inactive in normal genes. In the second type, single base changes lead to the creation of a new AG or GT dinucleotide in a sequence context that produces a new splicing site which is efficiently utilized.

The third type of splicing mutation consists of single base changes near, but not within, the GT dinucleotide at the 5' splice junction of IVS1. These mutations decrease the efficiency of normal splicing, and activate nearby cryptic 5' splice sites. Finally, single base changes near GT dinucleotides located in the appropriate sequence context can create a new 5' splice site. In summary, the analysis of a number of naturally occuring defects in splicing provide a well characterized set of mutations which could be invaluable in the analysis of the mechanisms of globin RNA splicing.

IN-VITRO ANALYSIS OF SPLICING MUTATIONS

The transient expression assay described above can be used to characterize the nature of splicing defects but it cannot be used to address the biochemical mechanisms of normal and abnormal splicing. In order to study these mechanisms we have established an in vitro system in which β-globin mRNA splicing can be studied in detail. The approach we are taking is based on the development of a procedure for the in vitro synthesis of β-globin pre-mRNA (6). Normal or mutant β-globin genes are inserted into a plasmid containing a promoter from the bacteriophage SP6. When this plasmid in linearized by digestion with an appropriate restriction enzyme and transcribed with SP6 polymerase, a synthetic β-globin pre-mRNA is produced which contains both intervening sequences and a small amount of 5' and 3' flanking sequences. Because these transcripts carry additional flanking sequences, they are not identical to the normal β-globin precursor. Nevertheless, they are accurately spliced when injected into Xenopus oocyte nuclei (6). The fact that this RNA is an active substrate for splicing in oocytes demonstrates that transcription and splicing are not obligatorily coupled, thus setting the stage for the development of an in vitro splicing system in which the synthetic pre-mRNA is added directly to a cell-free extract.

The presence of RNA splicing activities in cell-free extracts has been reported using both globin (7) and adenovirus (8,9,10) genes as transcription templates. In some studies both transcription and splicing are carried out in the same extracts (7,10), while in another transcripts are produced in one mammalian cell extract under conditions which prevent splicing, and then purified and added back to a second extract (9). Finally, in one case an unspliced RNA precursor is purified from viral-infected cells and then added to a cell-free extract (8). In all of these cases a homogeneous RNA precursor is difficult to obtain in sufficient amounts. The advantage of the SP6 system is that unlimited amounts of a biologically active pre-mRNA can be obtained for any cloned gene, facilitating the optimization of the splicing reaction and the purification of the necessary components.

Using the SP6-β globin pre-mRNA as a substrate, we have tested a number of cell-free extracts for splicing activity. The highest activity was observed with nuclear extracts prepared by a procedure originally developed for efficient in vitro transcription of the adenovirus major late promoter (11). By systematically varying several parameters including substrate structure, incubation time, and the concentrations of nuclear extract, substrate, ATP, and magnesium, we have established conditions in which IVS1 is accurately spliced in approximately 90% of the input pre-mRNA molecules. Preliminary studies indicate that IVS2 is also efficiently spliced.

We find that the products of the splicing reaction differ significantly depending on whether or not the synthetic pre-mRNA is capped in vitro with vaccinia virus guanylyltransferase prior to incubation with the extract. If the RNA is capped, IVS1 is precisely removed and exons 1 and 2 are joined in approximately 90% of the input RNA molecules. A small fraction of the RNA is cleaved at the IVS1 5' splice junction without concomitant cleavage at the 3' junction. However, we cannot detect any products which are cut at the 3' splice junction and not ligated to other sequences. If the synthetic pre-mRNA is not capped, only 40% of the input RNA is accurately spliced. Three other classes of processing products account for another 50% of the input RNA. First, we detect RNA products that are cleaved upstream of the normal 5' splice junction, at or near a cryptic splice site that is activated in vivo by several thalassemia mutations (5). Second, RNA products are produced that appear to be cleaved within IVS1 at or near a sequence that matches the consensus for 3' splice junctions. This sequence does not function in vivo as a 3' splice junction in transcripts from either normal or mutant β-globin genes. Neither of these two aberrant cleavage events observed in vitro gives rise to products that are ligated. Finally, the third class of aberrant processing products of uncapped substrates appears to result from cleavage at the normal 3' splice junction and ligation to one of three short as yet unidentified sequences. Presently we do not know if any or all of the aberrantly processed RNAs represent splicing intermediates or dead-end products.

We conclude that a 5' cap structure can influence both the efficiency and accuracy of splicing in vitro. However, experiments in which the pre-mRNA contains a non-hydrolyzable 5' nucleotide, which cannot be capped, definitively show that a 5' cap is not required for in vitro splicing. Furthermore, as was previously shown in microinjected oocytes (6), we find that a correct 3' end and poly A tail are not required for splicing. Thus, a transcript possessing 555 nucleotides of β globin sequences past the polyadenylation site is efficiently spliced in vitro. Likewise, transcripts with 86 nucleotides or 16 nucleotides of sequences 5' to the in vivo mRNA cap site are efficiently spliced.

A time course of the in vitro splicing reaction shows that there is a significant time lag before correctly spliced molecules are produced. However the kinetics of appearance differs for the various aberrant products, some of which appear almost immediately, and become less abundant as the reaction proceeds. In agreement with previous studies (9), we find that the splicing reaction requires ATP. Surprisingly, the cleavage reaction is ATP-dependent, in contrast to the well studied tRNA splicing endonuclease (12) as well as most other nucleases. Possible interpretations of this result include: (i) The pre-mRNA splicing endonuclease has an energy requirement for cleavage. (ii) The pre-mRNA splicing endonuclease has an energy requirement for locating the splice junction. (iii) There is an energy requirement for assembling a ribonucleoprotein structure that is the obligatory substrate for the splicing endonuclease. (iv) Cleavage and ligation are obligatorily coupled and the ATP-requirement is actually for ligation. (v) ATP is required not for energy but as a cofactor for either ribonucleoprotein assembly or cleavage. Experiments are in progress to distinguish between these various possibilities. Interestingly, in the absence of ATP the aberrant processing products are not generated either.

To test the specificity of β-globin splicing in vitro, we have examined the processing of transcripts derived from three thalassemic genes. We find that a single base change at position 1 of IVS1 completely abolishes correct splicing and results instead in the activation of three cryptic 5' splice sites, all of which are ligated to the correct 3' splice site. Single base changes at positions 5 and 6 of IVS1 do not abolish the correct 5' splice site, but also lead to the utilization of the same three cryptic sites. These results are qualitatively identical to those obtained with these mutants in a transient expression assay (5). When these mutant transcripts are not capped, they generate the same aberrant products as the wild type SP6 β-globin RNA, with the important exception that cutting at or near the normal 5' splice site is absent when the IVS1 position 1 mutant is used.

In summary, the analysis of the structure of cloned β-thalassemia genes and the expression of these genes after transfection into mammalian cells in culture, has established the molecular basis of a number of different thalassemias. In addition these studies have provided new information regarding the sequences required for RNA splicing. The availability of a well characterized set of splicing mutants, the ability to produce virtually unlimited amounts of synthetic pre-mRNA, and the high efficiency of in vitro splicing of this pre-mRNA should make it possible to study the mechanism of splicing and to fractionate the necessary components for the splicing reaction.

REFERENCES – (1) Maniatis,T., Fritsch, E.F., Lauer, J. and Lawn, R.M. (1980) Ann. Rev. Genet. 14, 145; (2) Orkin, S.H. and Nathan, D.G. (1981) Adv. in Hum. Genet. 11, 233; (3) Banerji, J. and Schaffner, W. (1983) in 'Genetic Engineering' J.K. Setlow and A. Hollaender eds., Plenum Press, New York, Vol 5; (4) Treisman, R., Orkin, S. and Maniatis, T. (1983) in 'Hemoglobin Switching' G. Stamatoyannopoulos and A. Nienhuis eds., Alan Liss, New York (in press); (5) Treisman, R., Orkin, S. and Maniatis, T. (1983) Nature 302, 591; (6) Green, M.R., Maniatis, T. and Melton, D.A. (1983) Cell 32, 681; (7) Kole, R. and Weissman, S.M. (1982) Nucl. Acids Res. 10, 5429; (8) Goldenberg, C.J. and Hauser, S.D. (1983) Nucl. Acids Res. 11, 1337; (9) Hernandez, N. and Keller, W. (1983) Cell (in press). (10) Padgett, R.A., Hardy, S.F. and Sharp, P.A. (1983) Proc. Nat. Acad. Sci. USA 80, 5230; (11) Dignam, J.D., Lebovitz, R.M. and Roeder, R.G. (1983) Nucl. Acids Res. 11, 1475; (12) Peebles, C. L., Gegenheimer, P. and Abelson, J. (1983) Cell 32, 525.

HUMAN GENETIC LINKAGE STUDIES WITH DNA MARKERS
R. L. White, M. Leppert, D. Drayna, R. Leach and D. Barker

Department of Cellular, Viral and Molecular Biology and Howard Hughes Medical
Institute, University of Utah Medical School, Salt Lake City, Utah 84132

Thanks to modern in vitro technologies, the human as an experimental system
is falling prey to molecular biologists. Cells can be grown, systems reconstruc-
ted and genes sequenced all with a minimal invasion of a human subject. These
developments are very important since the human is a peculiarly awkward system
for direct experimental manipulation. It is perhaps the only system where the
experimental system has its own point of view. Although molecular biology has a
number of approaches, genetics has always been perceived as a very significant
part of the molecular biology of any system. Since my own background and inclina-
tions agree, we have stressed genetic approaches in our own work.

The human system actually offers many advantages to the investigator. Because
of an exquisitely refined screening program, related to the fact that this system
is one of the few from which individuals will actively complain about their phenotype, many important mutants have been characterized and a wealth of important
cytogenetic observations have accumulated on both constitutional (inherited genotype) and somatic cell materials in the case of tumor cytogenetics. If you read
even Time magazine, the recent congruence of oncogene studies with studies of
tumor translocations cannot have escaped notice.

I should not, however, leave you with the impression that the human is a per-
fect research subject. The study of the genetics of the human does have its own
specific problems. In general, genetic approaches require the examination of
specific hypotheses in strains or organisms of known genotype and the approach
is of the form, "If we construct a strain of this specific genotype, then we
would expect to make the following observation under these conditions." In fact,
the construction of strains of specific genotype is often the major part of a
genetic experiment. Strain construction is not possible with the human.

An approach to this problem has been suggested (1). In principle, restriction enzyme diagnosis can detect a very large number of polymorphisms in DNA
sequence. This could create a very large and dense set of genetic markers for
the human and make possible the identification of individuals of known genotype
at specific loci within large families. The scheme is illustrated in Figure 1.
DNA sequence variation will sometimes affect a restriction site and be detected
as a change in pattern on a Southern transfer probed with a cloned DNA segment
which defines a specific locus. The resultant gel patterns become genetic
markers with codominant alleles for the locus. Since these markers can be
determined from only a few milliliters of blood sample it is possible to make
genetic determinations on individuals with little invasion.

An example of this approach is shown in Figure 2. We wanted to determine
whether inheritance of a mutant oncogene might be the cause of a genetic predisposition to colon cancer found in families with Gardner syndrome (2). The
loci for the Kirsten ras gene and the Harvey ras gene were defined with probes
from Weinberg (3) and Wigler (4), respectively. Polymorphism was found with
the TaqI enzyme at both loci. Wigler had already reported polymorphism at the
Harvey locus. Since the disease is known to be due to a rare autosomal dominant
mutation, an affected individual will be heterozygous at the disease locus. If
the individual is also heterozygous at the oncogene locus and one of the two
oncogene alleles is responsible for the disorder, then the disease should co-
inherit with one of the oncogene alleles. As can be seen in Figure 2, this is
not the case. Affected individual 6454 must have inherited Kirsten allele 2
from her affected father; however, affected individual 6459 inherited Kirsten
allele 1 from her affected parent. In a similar manner, the Harvey ras locus
was shown to be unlinked to the Gardner locus. These data permit the exclusion
of these two oncogenes as the cause of this inherited predisposition to colon
cancer.

For many genetic diseases, it would be a step forward to know their map
position. In order to do general mapping of disease loci, it is a considerable
advantage to have a good map of the human genome, defined by evenly spaced
genetic loci. It is believed that some 75 markers spaced 40 centimorgans apart
would span the human genome. Such a marker set would likely be derived from a
much larger initial set. A large number of DNA markers now exist for the human;
over 200, in fact, including both real and pseudo genes as well as anonymous sites
(5). These vary considerably in quality, however, with less than 20 reflecting
good multi allelic loci.

Multi allelism is important since we depend on natural matings for our heterozygotes and a two allele system with a rare minor allele gives few heterozygotes.
The best multi allelic markers consist of families of fragment lengths defined by a
single enzyme such as we have previously characterized (6). A handful of analogous
multi allelic markers such as insulin and Harvey ras have now been characterized as
due to variations in number of sets of tandem repeats of 14 to 36 base pairs (7,8,9).
Multi allelic systems can also be constructed by stringing together several restriction site variants at the same locus as has been done with beta globin (10) and an
anonymous locus, ADJ762 (11). Multiple polymorphic MspI and TaqI sites as well as
a polymorphic BclI site are found at this locus. We are not surprised at the
multiple TaqI and MspI polymorphisms since these have been found to be hotspots for
polymorphism in the human due to the CpG dimer sequence in the recognition sites
(12). We believe the methylated cytosine residues found in this sequence are hotspots for mutation in the human. This kind of polymorphic locus is somewhat more
laborious to build and score, however.

Since four good multi allelic DNA markers, Harvey ras, insulin, ADJ762 and beta
globin, had been shown to map to the short arm of chromosome 11 by physical methods
and, therefore, should be genetically linked, these seemed a good choice to initiate
a linkage map. However, appropriate families first had to be ascertained and sampled.

Since controlled matings are not possible in the human, one of the major diffi-
culties is the determination of phase, how the alleles of the several loci distribute
on the two chromosomes. This is important, since the choice of parental phase deter-
mines whether a progeny chromosome is to be scored as recombinant or nonrecombinant.
However, genotypic information from the grandparents of the sibship can often resolve
this issue. Given that we now have to score grandparents as well as parents, it is
efficient to be able to score as many progeny chromosomes as possible from such a
mating. We have therefore ascertained a number of Utah and Idaho families of optimal
structure, consisting of four living grandparents and sibships of 7 or 8.

Using these families, we have been able to obtain a high resolution linkage map
for the four chromosome 11 loci which is shown in Figure 3A. For each interval 100 to
200 chromosomes have been scored so that the variance on the determinations is less
than 20%. Furthermore, and importantly we think, the gene orders have been confirmed
by the multiply heterozygous three and four factor crosses which occur within the
sample set. With the gene order Harvey ras – insulin – ADJ762 – beta globin, in no
case do we require more than a single recombination event in order to explain the
data set.

With the same set of families, data has been gathered by Dennis Drayna with a set
of probes from the X chromosome (13). As seen in Figure 3B, although the map of X is
not yet complete, we can see that the total length will exceed 200 centimorgans,
somewhat more than expected. Figure 3C shows the distal long arm region in more
detail and again we are able to obtain a high resolution map requiring, in this case,
only one double exchange with multiply marked crosses. It should be noted that two
of these distal markers are very close to the locus of a very important genetic
disorder, the fragile site associated with X-linked mental retardation (14).

With the same set of families, Robin Leach has constructed a linkage map of the
short arm of chromosome 6. As seen in figure 3D, the map still has a few holes but
seems well on the way to usability.

As data accumulates within this set of families, it will be possible to quickly
identify the approximate chromosomal location of new markers by a method analogous
to that used with mouse recombinant inbred lines. Since we very often know the
parental and grandparental origin of each marker in each progeny chromosome, we will
be able to develop a binary signature for each locus as illustrated in Figure 4. The
two loci known to be linked on chromosome 11 show only one discrepancy with each
other, while the others, known to be on different chromosomes, show multiple discrep-
ancies. As the binary string characterizing each locus is expanded to several
hundred progeny chromosomes, the resolution afforded by this method should be
excellent.

References--(1) Botstein, D., White, R., Skolnick, M. and Davis, R. (1980) Am.J.Hum.
Gen. 32, 314-331. (2) Barker, D., McCoy, M., Weinberg, R., Goldfarb, M., Wigler, M.,
Burt, R., Gardner, E. and White, R. (1983) Molec.Biol.and Med., in press. (3) Shih,
C. and Weinberg, R. (1982) Cell 29, 1y1-169. (4) Goldfarb, M., Shimizu, K., Perucho,
M. and Wigler, M. (1982) Nature 296, 404-409. (5) White, R., Leppert, M., Bishop,
T., Barker, D., Berkowitz, J., Brown, C., Callahan, P., Holm, T. and Jerominski, L.
(1983) Paper presented to VII Internatl.Gene Mapping Workshop, Los Angeles. (6) Wyman,
A. and White, R. (1980) Proc.Nat.Acad.Sci.USA 77, 6754-6758. (7) Bell, G., Karam,
J. and Rutter, W. (1981). Proc.Nat.Acad.Sci.USA 78, 5759-5763. (8) Proudfoot, N.,

88

Gil, A. and Maniatas, T. (1982) Cell 31, 553-563. (9) Chapman, B., Vincent, K. and Wilson, A. (1983) Submitted. (10) Kazazian, H., Antonarakis, S., Cheng, T., Boehm, C. and Waber, P. (1983) In Banbury Report 14: Recombinant DNA Applications to Human Disease (Cold Spring Harbor Labs., New York). (11) Barker, D., Holm, T. and White, R. (1983) In preparation. (12) Barker, D., Schafer, M. and White, R. (1983) Submitted. (13) Davies, K. and Drayna, D., personal communication. (14) Davies, K. and Drayna, D., personal communication.

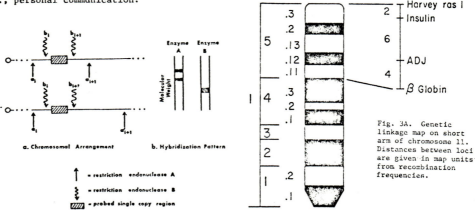

Fig. 3A. Genetic linkage map on short arm of chromosome 11. Distances between loci are given in map units from recombination frequencies.

FIG. 1. —a, Cuts made in pair of homologous chromosomes by enzyme A and enzyme B; b, hybridization pattern of enzymes A and B given cuts of a.

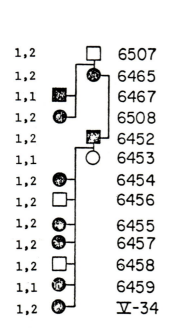

Fig. 2. The alleles of the Taq I polymorphism at the c-Ki-ras2 locus in individuals from an informative portion of Kindred 109.

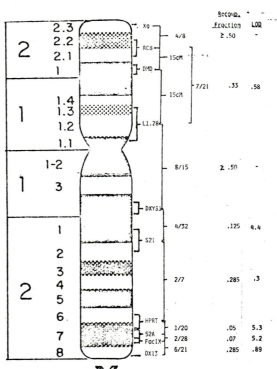

Fig. 3B. Genetic map of the X chromosome: DMD is the locus for Duchenne Muscular Dystrophy, FacIX is the site of Factor IX deficiency in hemophilia, and Xg is a red blood cell antigen. All other loci are RFLP sites.

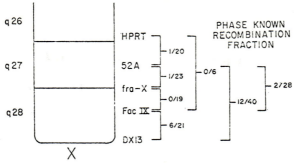

Fig. 3C. Fine structure mapping of distal portion of Xq. Fra-X is the site for fragile X-linked mental retardation. Physical locations are approximate.

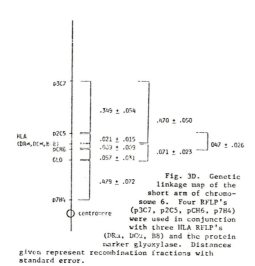

Fig. 3D. Genetic linkage map of the short arm of chromosome 6. Four RFLP's (p3C7, p2C5, pCH6, p7H4) were used in conjunction with three HLA RFLP's (DRα, DCα, B8) and the protein marker glyoxylase. Distances given represent recombination fractions with standard error.

chromosome number

locus	1	2	3	4	5	6	7	8	9	10	11	12	13	14	15	16	17	18	19	20	21	22	23	24	25	26	27	28	29	30	31	32	33	34	35	36
DCHI	0	0	0	0	1	0	1	1	1	0	0	1	0	1	1	0	0	0	1	0	1	1	0	0	1	0	0	0	0	0	1	0	0	1	0	0
IF8	1	0	0	0	1	0	1	0	-	-	1	1	1	1	1	0	1	1	1	-	-	0	-	1	0	-	-	-	-	-	-	-	-	-	-	-
Insulin	1	1	1	0	0	0	1	0	-	-	0	0	1	0	0	0	0	0	0	0	1	1	0	0	1	0	0	1	1	1	0	1	0	1	0
D11S12	1	1	1	1	0	0	1	-	-	-	-	-	0	0	0	0	0	0	-	-	-	-	-	-	-	-	1	1	1	1	0	1	0	1	0

Fig. 4. Chromosome distribution patterns. Genotypes at four loci for a sample of 36 progeny chromosomes. These issue from parents whose allele distribution is certain. DCHI is a locus on chromosome 6, IE8 is a locus on chromosome 13, and Insulin is a locus on chromosome 11 as is D11S12.

THE CHARACTERIZATION AND CORRECTION OF LESCH-NYHAN GENE DEFECTS BY RECOMBINANT DNA TECHNIQUES.

C. Thomas Caskey, Thomas P. Yang, Pragna I. Patel, J. Timothy Stout and A. Craig Chinault

Departments of Medicine and Biochemistry, Baylor College of Medicine and Howard Hughes Medical Institute, Houston, Texas

Hypoxanthine-guanine phosphoribosyltransferase (HPRT) plays an important role in the metabolic pathway for the salvage of purines. HPRT deficiency results in two clinical syndromes: gouty arthritis and Lesch-Nyhan syndrome. Mutational alterations leading to these X-linked disorders are now amenable to molecular analysis by recombinant DNA methods.

Recombinant plasmids containing sequences complementary to mouse HPRT mRNA were identified at a frequency of 1 in 10,000 in libraries constructed by standard cDNA cloning techniques (1) using mRNA from a neuroblastoma cell line which had amplified copies of the functional HPRT gene (2). A mouse HPRT probe was then used to identify hamster and human HPRT cDNA recombinants in fibroblast and liver cDNA libraries, respectively, at a frequency of 1 in 50-75,000. Comparison of cDNA sequences (3,4) indicates a high degree (95%) of sequence homology within the protein coding region and divergence in both 3' and 5' non-coding regions. An open reading frame in each cDNA recombinant predicts a protein of 218 residues which is in agreement with the protein sequence determined for human HPRT (5) except that the initiator methionine is apparently removed in a post-translational modification step.

The molecular organization of the mouse HPRT gene has been determined by characterization of overlapping lambda genomic recombinants. The mouse gene is 34 kb in size with 8 introns. The exons and intron donor and acceptor sites have been established by DNA sequencing (6). Our current knowledge of the human HPRT gene indicates it is at least as large as the mouse gene. DNA sequence analysis of the human gene indicates the first three exons and the 9th exon are identical to those in the mouse gene. Based on this early characterization of the human HPRT gene we have assumed that the remaining human exons will show exon divisions similar to those found for the mouse gene. Additional DNA sequencing is needed to confirm this assumption.

A systematic study of DNA from Lesch-Nyhan patients has been undertaken to study the nature of mutation(s) at the HPRT locus. In order to delineate the region of the gene bearing the alteration, we have determined for the normal gene those restriction endonuclease fragments which correspond to specific exons. Exon assignments to DNA fragments were determined on the basis of their hybridization to cDNA subfragments chosen to represent specific regions of the gene. Any alterations found for Lesch-Nyhan patients can be compared to this data and thus their site of gene alteration identified. The restriction endonuclease gene fragments produced with BamHI, BglII,

PstI, and MspI have been examined by Southern analysis using full-length cDNA probes and the results are summarized in the following Table where "+" indicates the detection of an abnormal pattern.

LESCH-NYHAN SURVEY - SOUTHERN BLOT PATTERNS

Pattern		Restriction Enzymes		
	BamHI	BglII	PstI	MspI
Normal Southern Blot (42%)	0	0	0	0
X-linked Polymorphisms (23%)	+	0	0	0
Autosomal Polymorphism (33%)	0	0	0	+
Gene Alterations (20%):				
RJK 849	+	0	+	0
GM 3467	+	+	+	0
GM 2227	0	+	+	+
GM 1662	+	+	0	0
MA	+	+	+	+

Forty-two percent of the individuals examined have shown no variation in their restriction endonuclease fragment patterns compared to normal. These patients are presumed to possess mutations which are undetectable by Southern analysis, such as point mutations and small deletions or insertions. Alternatively, a major gene alteration may be present which is not detectable with the set of endonucleases used. A large fraction of the pattern alterations observed represent restriction fragment length polymorphisms and are not directly related to gene mutation. The 23% frequency of X-linked BamHI polymorphism for Lesch-Nyhan patients that was observed is identical to that reported earlier for a control population (7). The frequent 3.6 kb MspI polymorphism is observed in 33% of Lesch-Nyhan patients and controls. This RFLP is associated with an autosomal pseudogene mapped to chromosome 5. Twenty percent of Lesch-Nyhan patients have shown restriction endonuclease DNA fragment patterns indicating major gene alterations. Such changes include loss of fragments, loss of fragments associated with the gain of new fragments and shift of fragments to higher or lower molecular weight positions. We have studied most intensively five patients: GM 1662, GM 3467, GM 2227, RJK 849, and MA. The types of DNA changes seen in each patient is unique, suggesting Lesch-Nyhan disease arises by a heterogeneous group of mutations. A summary of our current knowledge of the HPRT gene organization and the current understanding of several Lesch-Nyhan cases is given in Figure 1.

RJK 849 is missing exons 7,8 and 9 and most bands associated with exons 4,5 & 6. Exons 1,2 & 3 were present. Since no new DNA fragments were detected we believe this patient has a partial gene

Figure 1

HPRT GENE STRUCTURE AND MUTANT ANALYSIS

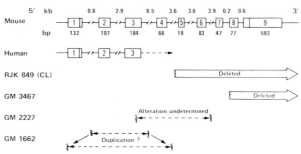

deletion initiating in exons 4,5 or 6 and extending through the 3'
end of the gene. Analysis of GM 3467 reveals a partial gene deletion
starting within the region coding for exons 7,8 & 9 and extending 3'
of the last exon. An additional patient (MA) has been identified
with a total deletion of the HPRT gene (not shown). GM 2227 represents a mutant with Southern alterations associated with exons 3,4,5
and/or 6. The exact nature of this alteration has not been determined. GM 1662 represents an unusual alteraton at the HPRT locus.
Evidence from Southern analysis suggests this mutation is a partial
gene duplication which involves exons 2 and 3. Efforts are currently
underway to construct and screen genomic lambda libraries for the
purpose of characterizing these mutations in detail.

The analysis of Lesch-Nyhan mutant gene expression by analysis
of their mRNA size and content has been carried out by Northern analysis. As anticipated, none of the three deletion mutants produces
mRNA. Two patients which have normal Southern patterns have a normal
size mRNA and are presumed to represent point mutations whereas a
third patient with a normal Southern study has no detectable mRNA.
The mutant GM 1662 has mRNA larger than normal HPRT mRNA in keeping
with the proposed partial gene duplication.

Recombinant DNA techniques now offer an opportunity for accurate
and simple methods for carrier detection of X-linked inherited disorders. Lesch-Nyhan disease is an excellent example of this improvement.
Previous carrier detection methods for this disorder involved the
clonal isolation of cultured fibroblasts from suspected carrier
females or quantitation of enzyme activity in hair follicles. Each
is influenced by the chance occurrence of X-inactivation by the
mechanism of lyonization. Since recombinant methods examine DNA
structure, not expression, any alteration associated with the disease gene can be used to detect carriers. We have used DNA isolated
from peripheral blood specimens for the purpose of carrier detection
in families with RFLP (BamH1) and gene alterations detectable by
Southern analysis. Presently, 43% of Lesch-Nyhan families are

amenable to carrier studies by recombinant DNA methods and we can anticipate further improvement in these methods.

The ability to select HPRT$^+$ cells in HAT medium is an important genetic feature of this locus which aids in the development of in vitro gene transfer. We have prepared three expressing vectors for human HPRT sequences (7) which are diagrammed in Figure 2. Each of the recombinants contains the human cDNA coding sequences and one of three different promoters. These include a viral LTR, the mouse HPRT natural promoter and the metallothionein promoter. Each recombinant has been successfully used to introduce functional HPRT sequences into either rodent or Lesch-Nyhan cells by DNA-mediated gene transfer. These cell lines are transfected at a frequency of 10^{-4} by the above method with incorporation of 1-50 copies into the genome. The level of expression ranges from low to normal in the cells rescued in HAT. We are presently constructing defective retroviral particles which possess each of these minigenes.

Figure 2

HPRT EXPRESSION VECTORS

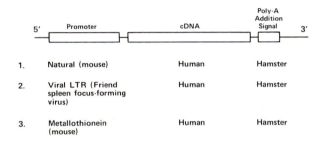

References. (1) Brennand, J., Chinault, A.C., Konecki, D.S., Melton, D.W. and Caskey, C.T. (1982) Proc. Natl. Acad. Sci. USA 79, 1950-1954; (2) Melton, D.W. (1981) Somatic Cell Genet. 7, 331-344; (3) Konecki, D.S., Brennand, J., Fuscoe, J.C., Caskey, C.T. and Chinault, A.C. (1982) Nucleic Acids Res. 10, 6763-6775; (4) Jolly, D.J., Okayama, H., Berg, P., Esty, A.C., Filpula, D., Bohlen, P., Johnson, G.G., Shively, J.E., Hunkapillar, T. and Friedman, T. (1983) Proc. Natl. Acad. Sci. USA 80, 477-481; (5) Wilson, J.M., Tarr, G.E., Mahoney, W.C. and Kelley, W.N. (1982) J. Biol. Chem. 257, 10978-10985; (6) Melton, D.W., Konecki, D.S., Brennand, J. and Caskey, C.T. (1983) submitted; (7) Nussbaum, R.L., Crowder, W.E., Nyhan, W.E. Caskey, J., Konecki, D.S. and Caskey, C.T. (1983) J. Biol. Chem. 258, 9593-9596.

RANDOM GENE PROBES AND THE MAPPING OF MUSCULAR DYSTROPHY AND SIMILAR INHERITED DISEASES

Robert Williamson, Conrad Gilliam, Steve Hodgkinson, Caroline Ingle, Mark Blaxter and Kay Davies

Department of Biochemistry, St.Mary's Hospital Medical School, University of London, W2 1PG, England.

Using recombinant DNA techniques, the molecular biologist can isolate human structural genes which then can be identified by sequence or product and prepared in complete purity and unlimited amount. Several dozen genes coding for proteins involved in disease processes have been isolated (Table), and by the end of 1984 approximately 300 human genes will have been characterised. The study of human genetics is shifting from the indirect study of phenotype to the direct study of gene sequence, organisation, expression and inheritance (1).

DISEASE	PROBE
α-thalassaemia	α-globin
β-thalassaemia	β-globin
sickle cell disease	β-globin
emphysema	α- 1 antitrypsin
hereditary dwarfism	human growth hormone
Lesch-Nyhan syndrome	HPRT
phenylketonuria	phenylalanine hydroxylase
osteogensis imperfecta (some)	collagen
analbuminaemia	albumin
hypercholesterolaemia	various apolipoprotein genes
thyroid medullary carcinoma	calcitonin
Christmas disease	factor IX

HUMAN GENE PROBES AVAILABLE TO DEFINE MOLECULAR PATHOLOGY

If the biochemical defect causing a genetic disease is known, the definition of the molecular pathology becomes the relatively simple task of obtaining a gene probe for the mutated coding sequence. The molecular biologist will usually attempt to obtain a cDNA clone from a purified, or partially purified, messenger RNA and then screen a genomic library with this clone to obtain nuclear DNA. However, for diseases where a protein is expressed differentially in patient and control, it is also possible to prepare a library of cDNAs in a suitable host-vector system, in which case this library becomes a representative resource specific for the individual as well as the tissue from which it has been prepared.

Since all genetic diseases involve heritable changes in genomic DNA, in principle any hereditary disease (or, for that matter, any inherited phenotype) can be analysed at the level of the gene. The alleles of a single gene that malfunctions because of mutation can be cloned and then studied in detail. I will not dwell on the well-known ways in which this has been applied to the haemo-globinopathies and other biochemically characterised human diseases caused by a mutation in a single gene, other than to note that a specific gene probe for the mutation in such a case is also a disease-specific probe (2). Therefore the probe can be used to study gene structure directly (by restriction site analysis), to isolate patient-specific genomic clones, to study gene function using "Northern blots" and in vitro transcription, and can be sequenced to give total information on molecular structure.

DISEASES WHERE THE DEFECT IS NOT UNDERSTOOD

There are other diseases which are known by family studies to be caused by a defect at a single gene locus, but where the biochemistry of the mutation is totally unknown. Examples include Duchenne muscular dystrophy, myotonic dystrophy, cystic fibrosis and Huntington's chorea. There are other localised single gene "phenomenae" which cause profound phenotypic effects of a cellular, or structural, kind, such as the mutations causing X-linked mental retardation, aniridia, retino-blastoma or Wilms' tumour. Transpositions, which can be inherited or acquired, are sometimes associated with tumours (as between chronic myelogenous leukaemia and "Philadelphia chromosome"). These are all examples of single locus events associated with major pathology where a known biochemical effect has not been identified.

How can the "new technology" of recombinant DNA analysis help in such cases? One possibility is that the affected gene is expressed in a particular tissue in normal people, but not for persons affected clinically (as for the globin gene in most cases of thalassaemia). Complementary DNA libraries from messenger RNA (which are both tissue-specific and person-specific) can be prepared from patient and control, and compared for differences, looking for sequences absent from the patient. These would be "candidates" for genes affected by the mutation. Complete libraries from messenger RNA (via cDNA) exist for several normal human tissues: lymphocytes, fibroblasts, fetal and adult muscle, liver and brain (3). These are not only a primary resource for the isolation of genes which are expressed in a particular tissue, but also useful for tissue/tissue and patient/control comparisons.

For diseases such as cystic fibrosis, there is every reason to think that the pathology is caused by a protein defect, and its expression can be studied using populations of mRNA in appropriate tissues such as sweat glands and pancreas.

One problem in this approach is that it is very difficult to detect genes that are expressed at only low levels. There are also some mutations (such as those causing a single amino acid substitution, as in sickle cell anaemia) which can affect the function of a protein, yet not affect the level or hybridisation of mRNA.

In this case, or for a disease which is caused by a mutation in a control sequence or otherwise not expressed as mRNA, then comparison of cDNA libraries will not be helpful. It is necessary to turn to genomic libraries. In principle, it would be possible to compare the DNA sequences of two people in extenso, and to determine all differences, and attempt to relate these to disease. However, this is impracticable technically (there are 3×10^9 base pairs in the human haploid genome). It is also impossible scientifically, since base changes are very common even between normal individuals - Jeffreys (4) has estimated that random base changes, many in the non-coding sequences, occur one in every 200 base pairs along a chromosome between two individuals. Therefore sequence differences are not usually a cause of dysfunction, but part of the normal genetic variation which allows for both differences between individuals and for evolutionary change.

LINKAGE ANALYSIS

This normal variation provides a new tool for the study of inheritance. Since base changes are, to a first approximation, distributed randomly throughout the genome, some will occur (at random) in sites recognised by bacterial restriction enzymes. Where a base change causes a site to disappear from only one chromosome of the pair in each cell, and not from the other, then the two sequences can be distinguished by the size of gene fragment that is obtained after digestion. All that is required is that a hybridisation probe recognises the DNA sequence within the fragment containing the site.

The first example of a single base change causing a fragment length polymorphism was demonstrated by us for the mutation giving rise to a mutant beta-globin chain, haemoglobin O-Arab (5). Shortly afterwards, Kan and Dozy (6) showed that a polymorphism occurring approximately 5,000 base pairs to the 3' side of the β^S-globin gene is in linkage disequilibrium with the mutation causing sickle cell disease. Even though the polymorphism occurs in a sequence remote from the gene lesion (and has nothing whatever to do with the disease) it is possible to carry out gene analysis and antenatal diagnosis using the restriction site. The absence of the restriction site is usually associated with the gene defect. This approach can also be used for analysis of thalassaemia, and finds practical application for fetal diagnosis, particularly using DNA obtained by chorion biopsy.

Since crossover during meiosis is a relatively rare event, Solomon and Bodmer (7) predicted that it should be possible to construct a genetic linkage map of the entire human genome with as few as approximately 500 such chromosome-specific variant loci. Provided that these have been assigned to chromosomes, and lie in known relationship to one another, it will be possible to determine whether "loose" linkage exists between any of these loci and a given monogenic disease of unknown autosomal localisaton. This approach is applicable to all monogenic diseases whether they are dominant or recessive, and the method is independent of the nature of the dysfunction at the DNA level. Once close linkage is established, heterozygote as well as homozygote status can be assigned unequivocally for an individual in an informative family.

The most direct way of isolating chromosome-specific single-copy DNA probes for linkage analysis is to select them from chromosome-specific libraries. Whenever the chromosomal assignment of the disease is already established, a strategy involving the purification and cloning of chromosomes is invaluable. We have cloned a representative set of sequences derived from the human X chromosome using a fluorescence activated cell sorter (FACS-II) for the study of sex-linked diseases, such as Duchenne muscular dystrophy (8). Two clones have been studied which contain X-specific sequences from the middle of the short arm, and it has been shown that these flank either side of the mutation causing DMD (9). Our colleagues in Cardiff have shown that Duchenne and Becker muscular dystrophies behave as if allelic using these probes (10). Even with probes loosely linked to the mutation, we have found it possible to improve carrier prediction over that obtained using CPK levels alone (11), and when more and closer probes are available, fetal diagnosis will also be possible (12).

Similar approaches are possible for autosomal gene mutations, even where the biochemical defect is not known.

Using segregation analysis, we have recently demonstrated that complement 3 is not the mutation causing cystic fibrosis (13). We have also confirmed the linkage between the gene for C3 and myotonic dystrophy by studing linkage in a number of kindreds. It is heartening to all who use these techniques to know that a firm linkage has been established by a group working in Boston between a random gene probe and the autosomal dominant disease Huntington's chorea, as this condition was felt to be one defying analysis at the biochemical level by any other techniques.

MULTIFACTORIAL DISEASES WHERE SEVERAL GENES MAY BE INVOLVED

It is hard to think of any genetic disease, even the most simple, where the effect of the mutation cannot be modified by other genes or by the environment. For β^0-thalassaemia, for instance, the expression of the phenotype can be modulated in an individual who also possesses a mutation at the α-globin locus. The severity of the disease can be markedly affected, to give transfusion-independent thalassaemia intermedia rather than thalassaemia major. This illustrates that the combined effects of two mutations, each deleterious in itself, may not be additive but may even cancel each other to some extent.

Our ability to determine the contribution of specific genes involved in multifactorial inheritance of disease will depend upon three resources: a set of candidate genes where there are good reasons for suspecting involvement; large families in which inheritance can be studied; unequivocal clinical diagnosis, preferably with a numerical parameter which indicates risk or severity of the disease. These resources are, in our view, best met by the genetic component of the risk of early coronary heart disease, and several groups (including our own) are now studying the genes coding for the apolipoproteins, cell receptors, insulin, clotting factors and lipid metabolism enzymes to determine whether, and to what extent, each may be involved in lipidaemia and atherosclerosis.

REFERENCES AND FURTHER READING

(1) Williamson R, Clarke B, Crampton J, Davies K E, Hartley D, Hill M, Murray J, Taylor P, Polkey A, Woods D (1982) Human Gene-Specific and Chromosome-Specific Probes. in Human Genetics Congress, Part A:The Unfolding Genome, 23-28, Alan Liss, New York

(2) Davies K E (1981) The Application of DNA Recombinant Technology to the Analysis of the Human Genome and Genetic Disease. Human Genetics, 58:351-357.

(3) Woods D, Crampton J, Clarke B, Williamson R (1980) The Construction of a Recombinant cDNA Library representative of the poly(A)+ mRNA Population from normal human lymphocytes. Nucleic Acids Res, 8:5157-5168

(4) Jeffreys A J (1979) DNA sequence variants in Gγ -, Aγ-, δ - and β-globin genes of man. Cell, 18:1-10.

(5) Flavell R A, Kooter J M, DeBoer E, Little P F R, Williamson R (1978) Analysis of the β-,δ-globin gene loci in normal and Hb Lepore DNA: direct determination of gene linkage and intergene distance. Cell, 15:25-41.

(6) Kan Y W, Dozy A M (1978) Polymorphism of DNA sequences adjacent to human β^S-globin structural gene:relationship to sickle mutation. Proc Natl Acad Sci USA, 75:5631-5635.

(7) Solomon E, Bodmer W F (1979) Evolution of sickle variant gene. The Lancet, I:923.

(8) Davies K E, Young B D, Elles R G, Hill M E, Williamson R (1981) Cloning of a representative genomic library of the human X chromosome after sorting by flow cytometry. Nature, 293:374-376.

(9) Davies K E, Pearson P L, Harper P S, Murray J M, O'Brien T, Sarfarazi M, Williamson R (1983) Linkage analysis of two cloned DNA sequences flanking the Duchenne muscular dystrophy locus on the short arm of the human X chromosome. Nucleic Acids Research, 11:2303-2312.

(10) Kingston H M, Thomas N S T, Pearson P L, Sarfarazi, Harper P S (1983) Genetic linkage between Becker muscular dystrophy and a polymorphic DNA sequence on the short arm of the X chromosome. J Med Genet, 20:255-258.

(11) Harper P S, O'Brien T, Murray J M, Davies K E, Pearson P, Williamson R (1983) The use of linked DNA polymorphisms for genotype prediction in families with Duchenne muscular dystrophy. J Med Genet, 20: 252-254.

(12) Elles R G, Williamson R, Niazi M, Coleman D, Horwell D (1983) Absence of maternal contamination of chorionic villi used for fetal-gene analysis. New England J Med, 308:1433-1435.

(13) Davies K E, Gilliam T C, Williamson R (1983) Cystic Fibrosis is not caused by a Defect in the Gene coding for Human Complement 3. Molec Biol Med, 1, in press.

(14) Davies K E, Jackson J, Williamson R, Harper P, Ball S, Sarfarazi M, Meredith L, Fey G (1983) Linkage analysis of myotonic dystrophy and sequences on chromosome 19 using a cloned complement 3 gene probe. J Med Genet, 20:259-263.

Acknowledgements: This work was supported by the Cystic Fibrosis Research Trust, Muscular Dystrophy Group (U.K.), Muscular Dystrophy Association (U.S.A.) and the Medical Research Council. This manuscript is modified from one presented to a meeting of the Royal College of Obstetrics and Gynaecology, London, September 1983.

THE CLONING OF BLOOD COAGULATION FACTORS

Earl W. Davie, Dominic W. Chung, Sandra J. Friezner Degen,
Kotoku Kurachi, Mark W. Rixon, and Shinji Yoshitake

Dept. of Biochemistry, Univ. of Washington, Seattle, WA 98195

The coagulation of mammalian blood involves about a dozen proteins and most of these are synthesized in the liver (1). Many of
these coagulation factors are present in plasma in precursor forms
to serine proteases, including prothrombin, factor VII, factor IX,
factor X, factor XI, factor XII, and prekallikrein. Since these
proteins are secreted, they are synthesized with a leader sequence
and pass through the rough and smooth endoplasmic reticulum and the
Golgi apparatus on their way to the blood. During this time, they
undergo considerable processing, such as the removal of their signal
peptide and sometimes a pro peptide, addition of carbohydrate, modification of several amino acids, and occasionally the assembly of
more than one polypeptide into a mature protein. Amino acid modifications include the formation of γ-carboxyglutamate via the car-
boxylation of glutamic acid, formation of β-hydroxyaspartic acid
from aspartic acid, and phosphorylation of tyrosine (2-4).

In recent years, we and others have focused much of our research
activity on the cloning of the cDNAs and the genes for individual
clotting factors. Initially, these studies were directed toward
fibrinogen (5-8), prothrombin (9), and factor IX (10-12). Fibrinogen
is a large glycoprotein that participates in the final stages of the
clotting cascade (13). It has a molecular weight of 340,000, and
each molecule consists of two sets of three different polypeptide
chains. These chains have been designated α, β, and γ, with molecular weights of 67,600, 54,800, and 48,900, respectively. Fibrinogen
contains four carbohydrate chains, including one on each of the β
chains and one on each of the γ chains. The α chain is free of
carbohydrate even though it contains two potential binding sites
(Asn-X-Ser) for carbohydrate chains. The three pairs of polypeptide
chains in fibrinogen are held together by 29 disulfide bonds and
form long, slender structures that appear as trinodular structures
in the electron microscope. During the coagulation process, fibrinogen is converted by limited proteolysis from a soluble form to an
insoluble fibrin clot. This reaction involves the cleavage of
fibrinopeptides A and B from the amino-terminal region of both α and
β chains. In our studies on the cloning of fibrinogen, we employed
a bovine liver that had been stimulated by an acute phase reaction
in order to elevate the level of fibrinogen mRNA. In these experiments, the polyribosomal fraction containing mRNA for each of the
three fibrinogen chains was enriched by immunoprecipitation. cDNA
clones for the α and β chains of bovine fibrinogen were then isolated
and employed as probes for screening a human liver cDNA library. A
large number of cDNAs coding for both the α and β chains of human
fibrinogen were then identified by colony hybridization (5,6). Clones
for the γ chain were identified by screening the human cDNA library
with a synthetic nucleotide that corresponded to the unique amino

acid sequence of Trp-Trp-Met-Asn-Lys that is present in the carboxyl region of the γ chain (7). Plasmids with the largest cDNA inserts for each chain were then isolated and studied in greater detail. In the case of the α chain, a cDNA of over 2200 base pairs was identified (5). It included a short noncoding region at the 5' end followed by a region coding for a signal peptide of 19 (or 16) amino acids and a mature polypeptide of 625 amino acids. This clone was particularly interesting in that it contained 8 internal tandem repeats of 39 base pairs starting with amino acid residue 270 and ending with amino acid residue 372. Considerable nucleotide and amino acid identity was noted in these 8 tandem repeats. The clone for the α chain was also of interest in that the amino acid sequence predicted from the cDNA was 15 amino acids longer at the carboxyl-terminal end than that of the α chain isolated and sequenced from plasma fibrinogen. This indicates that minor proteolysis has taken place on the carboxyl-terminal end of the α chain during the assembly, secretion, or during the circulation of fibrinogen in blood.

The largest cDNA that was identified for the β chain of fibrinogen was a little over 1900 base pairs in length (6). It also coded for 461 amino acids present in the mature polypeptide chain. The largest cDNA for the γ chain was more than 1600 base pairs and coded for a leader sequence, as well as 1233 base pairs coding for 411 amino acids present in the mature γ chain (7). Considerable sequence identity in the DNAs was noted for the β and γ chains in both the coding and noncoding regions. There was limited homology, however, in the DNA sequence for the signal peptides for the α, β, and γ chains. The three different cDNAs have also been employed as probes for screening a λ phage library containing human genomic DNA. Positive phage have been identified for each of the genes for the α, β, and γ chains of human fibrinogen. At the present time, a major portion of the DNA sequence for the β and γ chains has been completed. The gene for the β chain contains 7 intervening sequences, the largest occurring at the 5' end between amino acid residues 8 and 9. These amino acids are present in the fibrinopeptide B. The gene for the γ chain contains 9 intervening sequences, the last of which is about 400 base pairs. This intervening sequence is of particular interest since it provides a coding region for about 15% of the mRNAs for the γ chain. This gives rise to variant forms of the γ chain, referred to as γ'. The γ' chain differs in size, charge, and sialic acid content from the more predominant γ chain. More recently, a carboxyl-terminal extension has been found in the γ' chain and sequenced by conventional amino acid sequencing techniques. The last four residues in the γ chain were replaced by 20 additional amino acids ending in leucine. In our experiments, we find that the 20 new amino acids on the carboxyl-terminal end of the γ' end are encoded by DNA present in the last intervening sequence. This suggests that the processing at the 3' end of the γ chain mRNA results in two (or more) polyadenylation sites, giving rise to a γ and a γ' mRNA. Whether these variant forms of fibrinogen with γ and γ' chains have any physiological significance is not known at the present time.

As previously noted, fibrinogen is converted to fibrin in the

presence of thrombin. Thrombin occurs, however, in plasma in a precursor form called prothrombin. Prothrombin is a vitamin K-dependent
protein that is converted to thrombin by minor proteolysis. This
reaction is catalyzed by factor X_a in the presence of factor V_a,
calcium ions, and phospholipid. The amino acid sequences for bovine
and human prothrombin have been established by classic techniques
of protein sequencing. Each protein contains 8-10% carbohydrate,
including 10 residues of γ-carboxyglutamic acid. Prothrombin also
contains two regions of internal homology that appear in tandem,
called kringle structures (14). These structures occur in the amino-
terminal region of the protein. In our studies on the cloning of
prothrombin, we have carried out enrichment of the mRNA by immunoprecipitation employing bovine liver polyribosomes. We were then
able to isolate a cDNA coding for bovine prothrombin and employ this
cDNA as a probe for the isolation of a human cDNA. The largest human
cDNA that we identified in our human cDNA library was about 2000 base
pairs in length (9). It coded for a portion of a signal sequence for
human prothrombin, in addition to 579 amino acids present in the
mature protein. The last two residues in the leader sequence (positions -2 and -1) were found to be arginine. These residues occur
just prior to the amino-terminal alanine which is present in the
mature protein circulating in plasma. Since the Arg-Ala bond is not
a typical cleavage site for signal peptidase, it appears likely that
the newly synthesized prothrombin in liver contains a pro leader
sequence analogous to factor IX (see below) and other plasma proteins,
such as serum albumin. This suggests that the signal peptidase actually cleaves at a peptide bond further upstream from the Arg-Ala
sequence, such as the Ser-Leu sequence at positions -8 and -7. The
10 glutamic acid residues that are present in the amino-terminal
region of prothrombin and converted to γ-carboxyglutamic acid in the
mature protein were found to be coded only by GAG.

The prothrombin cDNA has also been employed for the screening of
a human fetal liver genomic DNA library, and a number of positive
phage have been identified and sequenced. Thus far, we have found
13 intervening sequences in the gene for human prothrombin. Of
particular interest is the fact that the intervening sequences contain at least 10 copies of the AluI repetitive DNA. AluI repetitive
sequences have also been reported in the intervening sequences of
other genes, such as those for chicken $\alpha_{2(1)}$ collagen, chicken con-
albumin, and rat prolactin. Rat growth hormone and human cortico-
tropin-β-lipoprotein precursor genes have also been shown to contain
Alu repetitive DNA sequences.

We have also cloned a second vitamin K-dependent clotting factor,
called factor IX (10). This protein participates in the middle phase
of blood coagulation. In contrast to fibrinogen and prothrombin, the
gene for this protein is present on the X chromosome. Factor IX is
a single-chain glycoprotein containing 12 γ-carboxyglutamic acid
residues in the amino-terminal region of the protein. During the
coagulation process, factor IX is converted to factor IX_a by factor
XI_a in the presence of calcium ions. We have identified a cDNA
coding for human factor IX by screening the human cDNA liver library
with a single-stranded DNA prepared from enriched mRNA for baboon

factor IX, in addition to a synthetic oligonucleotide mixture. A plasmid containing a cDNA insert of more than 1400 base pairs has been identified for factor IX. This cDNA also codes for an amino-terminal leader sequence, in addition to the mature protein. The leader sequence in factor IX contains 46 amino acids and includes both a signal sequence and a pro sequence for the mature protein that circulates in plasma. This is analogous to prothrombin where there is also a pre-pro leader sequence. The 12 glutamic acid residues present in factor IX and converted to γ-carboxyglutamic acid in the mature protein are coded for by both GAA and GAG.

We have also employed the cDNA for factor IX as a probe for screening the human genomic DNA library and a number of positive phage have been identified. Thus far, we have sequenced a major portion of the 5' end of the gene. It is of particular interest to note that the first three intervening sequences in the gene for factor IX are in positions analogous to the first three intervening sequences in the gene for human prothrombin. Furthermore, considerable DNA and amino acid sequence homology exists between these two proteins for the first 50 amino acid residues in the mature proteins. Additional DNA sequencing, however, must be carried out to determine the degree of similarity in the remaining portions of these two human genes.

References. (1) Davie, E. W., Fujikawa, K., Kurachi, K. and Kisiel, W. (1979) Adv. Enzymol. 48, 277-318; (2) Stenflo, J., Fernlund, P., Egan, W. and Roepstorff, P. (1974) Proc. Natl. Acad. Sci. USA 71, 2730-2733; (3) Drakenberg, T., Fernlund, P., Roepstorff, P. and Stenflo, J. (1983) Proc. Natl. Acad. Sci. USA 80, 1802-1806; (4) McMullen, B. A., Fujikawa, K., Kisiel, W., Sasagawa,T., Howald, W. N., Kwa, E. Y. and Weinstein, B. (1983) Biochemistry 22, 2875-2884; (5) Rixon, M. W., Chan, W.-Y., Davie, E. W. and Chung, D.W. (1983) Biochemistry 22, 3237-3244; (6) Chung, D. W., Que, B. G., Rixon, M. W., Mace, M., Jr. and Davie, E. W. (1983) Biochemistry 22, 3244-3250; (7) Chung, D. W., Chan, W.-Y. and Davie, E. W. (1983) Biochemistry 22, 3250-3256; (8) Kant, J. A., Lord, S. T. and Crabtree, G. R. (1983) Proc. Natl. Acad. Sci. USA 80, 3953-3957; (9) Degen, S. J. Friezner, MacGillivray, R. T. A. and Davie, E. W. (1983) Biochemistry 22, 2087-2097; (10) Kurachi, K. and Davie, E. W. (1982) Proc. Natl. Acad. Sci. USA 79, 6461-6464; (11) Choo, K. H., Gould, K. G., Rees, D. J. G. and Brownlee, G. G. (1982) Nature 299, 178-180; (12) Jaye, M., de la Salle, H., Schamber, F., Balland, A., Kohli, V., Findeli, A., Tolstoshev, P. and Lecocq, J.-P. (1983) Nucl. Acids Res. 11, 2325-2335; (13) Marder, V. J., Francis, C. W. and Doolittle, R. F. (1982) in Hemostasis and Thrombosis (Colman, R.W. et al., eds.) pp. 145-163; (14) Magnusson, S., Petersen, T. E., Sottrup-Jensen, L. and Claeys, H. (1975) in Proteases and Biological Control (Reich, E. et al., eds.) pp. 123-149.

GENETIC DEFECTS IN LIPOPROTEIN RECEPTORS: A COMMON CAUSE OF
ATHEROSCLEROSIS IN MAN

Michael S. Brown and Joseph L. Goldstein,
Department of Molecular Genetics, University of Texas Health
Science Center at Dallas, Dallas, Texas 75235.

The concept of the low density lipoprotein (LDL) receptor was
formulated in 1973 to account for observed abnormalities in the
regulation of cholesterol metabolism in cultured fibroblasts from
patients with familial hypercholesterolemia (FH), an autosomal
dominant disorder that is a frequent cause of heart attacks.

LDL is a cholesterol-carrying plasma lipoprotein that
supplies cholesterol to cells. The LDL receptors are located in
regions of the plasma membrane that are indented and coated on
their cytoplasmic surface by a protein, clathrin; hence, their
designation as coated pits. Within minutes of their formation
coated pits invaginate into the cell and pinch off to form coated
endocytic vesicles which rapidly shed their coats to form
endosomes. From the endosomes the receptor-bound LDL is
eventually transported to lysosomes, where the LDL is degraded,
liberating its bound cholesterol for use by the cell.

The LDL receptor is but one example of a general class of
cell surface receptors that carry macromolecules into cells via
coated pits. Other members of this class are receptors for other
plasma transport proteins (transferrin, transcobalamin);
asialoglycoproteins; lysosomal enzymes; growth factors and
hormones (epidermal growth factor, platelet-derived growth factor,
insulin, chorionic gonadotrophin) and lipid-envelope viruses
(vesicular stomatitis virus, Semliki forest virus).

The structure, biosynthesis, and posttranslational processing
of the LDL receptor are coming to be understood. The receptor is
synthesized as a 120,000-dalton precursor that undergoes an
interesting form of processing: 30 min after synthesis its
apparent mol. wt. increases suddenly from 120,000 to 160,000, as
it travels from the endoplasmic reticulum to the cell surface.
This change is attributable to the elongation of 9 to 18 O-linked
carbohydrate chains, in addition to the processing of one or two
N-linked carbohydrate chains, on the receptor.

We have identified 8 mutant alleles at the receptor locus
that disrupt synthesis, processing, or transport of the receptor
to the surface of fibroblasts from 80 subjects with a clinical
disease called homozygous FH. Studies of the heterozygous parents
reveal that many of the FH "homozygotes" are genetic compounds
with 2 different receptor alleles.

One in every 500 people in the United States has the heterozygous form of FH. These individuals have one mutant gene and one normal gene at the LDL receptor locus. These subjects have a 50% deficiency of functional LDL receptors and a 2-fold increase in plasma LDL levels owing to inefficient uptake of LDL by the liver. An ideal therapy for FH heterozygotes would be a drug that stimulates their single normal receptor gene to produce an increased number of LDL receptors. The possibility of attaining this goal has emerged from the observation that the production of LDL receptors is under feedback regulation. Drugs that inhibit cellular cholesterol synthesis stimulate the synthesis of LDL receptors, enhance catabolism of LDL by the liver, and lower plasma LDL-cholesterol levels. Thus, a genetically dominant disease can be effectively treated by drugs that take advantage of built-in regulatory mechanisms to stimulate the single normal gene to increase production of the normal gene product.

Hybridization, Immunological and Enzymic Techniques

QUANTITATION OF SPECIFIC GENE EXPRESSION IN HUMAN DISEASES BY QUICK-BLOT

David H. Gillespie and Joel Bresser

Department of Hematology/Oncology, Hahnemann University, Broad and Vine, Philadelphia, PA 19102

Most human diseases involve aberrant gene regulation at some stage. Some diseases are consequences of germline mutations. Sickle cell anemia, thallasemias, and Down's syndrome are but three examples from a rather long list. Others are primarily consequences of somatic mutations. Cancer is the best example of this category, although the category may encompass atherosclerosis and coronary artery disease; diabetes; rheumatoid arthritis, systemic lupus erythematosus and other autoimmune diseases; neurological disorders such as multiple sclerosis and amyotrophic lateral sclerosis; etc. In diseases based on germline or somatic mutations environmental factors and genetic "predispositions" may aggravate, accelerate or delay clinical symptoms.

Diseases based on germline mutations are amenable to evaluations based on DNA structure. This is elegantly demonstrated by the restriction enzyme test for sickle cell anemia already in commercial kit form. Some diseases based on somatic mutations will also be amenable to evaluations based on DNA structure. Oncogene alterations offer a promising way to identify some persons with or at risk for cancer.

However, most human diseases will elude DNA structure analysis so that evaluations of mRNA quantity and structure will become preferred. We report here efforts to develop such an mRNA assay; one appropriate for large numbers of measurements yet retaining the sensitivity and accuracy required to reliably measure relatively small quantitative differences and one yielding results quickly and economically. The method dubbed "Quick-blot", involves the selective immobilization of mRNA onto nitrocellulose (NC), starting from cells which have been exposed to detergent and dissolved in NaI (Bresser, Doering and Gillespie, DNA 2:243-254, 1983). The procedure results in the immobilization of over 85% of mRNA, under 1% of rRNA, tRNA and tRNA and under 0.1% of protein. Irreversible binding is immediate and the mRNA-NC can be immediately used for a variety of purposes.

Figure 1, illustrates the Quick-blot technique as used in evaluation of mRNA quantity. In the left lane myc oncogene mRNA levels were measured in blood cells of a normal individual and referenced to the number of myc DNA sites in the same collection of cells. The myc RNA results were also referenced to total mRNA by hybridization of mRNA on a duplicate filter with a radioactive poly(T) probe and referenced to other selected mRNAs, using the remaining 22 replicate filters. Finally, the results were referenced to myc RNA levels in blood and marrow cells from several

Figure 1
myc gene expression in blood cells of a normal individual

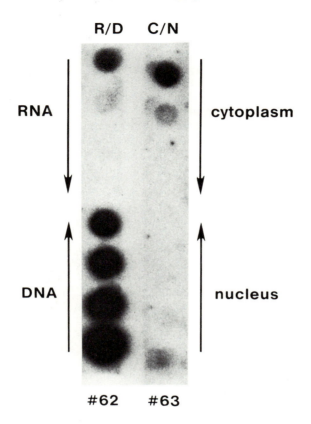

R/D   C/N

RNA   cytoplasm

DNA   nucleus

#62   #63

Figure 1 MRNA and DNA were immobilized from whole cells (R/D row). RNA was immobilized on the top four dots from progressively greater dilutions, top toward middle.   DNA was immobilized on the bottom four dots from progressively greater dilutions, bottom toward middle.

MRNA was also immobilized from cytoplasmic and nuclear fractions of the same cells (C/N row).   MRNA was immobilized on the top four dots from a cytoplasmic fraction.   The direction of dilution is top toward middle.   MRNA was immobilized on the bottom four dots from a nuclear fraction.   The direction of dilution is bottom toward middle.   Molecular hybridization was carried out with 10^6 cpm/ml of nick-translated myc oncogene probe at 42^0 in the 50% formamide system.   Radioautography was at -70^0 for 20 hr with an intensifying screen.

myeloproliferative disorder (MPD) and leukemia patients and normal
controls. In these contexts it is apparent that the myc gene is
expressed in some normal individuals and not others and that the
gene is overexpressed in some MPD and leukemia patients.

In the right lane the subcellular location of myc RNA was
determined. RNA was Quick-blotted from cytoplasmic and nuclear
fractions of the same cells used in the left lane and hybridized to
the myc gene probe. Note especially the lack of interaction with
nuclear material, graphically demonstrating the absence of
interference by DNA. This result originates from the specificity of
immobilization in the mRNA mode and from the fact that the Quick-
blot process contains no "baking" step which could cause DNA
denaturation.

Elimination of the baking step during mRNA immobilization
produced other, unexpected advantages. RNA immobilized by Quick-
blot can be reverse transcribed and translated into proteins
(Bresser, Hubbell and Gillespie, Proc. Nat. Acad. Sci. USA, in
press, 1983). Moreover, the RNA can be released from the filter and
further manipulated. These features provided the basis for a
battery of techniques for eluciding mRNA structure, for producing
DNA clones, clones corresponding to mRNA libraries from certain cell
types, and for rapidly producing an mRNA clone corresponding to a
specific mRNA.

MRNA Structure no. 1: Modified S1 Nuclease Assay

The structure of an immobilized mRNA can be determined by
measuring the size of a probe which has been hybridized to an
immobilized mRNA, digested with S1 nuclease, and released from the
filter. The experiment has been successfully accomplished by
hybridizing long single strands of labeled human DNA to Quick-
blotted nuclear RNA of leukemic leukocytes, digesting unhybridized
probe to nucleotides with S1 nuclease, releasing S1-resistant probe
from the filter and analyzing it by electrophoresis into a
polyacrylamide gel.

MRNA Structure no. 2: Modified Northern Transfer

In principle, mRNA can be released from NC with pure formamide,
fractionated by electrophoresis into polyacrylamide then transferred
to NC for hybridization with a radioactive probe. In practice, mRNA
has been released from NC, has been reverse transcribed and
translated and has been reapplied to NC for molecular hybridization,
but has not yet been successfully fractionated by electrophoresis
into agarose. In all instances so far examined the mRNA after
release from NC exhibited a lower electrophoretic mobility than
prior to immobilization. The reason for this is under
investigation.

After electrophoresis, mRNA can be transferred to NC either by Thomas' method using NaCl or by using NaI. Less convection occurs using NaCl, producing a sharper image on NC. MRNA transferred in NaI is biologically active and can be reverse transcribed or translated.

Cloning Copies of mRNA Populations in Cells

The construction of "mRNA" libraries from defined cell populations has become an important research tool. Since mRNA Quick-blotted from small numbers of cells can be reverse transcribed into full-length cDNA, a rapid cloning procedure is possible. A problem existed in low efficiency of transcription of Quick-blotted mRNA, but the efficiency of reverse transcription has been increased significantly by eliminating the EtOH and acetic anhydride soaks which are part of the "Standard mRNA Quick-blot"; eliminating salt during mRNA-filter prewashes; and using NH_4Ac during precipitation. Second strand synthesis on immobilized mRNA has not been proven, but is indicated from the fact that cDNA is released from the filter when Actinomycin D is not included in the synthesis mixture.

Cloning of purified mRNA by Quick-blot technology

Cloning of specific mRNAs from different cells provides a reagent for explaining exactly the differences in the regulation of the relevant mRNAs. The outline for this procedure is:

* Fractionate mRNA electrophoretically in polyacrylamide
* Transfer the mRNA to NC in NaI
* Locate the relevant mRNA species by molecular hybridization
* Melt off the hybridized probe
* Reverse transcribe the relevant mRNA
* Clone the cDNA and screen recombinants

The method is in principle compatible with any method of mRNA purification. Clearly, the simpler the method of mRNA purification the more powerful the overall method will be. Ideally, the mRNA purification outlined above under "mRNA structure no. 2: Modified Northern Transfer" will yield suitable mRNA populations for this experiment.

The transfer of mRNA from polyacrylamide to NC must be done in NaI to preserve biological activity. Once the total cell mRNA has been transferred to NC the relevant mRNA species can be detected by molecular hybridization. The mRNA-containing band can then be cut precisely from the membrane and the probe can be removed if necessary by dipping the membrane in boiling dilute salt solution. Reverse transcription and cloning can follow the procedures outlined in the previous section. Overall, this approach provides an extremely rapid and efficient means of cloning DNA copies of specific mRNAs in instances where mRNA enrichment is useful.

THE USE OF IMMUNOTOXINS FOR THE THERAPY OF CANCER AND THE MODULATION OF THE IMMUNE RESPONSE

Jonathan W. Uhr and Ellen S. Vitetta

Dept. Microbiology, Southwestern Medical School, UTHSC, Dallas, TX

The term immunotoxin is used to designate a hybrid molecule, one portion of which is a toxic protein and the other portion of which is an antibody or antigen. There are three major ways that immunotoxins can be used for the therapy of cancer (1): 1) in vitro treatment of autologous bone marrow to delete cancer cells (or T lymphocytes in allogeneic marrow) as part of the bone marrow transplantation approach; 2) parenteral treatment of patients bearing cancers; 3) parenteral treatment of patients to modulate their immune response for therapeutic purposes.

In our own studies, we have used the plant toxin, ricin. We have coupled the toxic subunit of ricin (A chain) to monoclonal or affinity purified polyvalent antibodies directed against cell surface immunoglobulins in order to kill neoplastic or normal B lymphocytes.

The first approach employed was the use of immunotoxins to kill tumor cells in infiltrated bone marrow. We found that in a murine leukemia (BCL_1), in vitro treatment of tumor infiltrated marrow (10^6 cells containing 15% tumor cells) with A chain-containing immunotoxins (15 min. $4°$ C) killed all leukemia cells in the majority of cases. In this tumor model, injection of 1 BCL_1 cell results in leukemia by 12 weeks in 50% of mice. In this approach, tumor-specific antibody is unnecessary and the only specificity requirement is to use an antibody that reacts with the tumor cells and kills them but does not react with the pleuripotential stem cells which reconstitute the entire hematopoietic system.

We have extended these findings to studies with human bone marrow. The Burkitt's lymphoma B cell line (Daudi) was mixed with normal human marrow and a polyvalent anti-human Ig A chain immunotoxin was used in an attempt to kill the leukemic cells without killing stem cells. The results showed that treatment with immunotoxin killed 97-99% of colony-forming Daudi cells with no killing of myeloid/granulocyte colony-forming cells, erythroid burst-forming units, or erythroid colony-forming unit stem cells (2). Thus, the immunotoxin A chain approach may be useful for the removal of tumor cells from autologous bone marrow.

A second use of immunotoxins is to administer them systemically to tumor-bearing individuals. In contrast to the use of immunotoxins for the in vitro treatment of bone marrow, systemic administration demands much stricter tumor cell specificity (i.e., cross-reactivity with normal cells may not be acceptable). We have used anti-idiotype-A chain conjugates to treat mice bearing far-advanced BCL_1 tumors (10^{10} tumor cells/mouse). The strategy was to nonspecifically reduce the tumor mass by at least 95% (by total lymphoid irradiation and splenectomy) and try to kill the remainder of the cells with anti-idiotype-A chain conjugates. This treatment regimen produced a prolonged remission (that is, the mice appeared tumor-free 12 weeks later). Control animals treated with nontumor-reactive immunotoxins after nonspecific cytoreduction were all dead 7 weeks after completion of the total lymphoid irradiation and splenectomy. These results were reproduced with anti-δ A chain-containing immunotoxins (1). Therefore, anti-human δ-A chain immunotoxins might be useful in systemic immunotherapy of human B cell tumors that bear surface IgD.

The results also show that 3 months after treatment with anti-δ immunotoxin, normal levels of IgD$^+$ cells were present. They had been reconstituted from stem cells, pre-B cells or IgM$^+$ IgD$^-$ cells. In this particular instance, the price of killing BCL$_1$ cells, which was the killing of virtually all virgin B lymphocytes for a period of time, was acceptable. Serum antibodies and memory cells that lack surface IgD apparently provided the animals with sufficient immunity to survive during this interim period.

We have followed the animals described above for 25 weeks to determine if remission persisted and, if so, whether the animals were tumor-free. The answers are that the animals were disease-free but when cells from the tissues of such animals were transferred to normal recipients, they invariably caused tumor in the recipients. We conclude, therefore, that the mice in prolonged remission probably have mounted an immune response that keeps the small number of remaining viable tumor cells in check. This putative host immune response may be an anti-idiotypic one.

Although A chain-containing immunotoxins can be highly effective in killing cells bearing the relevant surface Ig determinants, A chain containing immunotoxins directed against determinants on other types of cells (e.g. T cells) are frequently less effective (3-5). In contrast, when antibodies are coupled to intact ricin, the potency in killing cells with the relevant determinant is significantly greater (3-5). Thus, B chains may facilitate the entry of A chains into the cytoplasm (3-5). It would be desirable, therefore, to develop a strategy in which the putative transport role of the B chain could be preserved while minimizing its function as a lectin. To this end, we have developed an approach which utilizes 2 types of immunotoxin. Antibodies reactive with human B lymphocytes are conjugated to either ricin A chain or ricin B chain; by affinity purification of the immunotoxins, free A and B chains are eliminated. Using the 2 immunotoxins, the 2 subunits of the ricin toxin are thereby delivered independently to the same target cell (6).

A representative experiment is shown in Figure 1. Daudi cells were treated with rabbit anti-human immunoglobulin A chain (RαHIgA) at a concentration at which little toxicity was observed. No concentration of rabbit anti-human Ig B chain (RαHIgB) was toxic. However, when the same concentration of RαHIgA was mixed with various concentrations of RαHIgB, there was significant cytotoxicity. In contrast, when RαHIgA was admixed with rabbit anti-ovalbumin B, there was no synergy. Hence, there was insufficient contaminating free B chains in the B chain-containing

114

immunotoxins to synergize with the A chain-containing immunotoxins. These experiments were performed in galactose-free media indicating that the galactose binding site of the B chain is insufficient to allow a B chain-containing immunotoxin of irrelevant specificity to synergize with an A chain-containing immunotoxin that is specific to the target cell. The results indicate that the target cell specificity of the antibody combining site of the immunotoxins is essential for synergy. The novelty of the present approach is the separate delivery of the A chain and the B chain to the target cells so that reassociation takes place on or in the target cell.

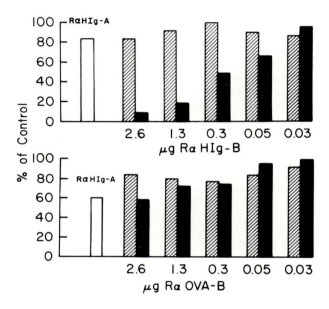

Figure 1. A and B chain-containing immunotoxins synergize in their ability to kill Daudi cells. Top panel: Daudi cells were treated with rabbit anti-HIg-A, 0.3 µg/ml. Different amounts of rabbit anti-HIg B (hatched bar) or rabbit anti-HIgA, 0.3 µg mixed with different amount of rabbit anti-HIgB (black bar). Lower panel: Same as above except that rabbit anti-OVAB was used in place of rabbit anti-HIgB.

Variations of this strategy that might be desirable include using 2 antibodies directed against different surface antigens on a single target cell. This maneuver could be utilized to increase the specificity of killing of the target cell since maximum killing would only occur if both antigens were present on the target cell. Another possibility is to use an Fab-A chain immunotoxin specific for the target cell and subsequently to administer a B chain-containing immunotoxin with specificity for the Fab fragment. If used _in vivo_, this approach could allow for clearance of excess Fab-A immunotoxin from the systemic circulation with retention of cell bound Fab-A immunotoxin until administration of the second immuntoxin. This maneuver might minimize nonspecific toxicity to the reticuloendothelial system.

References. (1) Vitetta, E.S., Krolick, K.A., and Uhr, J.W. (1982) Immunol. Rev. 62:159-183. (2) Muirhead, M., Martin, P.J., Torok-Storb, B., Uhr, J.W. and Vitetta, E.S. (1983) Blood 62:327-332. (3) Jansen, F.K., Blythman, H.E., Carriere, D., Casellas, P., Gros, O., Gros, P., Laurent, J.C., Paolucci, F., Pau, B., Poncelet, P., Richer, G., Vidal, H., and Voisin, G.A. (1982) Immunol. Rev. 62:185-216. (4) Neville, D.M., Jr. and Youle, R.J. (1982) Immunol. Rev. 62:75-92. (5) Thorpe, P.E. and Ross, W.C.J. (1982) Immunol. Rev. 62:119-158.

THE T-CELL CIRCUIT - CLINICAL AND BIOLOGIC IMPLICATIONS

Stuart F. Schlossman, M.D.

Dana-Farber Cancer Institute, Harvard Medical School, Boston,
Massachusetts

The precise dissection of the cellular mechanisms and
interactions involved in the generation of the human T cell
response has been facilitated by recent developments in: 1)
methods for the characterization and identification of human T
lymphocyte surface antigens utilizing monoclonal antibodies; 2)
new techniques for the isolation of highly purified subclasses of
human T lymphocytes dependent on cell surface markers; 3) methods
to discriminate both the functional properties and interactions of
isolated subsets of T lymphocytes; 4) techniques for the cloning
of human T cells; and 5) the ability to correlate normal and
abnormal functional properties of T lymphocyte subpopulations in
vitro with in vivo disorders of the immune response. These
studies have influenced our understanding of the differentiation
and functional program of the human T lymphocyte.

During differentiation, T cells diverge into functionally
distinct subsets of cells programmed for specific antigen
recognition and for the respective effector and regulatory
functions (Figure 1). In man, the earliest lymphoid cells in the

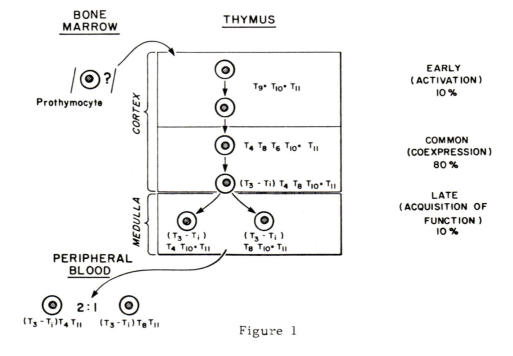

Figure 1

thymus lack mature T cell antigens but bear antigens found on cells of several lineages and activated T cells. This population accounts for approximately 10% of the total thymic pool and is reactive with several monoclonal antibodies including anti-T9 (transferrin receptor), anti-T10 and anti-T11 (the E rosette receptor). With further maturation, thymocytes lose T9, retain both T10 and T11 and acquire a thymocyte distinct antigen (the TL homolog in man). Concurrently, these cells express antigens defined by anti-T4 and anti-T8 (stage II). Thus, the majority of cortical thymocytes coexpress T4, T6, T8, T10 and T11 and accounts for approximately 70% of the total. With further maturation, thymocytes lose T6 and acquire T3 and a T cell idiotypic determinant (Ti). This T3/Ti complex appears late in cortical development and defines the T cell receptor in man. This cell coexpresses T3/Ti, T4, T8, T10, and T11 and appears to be the first cell in the thymus which is immunologically competent. With further maturation, the cells diverge into two major populations – the inducer population and the suppressor population which bear T4 and T8 respectively. These distinct nonoverlapping populations are seen in the medullary region of the thymus. Moreover, the unique cell surface glycoproteins appear to define the functional program of the T lymphocyte. The inducer cell, for example, bears a 62 KD glycoprotein termed T4 whereas the suppressor population bears the 76 KD molecule T8+. Both sets of cells recognize antigen with a specific antigen receptor termed the T3/Ti complex. The specific T cell receptor is a 90 K dalton heterodimer (Ti) comprised of a covalently linked 49 K α and a 43 K β chain which is membrane associated with the 20/25 K T3 molecule. Proteolytic cleavage and isoelectric focusing analysis of the Ti structure suggest sufficient peptide variability in the Ti molecules to account for an antigen specific recognition structure. Moreover, anti-Ti antibodies (anti-clonotypic) precisely mimic the antigen-like effects on specific T cells. This antigen recognition structure in association with the MHC restricting elements known as T4 for class II antigens and T8 for class I antigens makes up the major structure involved in T cell antigen recognition.

It should be noted that both the inducer and suppressor populations can be further divided into individual subsets of T lymphocytes. In this regard, individual T lymphocytes do not possess all of the effector and regulatory functions of the subset of cells to which they belong. It appears that each population within a given subset possesses a restricted functional program. Two subsets of inducer cells have been defined; one the T4+JRA+TQ1+ primarily functions as the inducer of the suppressor cell whereas the second population is T4+JRA-TQ1- and functions predominantly as the inducer of help. Immune homeostasis results from a delicate balance between these regulatory populations. Alterations and subset dynamics initiate a variety of immunopathologic disorders including autoimmunity,

118

immunodeficiency and malignant disorders. The application of this
new technology of cell surface characterization is expected to
have an important impact on our understanding of clinical
diseases. For example, it is now possible to define the
heterogeneity of T cell malignancies and relate this heterogeneity
to states of normal T cell differentiation. Moreover, disorders
of T cell maturation, diseases associated with losses of
subpopulations of cells, diseases associated with imbalances of T
cell subsets with restricted functions and lastly, diseases
associated with activation of T cell populations have been
described. It is believed that an understanding of both the
heterogeneity and functional repertoire of the human T cell as
well as the mechanisms and structures by which it recognizes
antigens and carries out its effector and regulatory programs
should provide new strategies capable of manipulating the immune
response to the benefit of the host.

General References

1. Reinherz EL, Schlossman SF. The differentiation and function of human T lymphocytes: A review. Cell 1980; 19:821-7.

2. Reinherz EL, Schlossman SF. The characterization and function of human immunoregulatory T lymphocyte subsets. Immunology Today 1981; 4:69-75.

3. Reinherz EL, Cooper MD, Schlossman SF, Rosen FS. Abnormalities of T cell maturation and regulation in human beings with immunodeficiency disorders. J Clin Invest. 1981; 68:699-705.

4. Reinherz EL, Morimoto C, Fitzgerald KA, Hussey RE, Daley JR, Schlossman SF. Heterogeneity of human T4+ inducer T cells as defined by a monoclonal antibody that delineates two functional subpopulations. J Immunol. 1982; 128:463-8.

5. Reinherz EL, Meuer S, Fitzgerald KA, Hussey RE, Levine H, Schlossman SF. Antigen recognition by human T lymphocytes is linked to surface expression of the T3 molecular complex. Cell 1982; 30:735-43.

6. Meuer SC, Fitzgerald KA, Hussey, RE, Hodgdon JC, Schlossman SF, Reinherz EL. Clonotypic structures involved in antigen-specific human T cell function. J Exp Med. 1983; 157:705-19.

7. Morimoto C, Reinherz EL, Borel Y, Schlossman SF. Direct demonstration of the human suppressor inducer subset by anti-T cell antibody. J Immunol. 1983; 130:157-61.

8. Acuto O, Meuer SC, Hodgdon JC, Schlossman SF, Reinherz EL. Peptide variability exists within α and β subunits of the T cell receptor for antigen. J Exp Med. 1983; 158:1368-1373.

ENZYME REPLACEMENT THERAPY USING LIPOSOMES OF NOVEL COMPOSITION

Kunio YAGI

Inst. of Applied Biochemistry, Yagi Memorial Park, Mitake,
Gifu 505-01, JAPAN

Many hereditary diseases are characterized by a deficiency in definite enzyme(s). Obviously such diseases are due to inborn errors in the gene, which cannot as yet be repaired. The sole treatment for the prevention or cure of these diseases would be the replacement of the lacking enzyme. For this purpose, several criteria should be met. Firstly, the enzyme should be incorporated into the site where the enzyme is lacking; however, the targeting of the enzyme to specific cells, organs, or tissues cannot be easily attained. Especially, the targeting of the enzyme into the brain has been impossible due to the presence of the blood-brain-barrier. Accordingly, hereditary diseases such as GM_1-gangliosidosis, Tay-Sachs, and Krabbe's disease, that are characterized by the lack of a definite enzyme in the brain, have never been cured. Secondly, the enzyme should act *in situ* without rapid decomposition; and, thirdly, the enzyme incorporated should not provoke any immunological reaction. To stabilize the enzyme as well as to reduce its immunogenicity, immobilization or modification of the enzyme would be a promising approach.

To incorporate enzyme into cells *in situ*, the mediation of liposomes, or artificial lipid vesicles (1-3), seems to be hopeful, since their incorporation into some cells has been achieved. For example, positively-charged liposomes were reported to be incorporated into mouse leukemia leucocytes (4) and Hela cells (5). Juliano and Stamp (6) reported that small liposomes were capable of reaching tumors more easily than larger liposomes. Gregoriadis and Neerunjun (7,8) conducted skillful experiments based on the insertion of anti-target-site (e.g., cell) IgG immunoglobulin into liposomes.

However, the incorporation of liposomes into the brain has never been achieved. To rectify this situation, we made extensive efforts and recently obtained successful results using liposomes of novel composition (9,10). The present communication summarizes the data which give us hope that enzyme replacement therapy in hereditary diseases of the brain may someday become a reality.

Enzymological study using D-glucose oxidase

To investigate liposomal systems capable of introducing enzyme into specific tissues, we entrapped D-glucose oxidase (β-D-glucose: O_2 1-oxidoreductase, EC 1.1.3.4) into liposomes as a marker and injected the enzyme-ladden liposomes intravenously into rats. After systematic investigation on the effect of lipid composition on the capability of liposomes to carry this enzyme to specific tissues, we found that the addition of lipids extracted from rat liver plasma membranes to a phosphatidylcholine-cholesterol system enabled the liposomes to penetrate into the brain, as shown in Fig. 1, I and II. To see which component of the lipids was responsible, the extracted lipids were fractionated into neutral lipids, glycolipids, and phospholipids; and it was found that the effect was due to the glycolipid fraction (see Fig. 1, III-V). Then, the effectiveness of a series of purified

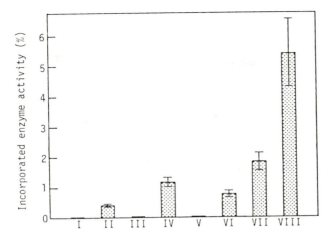

Fig. 1. The incorporation of D-glucose oxidase into rat brain by means of liposomes. The composition of liposomes was as follows: I, phosphatidylcholine-cholesterol (180.6 mg : 20.5 mg); II, I + lipids extracted from rat liver plasma membrane (20 mg); III, I + neutral lipid fraction from liver plasma membrane (20 mg); IV, I + glycolipid fraction from liver plasma membrane (20 mg); V, I + phospholipid fraction from liver plasma membrane (20 mg); VI, phosphatidylcholine-cholesterol-gangliosides (molar ratio, 7 : 2 : 1); VII, phosphatidylcholine-cholesterol-cerebroside (molar ratio, 7 : 2 : 1); VIII, phosphatidylcholine-cholesterol-sulfatide (molar ratio, 7 : 2 : 1). The incorporated enzyme activity was measured 30 min after injection and expressed as percent of the total activity injected. Mean ± SD is given (n=9).

glycolipids was examined, and sulfatide was found to be the most efficient, as shown in Fig. 1, VI-VIII. The incorporation of the enzyme into organs of the rat is summarized in Table I. It should be noted that at 30 minutes after the injection the amount of the enzyme incorporated into the brain exceeded the amount in the blood. The intracellular distribution of the incorporated enzyme was also investigated, and most of the enzyme activity was found in the soluble, cytoplasmic fraction.

TABLE I. INCORPORATION OF D-GLUCOSE OXIDASE INTO RAT ORGANS BY MEANS OF LIPOSOMES COMPOSED OF PHOSPHATIDYLCHOLINE-CHOLESTEROL WITH OR WITHOUT SULFATIDE

	Incorporated enzyme activity*	
	30 min	60 min
Liver	66.2 ± 2.2 (23.5 ± 1.6)**	58.9 ± 12.7 (21.7 ± 3.0)
Kidney	8.7 ± 0.6 (2.6 ± 0.5)	9.7 ± 0.3 (4.3 ± 1.0)
Spleen	5.9 ± 0.3 (1.0 ± 0.2)	5.3 ± 1.4 (6.0 ± 0.7)
Lung	4.1 ± 1.1 (1.7 ± 0.5)	6.0 ± 0.5 (2.4 ± 0.6)
Brain	5.4 ± 1.1 (0)	3.7 ± 0.6 (0)
Blood	3.7 ± 0.3 (1.4 ± 0.3)	3.8 ± 0.4 (1.4 ± 0.3)

 * The enzyme activity was expressed as percent of the total enzyme activity injected. Mean ± SD is given (n=9).
** The numbers in parentheses are the values obtained by means of liposomes without sulfatide.

122

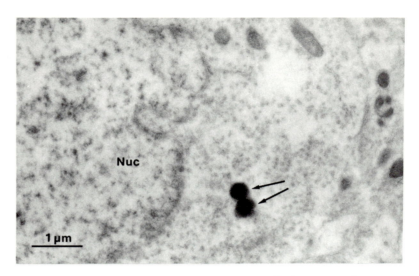

Fig. 2 Electron micrograph of *nucleus supraopticus* of the brain after the injection of the liposomes containing horseradish peroxidase. Arrows show the reaction products of high density in the cytoplasm close to the nucleus (Nuc). The specimen was observed without contrast staining.

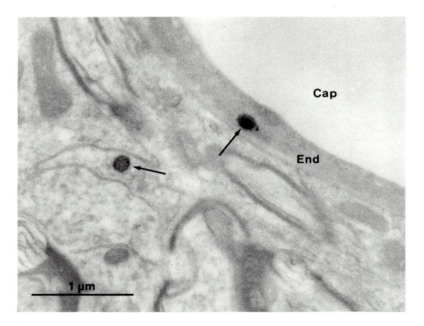

Fig. 3 Electron micrograph of *locus ceruleus* of the brain after the injection of the liposomes containing ferritin. Liposomes containing ferritin molecules in the endothelial cell (End) of the capillary (Cap) and the astrocyte are indicated by arrows. The specimen was observed without contrast staining.

Histochemical study using horseradish peroxidase

To confirm the incorporation of the enzyme into the brain tissue by means of the above-mentioned liposomes, we conducted a histochemical study. Horseradish peroxidase (donor: hydrogen-peroxide oxidoreductase, EC 1.11.1.7) was entrapped within liposomes having the composition of phosphatidylcholine, cholesterol, sulfatide (molar ratio, 7 : 2 : 1) and was injected intravenously into a rat. After 30 minutes, the animal was treated as described elsewhere (10) to visualize the enzyme by its enzymatic activity. Fig. 2 shows an electron micrograph of the *nucleus supraopticus* of the rat brain. Spots of high electron-density with a diameter of 0.3 μm are observable in a neuroglial cell. In the control brain, such spots were never observed. Judging from the shape and density of these spots, we ascribed them to the catalytic action of horseradish peroxidase. This indicates that the liposomes containing the enzyme were indeed incorporated into the brain. Since it is well known that the blood-brain-barrier is well developed in the *nucleus supraopticus*, it appears that the liposomes passed through the blood-brain-barrier.

Morphological study using ferritin

To demonstrate more directly this incorporation, we also used ferritin-ladden liposomes, since ferritin can be easily observed electron microscopically and liposomes containing it can be distinguished from the cellular background by the characteristic appearance of the ferritin molecule. Liposomes of the same composition as those used for horseradish peroxidase, but containing ferritin instead, were injected intravenously into a rat. After 1 hour, the animal was treated as described elsewhere (10). Fig. 3 shows an electron micrograph of the *locus ceruleus* of the brain, in which liposomes containing the distinctive ferritin marker are seen. One is in the endothelial cell of a blood capillary; another, in the cytoplasm of an astrocyte. It should be mentioned that the blood-brain-barrier is also well developed in the *locus ceruleus*.

From these results, it is concluded that our liposomes enable the enzyme to pass through the blood-brain-barrier and that our liposomes open up a possible avenue for the prevention or cure of hereditary diseases of the brain which involve enzyme deficiencies.

References— (1) Bangham, A. D., Standish, M. M., and Weissmann, G. (1965) J. Mol. Biol. 13, 253-259; (2) Sessa, G., and Weissmann, G. (1968) J. Lipid Res. 9, 310-318; (3) Bangham, A. D., Hill, M. W., and Miller, N. G. A. (1974) in Methods in Membrane Biology (Korn, E. D. ed.), Vol. 1, pp. 1-68, Plenum Press, New York; (4) Magee, W. E., and Miller, O. V. (1972) Nature 235, 339-340; (5) Magee, W. E., Goff, C. W., Schoknecht, J., Smith, M. D., and Cherian, K. (1974) J. Cell Biol. 63, 492-504; (6) Juliano, R. L., and Stamp, D. (1975) Biochem. Biophys. Res. Commun. 63, 651-658; (7) Gregoriadis, G. (1974) In Enzyme Replacement Therapy of Lysosomal Storage Diseases (Tager, J. M., Hooghwinkel, J. M., and Daoms, W. T. eds.) pp. 131-148, North-Holland Publishing Co., Amsterdam; (8) Gregoriadis, G., and Neerunjun, E. D. (1975) Biochem. Biophys. Res. Commun. 65, 537-544; (9) Naoi, M., and Yagi, K. (1980) Biochem. Int. 6, 591-596; (10) Yagi, K., Naoi, M., Sakai, H., Abe, H., Konishi, H., and Arichi, S. (1982) J. Appl. Biochem. 4, 121-125

Poster Session Reports

THE ISOLATION OF A CLONE CONTAINING THE COMPLETE HUMAN APRT GENE

Janet Arrand[ab], Elliot Drobetsky[c] and Anne Murray[b]
[a]BRL (UK) Ltd., P.O. Box 145, Science Park, Cambridge 4, England
[b]Department of Biochemistry, St. Mary's Hospital Medical School, London
W2, England [c]Laboratory of Molecular Genetics, Clinical Research
Institute of Montreal, Pine Avenue West, Montreal, Quebec, Canada.

INTRODUCTION

Several human chromosome libraries have been contructed (1) and
clones from these have been assigned both physical and genetic locations
(2,3) whilst their actual genetic function remains, for the most part,
obscure. Individual genes, such as B-globin, which are highly expressed
can be cloned using cDNA; most enzymes cannot be cloned in this way and
some form of enrichment is necessary for their isolation.

Enrichment can be achieved for genes for whose products there exists
both a positive selection and a cell line deficient in the relevant
activity (4). Few mutant human cell lines exist, whereas mouse and
hamster cell mutants are available, as are the respective cloned genes.
Provided that there is homology between the cloned rodent genes and their
human counterparts, the human genes can be selected from total genomic
libraries.

Here we report the isolation of the complete, transforming human aprt
gene from a human genomic library (5) by utilising its cross-hybridisation
with the cloned hamster gene (4).

RESULTS

Southern blots of restricted human DNA were hybridised with nick-
translated non-repetitive hamster aprt DNA (6) and were washed to various
stringencies. After 1 x SSC washing, human aprt-containing bands were
readily visible on autoradiograms.

The hamster probe was then used under these conditions to screen
1.4×10^5 plaques from the Maniatis human genomic library. 4 cross
hybridising plaques were isolated. Each contained a 17.4kb EcoRI insert,
whose restriction map is shown below:

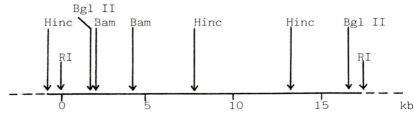

Transfection of the whole clone and isolated restriction fragments into
aprt⁻ hamster cells has localised the coding region of the gene to the
8.6kb HincII fragment. Human aprt-containing sequences have been detected
in the hamster aprt+ transformants. Smaller fragments tested showed no
transforming activity.

The 2.3kb Bam HI fragment of the human clone was shown by hybridisation to nick translated total human DNA, to contain few or no repetitive
sequences. This fragment was used to probe digests of randomly selected
human DNA samples. The chromosome region surrounding the aprt gene was
found to be highly polymorphic with respect to the TaqI restriction enzyme
site.

DISCUSSION

Our results show that selectable human genes can be successfully cloned by probing libraries with cloned hamster counterparts. This will facilitate the isolation of many more specific human genes, especially those involved in nucleic acid metabolism, where deficiencies cause diseases such as Lesh-Nyan (hgprt-).

The human aprt clone can be used for chromosome walking studies on chromosome 16, for the analysis of the polymorphic region surrounding the gene, and for familial studies on the human aprt- trait.

SUMMARY

We have isolated a lambda clone containing the complete human aprt gene, as shown by its transforming activity for aprt- cells. DNA fragments from this clone are being used to analyse the aprt locus on human chromosome 16.

BIBLIOGRAPHY

1. Young, B.D. and Davies, K. (1983) in "Progress and Topics in Cytogenetics". (in press)
2. Harper, M.E. and Saunders, G.R. (1981) Chromosoma 83 431.
3. Shows, T.B. and McAlpine, C.J. (1982) Cytogenet. Cell. Genet 32 221.
4. Lowy I. et al. (1980) Cell 22 817.
5. Maniatis, T. et al. (1978) Cell 15 687.
6. Meuth, M. and Arrand, J.E. (1982) Mol. Cell. Biol. 2 1459.

LACK OF POLYMORPHISM FOR C-TYPE RETROVIRUS SEQUENCES IN THE SYRIAN HAMSTER

Sally S. Atherton, Robert D. Streilein, and J. Wayne Streilein, Dept. of Cell Biology, University of Texas Health Science Center, Dallas, Texas   75235

INTRODUCTION. It has been suggested that the generation of poly-morphism at a major histocompatibility complex (MHC) and the subse-quent expression of class I antigens is related to the content and expression of C-type retrovirus sequences which have become integrated at or near the genes comprising the MHC (1). We have shown that the Syrian hamster (Mesocricetus auratus) lacks polymorphism for class I gene products as detected both serologically and biochemically (A. Darden and J.W. Streilein, manuscript in preparation). Our investiga-tions of the endogenous C-type retroviruses of the hamster led us to examine whether genetically diverse Syrian hamsters display polymorph-ism at the loci coding for these retrovirus sequences.

MATERIALS AND METHODS. Livers from adult mice and adult hamsters of selected strains were minced and dounce-homogenized. The nuclei were pelleted and washed 1X in 10mM Tris-HCl, pH 8.0, 10mM NaCl, 3mM $MgCl_2$ followed by lysis in 1% SDS and 50mM EDTA. Proteinase K was added to a final concentration of 100μg/ml, and the mixture was in-cubated at 50° C for 3 hr. The DNA was deproteinized by extraction with phenol:chloroform:isoamyl alcohol (50:50:1). The DNA was dial-yzed and quantitated spectrophotometrically. Aliquots of DNA (10-20μg) were digested according to the manufacturer's specifications and electrophoresed into 1% agarose gels made in Tris-acetate. The gels were blotted onto nitrocellulose (2) and hybridized under stringent conditions (3). The Moloney-MuLV probe (4) was kindly supplied by Dr. B. Ozanne, UTHSC-D. The probe was nick-translated (5) to a spe-cific activity of >1 X 10^8 CPM/μg.

RESULTS. In order to study C-type retrovirus sequences in the hamster genome, we compared hamster and mouse DNAs for (a) similarity of sequences between the two species and (b) the pattern of sequences found among selected mouse strains. Figure 1 shows that hamsters and

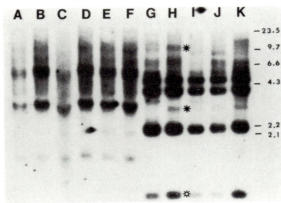

Figure 1. Comparison of Syrian hamster (Lanes A-F) and mouse (Lanes G-K) retro-virus sequences. Genomic DNAs were digested with Sst 1 and hybridized as described. Lane A-German, B-MHA, C-Murphy D-MIT, E-CB, F-LSH, G-T/t[w5], H-C57BL/6, I-C3H, J-A/J, K-BALB/c. Molecular weights (kilobase pairs) are indi-cated to the right of the figure.

mice differ markedly from each other in their retrovirus sequences. Moreover, there is considerable polymorphism of C-type retrovirus

sequences among the mouse strains tested. This polymorphism is reflected by either the addition of one or more bands (closed asterisks)
or by bands represented in different molar amounts (open asterisk).
We were also able to demonstrate (data not shown) that the degree of
murine polymorphism shown in Figure 1 was independent of the restriction enzyme used in these types of experiments. To determine whether
hamsters display polymorphism for insertion of retrovirus sequences,
we examined the DNA from several hamster strains. Figure 2 shows the

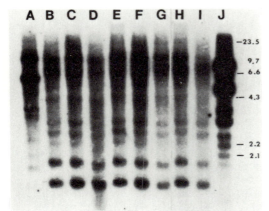

Figure 2. Pst 1 digests of
Syrian and Phodopus hamster DNA
demonstrating lack of polymorphism of endogenous retrovirus
sequences among Syrian hamsters.
Gels were blotted and hybridized
as described. Lane A-Phodopus,
B-UT1, C-MHA, D-Murphy, E-MIT,
F-LSH, G-LVG, H-CB, I-German J-
BALB/c (mouse). Molecular weight
(kilobase pairs) are indicated to
the right of the figure.

pattern obtained when ^{32}P-labeled Moloney-MuLV probe was hybridized
with DNA from several strains of Syrian hamster and another hamster
species, Phodopus songorus. Normal BALB/c mouse DNA was included as
a specificity control. All strains of Syrian hamster show an identical pattern of hybridization which is distinct from either that of
the mouse or that of the Phodopus hamster.

DISCUSSION. Our experiments have shown that although much homology (both in sequence and organization) exists between hamster and
mouse retrovirus genes, the insertion sites of the hamster retrovirus
genes are different than those of the mouse. Moreover, the hybridization data from genetically disparate hamster strains reveal no evidence for polymorphism of retrovirus sequences. The fact that lack of
polymorphism is found for both class I MHC genes and endogenous virus
sequences in hamsters provides circumstantial evidence in support of
the contention that the expression and function of these two sets of
genes are related.

REFERENCES. (1) Meruelo, D., and Edidin, M. (1980) Contemporary
Topics Immunobiol. 9, 231-253; (2) Southern, E.M. (1975) J. Mol. Biol.
38, 503-517; (3) Atherton, S.S., Sullivan, D., Dauenhauer, S.A.,
Ruyechan, W., and O'Callaghan, D.J. (1982) Virology 120, 18-32; (4)
Shoemaker, C., Goff, S., Gilboa, E., Paskind, M., Mitra, S.W., and
Baltimore, D. (1980) Proc. Natl. Acad. Sci. USA 77, 3932-3936; (5)
Rigby, P.W.J., Dieckmann, M., Rhodes, C., and Berg, P. (1977) J. Mol.
Biol. 113, 237-251.

SYNTHESIS, CLONING AND EXPRESSION OF GENES CODING FOR HUMAN EPIDERMAL GROWTH FACTOR AND RAT TYPE I TRANSFORMING GROWTH FACTOR IN E.COLI

Allen Banks*, Margery Nicolson+, David Hare*
*Amgen Development Inc., Boulder CO 80301
+Amgen Inc., Thousand Oaks, CA 91320

Human epidermal growth factor (hEGF) is a 53 amino acid polypeptide with the ability to stimulate mitosis of mammalian cells in vitro (1). All mammalian cells appear to have receptors for EGF (2), indicating that the in vivo requirements for EGF are probably extensive. Type I rat transforming growth factor (rTGF) is a 50 amino acid polypeptide described by Todaro and co-workers (3). Sequence alignment indicates distinct structural similarities between hEGF and rTGF especially in the positioning of cysteine residues. Both rTGF and hEGF compete equivalently with ^{125}I-labeled mouse EGF for EGF receptors on human A431 cells. Evidence using cells transformed with an oncogene suggests that EGF secretion is supplanted by TGF secretion in the transformed phenotype (4). Because the two molecules appear to be functionally equivalent we have undertaken further biological characterization of these peptides. In order to obtain material for these studies we have expressed genes for hEGF and rTGF in E.coli.

The synthetic structural genes for both hEGF and rTGF were designed as BamHI-SalI fragments. Since small polypeptides expressed in E.coli are often degraded, we allowed ourselves the option of either expressing the proteins directly or fused to a larger, more stable protein. Consequently, we designed a synthetic linker which allowed placement of the structural genes either behind a trp promoter, a synthetic T5/lac promoter, or fused to β-galactosidase. This linker, when cloned 5' to the structural gene in the appropriate vector system, allowed expression of the proteins fused to β-galactosidase, with 8 extra amino acids fused onto the amino terminus using the trp promoter, or with one extra amino acid on the amino terminus using the T5/lac promoter. The synthetic genes were designed using codons most frequently used in highly expressed proteins of E.coli. A unique SphI restriction site was introduced in the coding sequence at a point common to both genes which would allow interchange of gene modules to produce two different hEGF/rTGF hybrid proteins.

The genes were subdivided into oligomers for chemical synthesis. These oligomers, approximately 25 nucleotides in length, were synthesized using phosphoramidate chemistry in the standard 4 step procedure which uses both aqueous I_2 oxidation and acetic anhydride capping (5). Purified oligomers were then phosphorylated and ligated to give the final synthetic gene products, 175 bp for hEGF and 166 bp for rTGF.

The completed genes were cloned into M13 for sequencing and subsequently transferred into E.coli direct expression vectors. Both the hEGF and rTGF produced by these recombinant DNA methods are fully active in the EGF radioreceptor assay using human epidermoid carcinoma A431 cells, in the ^{3}H-thymidine uptake assay using human foreskin fibroblasts and in the soft agar colony forming assay using NRK cells (3). In addition, the hEGF is active in causing premature eyelid opening in neonatal mice (1).

hEGF/rTGF hybrids have been constructed and expressed in E.coli at levels similar to those of the natural proteins in E.coli. We anticipate that these hybrids will have novel biological properties which are reflective of their composite structural features. Comparison of these biological properties with those of the natural proteins may help identify those portions of the natural proteins which are associated with specific biological actions.

References - (1) Hollenberg, M.D. (1979) Vitamins and Hormones, Vol. 37, 69-111; (2) Adamson, E.D. and Rees, A.R. (1981) Molecular and Cellular Biochemistry 34, 129-152; (3) Marquardt, H., Hunkapiller, M.W., Hood, L.E., Twardzik, D.R., DeLarco, J.E., Stephenson, J.R. and Todaro, G.J. (1983) Proc Nat'l Acad Sci 80, 4684-4688 and: G. Todaro (1983) Eleventh Cold Spring Harbor Conference on Cell Proliferation and Cancer, presented at oncogene session; (4) Massague, J. (1983) Journal Biological Chemistry In Press. and Nakano, H., Yamamoto, F., Neville, C., Evans, D., and Perucho, M. (1983) Eleventh Cold Spring Harbor Conference on Cell Profileration and Cancer Abstracts p. 84; (5) Tanaka, T. and Letsinger, R.L. (1982) Nucleic Acids Research 10, 3249-3260.

Isolation and Characterization of Single Copy Sequences from the Human Chromosome 21 Library

D. J. Baro, S. M. McCutcheon and M. R. Cummings
Department of Biological Sciences and Institute for the
Study of Developmental Disabilities, University of Illinois
Chicago, Illinois.

The chromosome 21 library constructed by Krumlauff, et al (1) was screened for the presence of single copy sequences. A total of 840 plaques were examined by the method of Crampton, et al (2). Ten percent of the plaques showed no hybridization under conditions in which repetitive sequences (>50-100 copies) will hybridize (3). From these 84 plaques, 13 were selected at random for further study. Bulk lysates of clones were prepared according to Blattner, et al (4) and Maniatis et al (5), and phage DNA was purified as described by Yamamoto et al (6).

To determine the origin of the phage insert, each clone was cut with EcoRI, electrophoresed on 0.8% agarose gels and stained with ethidium bromide (Fig 1A). The DNA was then transferred to nitrocellulose (7), and probed with nick-translated λ DNA (Fig. 1B). The results indicate that all phage consist of the λ gtwes arms and an insert of human origin. The average length of the insert is 8.5 kb.

To further substantiate the idea that the inserts represent low copy number DNA, the following experiment was performed. JW102, a plasmid containing a 0.8 kb human cDNA β-globin clone (8) and the 12 putative low copy number phage were denatured and spotted onto nitrocellulose in increasing concentrations (1-25 μg). The dot blots were then hybridized to nick-translated genomic DNA with an average length of 300 nucleotides and a specific activity of 10^8 cpm/μg. By measuring the relative number of counts corrected for insert length, the results are consistent with the idea that most of the clones represent low copy number DNA.

To determine their genomic organizations, purified DNA from the clones was nick-translated and hybridized to Southern blots (7) containing EcoRI digests of genomic DNAs from the following fibroblastic cell lines: human trisomy 21, hamster-human hybrids containing only human chromosome 21, and a hamster cell line. Fig 2 shows the genomic digests probed with clone 21-5, which contains an 8.4 kb putative low copy insert. A single band identical in size to the cloned human insert is seen in the trisomic and hybrid lanes, with no visible hybridization in the hamster lane. The hybridization provides further evidence of the human origin of the insert since no hybridization is seen in the hamster lane. The band in the hybrid lane indicates that the insert is from a sequence on chromosome 21 and not another chromosome. Furthermore, because the hybridizing probe is the same size as the genomic fragment, it appears that no rearrangement of the insert occurred during the cloning process. The length of exposure necessary to visualize the hybridizing bands is consistent with that expected for single copy or low copy number DNA.

When the final screening of the more than 800 clones is completed, we will have isolated a significant fraction of the single copy DNA sequences on chromosome 21. Such sequences have been the primary tools in the detection of polymorphisms, duplications and deletions in population screenings and analysis of disease at the molecular level. We intend to use these clones for the identification of structural genes and the construction of regional chromosome maps.

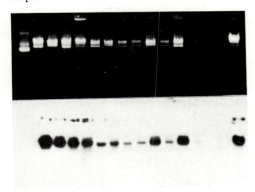

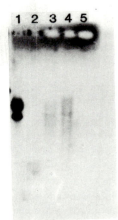

Fig. 1 (a) EtBr stained gel of EcoRI cut DNA, Lane 1: plasmid JW 102 containing β-globin cDNA. Lanes 2-15: 12 putative low copy phage. (b) Southern blot of (a) probed with λ DNA nick-translated to a specific activity of 2×10^6 cpm/μg.

Fig. 2. Southern blot of EcoRI digests of DNA hybridized to clone 21-5, (lane 1) clone 21-5; (lane 3) genomic DNA from a human cell line 47,XY + 21; (lane 4) genomic DNA from hamster-human hybrid cell line; (lane 5) genomic DNA from CHO cell line. The concentration of the probe was .2 μg/ml with a specific activity of 5×10^7. The hybridization was carried out for 18 hrs. The filter was exposed for 6 days at $-70°C$ with an intensifying screen.

REFERENCES. (1). Krumlauff, et al, 1982. Proc Nat Acad Sci 79:2971; (2). Crampton, et al, 1981. Nucl Acid Res 9: 3821; (3). Shen, Maniatis, 1980. Cell 15: 379; (4). Blattner, et al, 1977. Science 196: 161; (5). Maniatis, et al, 1978. Cell 15: 687 (6). Yamamoto, et al, 1970. Virology 40: 734; (7). Southern, 1975. J Mol Biol 98: 503: (8). Wilson, et al, 1978. Nucl Acid Res 5: 563.

Acknowledgements: We wish to thank Carol Jones for the hamster and hamster-human hybrid cell lines, Alan Kinniburgh for the clone JW 102 and Bryan Young for the chromosome 21 library.

STRUCTURE AND EXPRESSION OF MOUSE RENIN GENES

L.J. Beecroft, D.W. Burt, J.J. Mullins and D. Pioli

Dept. of Biochemistry, University of Leicester, Leicester, U.K.

SUMMARY: We report the detailed analysis and comparison of the two renin genes, Ren-1 and Ren-2, from the high producer DBA/2 mouse.

Introduction

Renin is an aspartyl protease that plays a key role in the maintenance of blood pressure in mammals. Although the juxtaglomerula cells of the kidney are the primary source of plasma renin, the enzyme is also synthesised in significant amounts in the submaxillary gland (SMG) of the mouse. The production of SMG renin is particularly interesting because it is under androgen regulation. In addition, inbred strains of mice can be divided into two distinct phenotypes according to the level of SMG renin activity expressed (1).

We have demonstrated the genetic basis of the phenotypic variation, analysed the structure of the genes, and are investigating the control mechanisms and basis of tissue specific expression.

Results

Mullins et al (2) demonstrated the existence of two renin genes in the high producer DBA/2 mouse by the isolation and characterisation of genomic clones. Restriction mapping revealed substantial homology between them, extending over at least 10kb of DNA and stretching well beyond the renin genes. Within the large duplicated region, 3kb of DNA was found, downstream of the Ren-2 gene, which must be the result of an insertion or deletion event.

The exon-intron structure of Ren-1 and Ren-2 was elucidated by heteroduplex analysis and confirmed by sequencing all exon-intron junctions. The 5' upstream region of Ren-1 was sequenced and analysed in detail, using S1-mapping, primer extension and in vitro transcription. Sequencing revealed three possible transcription starts, the most 5' having no TATAA box, and also an AG rich region.

Comparison of DNA sequences of exon VII from the Ren-1 and Ren-2 genes of DBA/2 with SMG mRNA sequences from the same strain showed that the SMG mRNA is transcribed from Ren-2 in DBA/2. The sequence of kidney mRNA from high producer Swiss strain (3) corresponds exactly to that of exon VII of DBA/2 Ren-1 gene, strongly suggesting that kidney renin is transcribed from the Ren-1 gene.

Sequence comparisons of Ren-1 and Ren-2 genes reveal a number of amino acid changes which are reflected in the different thermostabilities of SMG and kidney renins (4). Also, there are no potential glycosylation signals within the entire SMG polypeptide sequence, but there is at least one in the kidney enzyme. Inagami et al (5) have reported that kidney renin is glycosylated, whereas SMG renin is not.

These comparative studies indicate that Ren-1 and Ren-2 are both functional genes expressed in a tissue specific manner.

Discussion

We have confirmed that there are two renin genes in the high producer mouse, with grossly similar exon-intron structure. Upstream of the Ren-1 gene, three possible transcription starts have been identified. Experiments are under way to determine which is the most important. The significance of the 5' AG-rich region and the 3' 3kb insert is under investigation. Finally, we are studying the mechanism and control of tissue specific expression.

Bibliography

1) Wilson C.M., Erdos E.G., Wilson J.D. and Taylor B.A. (1978) Proc. Natl. Acad. Sci. USA, _75_, 5623-5626

2) Mullins J.J., Burt D.W., Windass J.D., McTurk P., George H. and Brammar W.J. (1982) EMBO J. _1_, 1461-66

3) Panthier J.J. and Rougeon F. (1983) EMBO J. _2_, 675-678

4) Wilson C.M. and Taylor B.A. (1982) J. Biol. Chem. _257_, 217-223

5) Inagami T., Murakami K., Yokosawa H., Matoba T., Yokosawa N., Takii Y. and Misono K. (1980) in "Enzymatic release of Vasoactive Peptides" ed. by Gross F. and Vogel H.G., Raven Press, NY, pp 7-30

A NEW RESTRICTION FRAGMENT LENGTH POLYMORPHISM CLOSELY LINKED TO THE HUMAN HYPOXANTHINE-GUANINE PHOSPHORIBOSYLTRANSFERASE (HPRT) LOCUS

Barbara A. Boggs, Robert L. Nussbaum and Richard A. Lewis

Depts. of Medicine and Ophthalmology, Baylor College of Medicine and Howard Hughes Medical Institute, Houston, TX.

Restriction fragment length polymorphisms (RFLPs) can be used to construct a linkage map of the entire human genome or a particular chromosomal region of interest. We have isolated a 1.4 kb Hind III sequence (6A-1) from an X-chromosome sorted library (1) that maps to Xq26-qter using two independent somatic cell hybrids (2).

Southern analysis of 20 female DNAs digested with Taq I reveals a constant 3.5 kb fragment with either a 5.0 kb fragment, a 7.0 kb fragment or both. The allele frequency of the 7.0 kb fragment is 1/3 and of the 5.0 kb fragment is 2/3 with an average heterozygosity of 44%. Inheritance of this polymorphism was studied in two families, one of which is segregating for the Lesch-Nyhan syndrome and the other segregating for both X-linked choroideremia (McK 30310) and the Bam HI RFLP at the HPRT locus (2). The Southern pattern seen in Fig. 1 is from a family with one affected male with Lesch-Nyhan syndrome (GM 2226) in which the mother is heterozygous for the 5.0 and 7.0 kb fragments. The affected boy and his carrier sister inherited the 7.0 kb fragment and the unaffected boy inherited the 5.0 kb fragment from the mother.

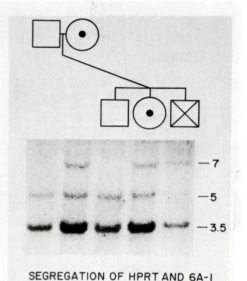

SEGREGATION OF HPRT AND 6A-I

Fig. 1 Segregation of 6A-1 restriction fragment length polymorphsim with Lesch-Nyhan syndrome. Pedigree shows affected male ⊠ and carrier female ⊙. The lane of the Southern blot below each individual contains his Taq 1 digested DNA probed with 6A-1 and shows either the 5 kb or 7 kb allele in addition to a constant 3.5 kb fragment.

Fig. 2 shows an extensive family pedigree with X-linked choroideremia where the alleles for the HPRT and 6A-1 are shown segregating. No recombination events have been observed between HPRT and 6A-1 in 13 informative meioses with the phase known in 10. In Table 1 is shown the maximum likelihood of recombination Θ between the three loci. No measurable linkage is seen between choroideremia and either HPRT or 6A-1.

In summary, a new RFLP has been found closely linked to the HPRT locus which should prove useful for gene mapping in this region of the X-chromosome. Should this close linkage persist after more extensive

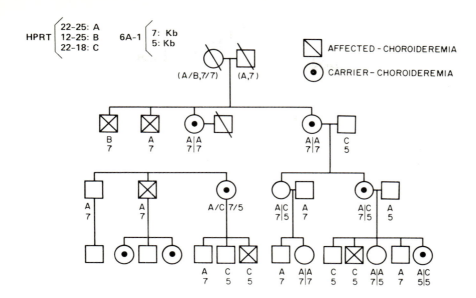

Fig. 2 Segregation of RFLP's for HPRT and 6A-1 in a family also segregating for chorideremia. Phase-known genotypes for HPRT and 6A-1 are shown with the coupled alleles on the same side of a vertical line. Phase-unknown genotypes are shown as pairs of alleles separated by a comma. Inferred genotypes are in parentheses.

analysis, it would prove a useful addition to the Bam HI RFLP for the prenatal diagnosis and carrier detection of the Lesch-Nyhan syndrome.

TABLE 1

LOCI	MAXIMUM LIKELIHOOD RECOMBINATION DIST.	95% CONFIDENCE LIMITS	LOD SCORE
HPRT/6A-1	0 cM	$0<\theta<20$	3.61
HPRT/CHOROIDEREMIA	50 cM	$30<\theta<50$	----
6A-1/CHOROIDEREMIA	50 cM	$25<\theta<50$	----

References. (1) Kunkel, L. M., Tantravahi, U., Eisenhard, M., Latt, S. A. (1982) Nucleic Acids. Res. 10, 1557-1577; (2) Nussbaum, R. L., Crowder, W. E., Nyhan, W. L., Caskey, C. T. (1983) Proc. Natl. Acad. Sci. USA 80, 4035-4039.

Acknowledgements. This research was supported by the Retinitis Pigmentosa Center Grant, Muscular Dystrophy Association (Project 11, Jerry Lewis Neuromuscular Diseases Research Center, Baylor College of Medicine), and the Howard Hughes Medical Institute. We wish to thank L. Kunkel and S. Latt for providing us with the X-chromosome library.

A cDNA CLONE FROM AN ABUNDANT NONRIBOSOMAL 35S RNA IN SALIVARY GLANDS OF CHIRONOMUS TENTANS

John R. Bower and Steven T. Case
Dept. of Biochem., The Univ. of MS Med. Ctr., Jackson, MS 39216

Salivary glands in Chironomus tentans larvae provide a model system whereby tissue-specific gene expression can be studied (1,2). While studying the transport of RNA from the nucleus to the cytoplasm, Egyhazi (3,4) detected a radiolabeled 35S RNA. We became interested in 35S RNA because its relative abundance in salivary glands suggests that it may be a tissue-specific mRNA.

When extracts of total salivary gland RNA are fractionated on 0.75% agarose gels in the presence of methyl mercury and stained with ethidium bromide, several discrete bands can be seen which migrate slower than mouse 28S rRNA (Fig. 1A and 1B). Since these bands were approximatley the size of nuclear precursors to C. tentans rRNA (5), we wanted to determine if they had any sequence homology to cloned rDNA. Thus, individual stained bands were excised from one gel, rerun in parallel lanes on a second gel, blotted onto nitrocellulose and hybridized with various genomic rDNA clones labeled by nick-translation. Autoradiograms (Fig. 1C - 1F) demonstrated that 38S and 30S RNA bands were the predicted (5) rRNA precursors and that 35S RNA was a nonribosomal RNA.

35S RNA was subsequently purified from agarose gels and used as a template for randomly primed synthesis of cDNA. The cDNA was copied into double-stranded DNA and inserted into the Pst I site of pBR322 via homopolymeric tailing. Recombinant plasmids were detected by antibiotic resistance and screened by colony hybridization with radiolabeled 35S RNA. Final identification of clones with inserts complementary to 35S RNA was obtained by hybridizing radioactive recombinant plasmid DNA to Northern blots

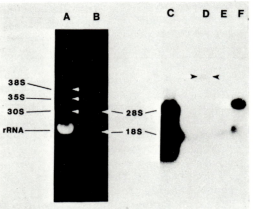

Fig. 1. Demonstration that salivary gland 35S is a nonribosomal RNA. Total salivary gland RNA (A) and total mouse RNA (B) were fractionated on 0.75% agarose gels containing methyl mercury and stained with ethidium bromide. Upon denaturation C. tentans 28S rRNA is converted into two molecules that comigrate with 18S rRNA at a position designated as "rRNA." A Northern blot containing mouse RNA (C) and gel purified fractions of C. tentans 38S RNA (D), 35S RNA (E) and 30S RNA (F) was hybridized with radioactive genomic clones of mouse rDNA. Small arrows indicate bands visible on the original photographs.

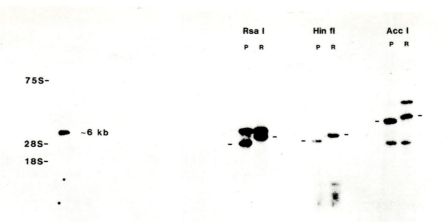

<table>
<tr><td></td><td colspan="2">Rsa I</td><td colspan="2">Hin fI</td><td colspan="2">Acc I</td></tr>
<tr><td></td><td>P</td><td>R</td><td>P</td><td>R</td><td>P</td><td>R</td></tr>
</table>

75S-

~6 kb

28S-

18S-

Fig. 2. Hybridization of radioactive pCt35 to a Northern blot of total salivary gland RNA. The position of salivary gland (75S; ref. 6) and mouse (18S and 28S) RNA markers was determined by hybridization of appropriate cloned probes to blots of parallel lanes.

Fig. 3. Autoradiogram showing selected restriction enzyme cleavage patterns of radiolabeled pBR322 (P) DNA compared to the recombinant (R) pCt35. Small bars indicate bands that represent restriction fragments which contain the Pst I site used to insert the cDNA sequences. Electrophoresis was in a 1.5% agarose gel.

containing total salivary gland RNA. The first clone we are characterizing, pCt35, hybridizes to a single discrete band which comigrates with 35S RNA and is apparently 6 kb in length (Fig. 2).

Restriction enzyme cleavage patterns of pCt35 indicate that the plasmid has a 400 to 500 bp insert within the restriction fragments of pBR322 known to contain the Pst I site (Fig. 3). Experiments currently in progress will determine the sequence of the pCt35 insert, its location within the 6 kb transcript, its relationship to other 35S RNA cDNA clones, and the location of its gene on polytene chromosomes.

References - (1) Case, S.T. and Daneholt, B. (1977) Int. Rev. Biochem. 15, 45; (2) Grossbach, U. (1977) Res. Prob. Cell Diff. 8, 147; (3) Egyhazi, E. (1976) Cell 7, 507; (4) Egyhazi, E. (1978) Chromosoma 65, 137; (5) Ringborg, U. et al. (1970) J. Mol Biol. 51, 327; (6) Case, S.T. and Daneholt, B. (1978) J. Mol. Biol. 124, 223.

Acknowledgment - This project was supported by Biomedical Research Support Grant 5-SO7-RRO5386.

MOLECULAR CLONING AND NUCLEOTIDE SEQUENCE ANALYSIS OF HUMAN c-sis/PLATELET-DERIVED GROWTH FACTOR GENE

Ing-Ming Chiu, Steven R. Tronick, Hisanaga Igarashi, E. Premkumar Reddy, Keith C. Robbins and Stuart A. Aaronson

Laboratory of Cellular and Molecular Biology, Building 37, Room 1A07, National Cancer Institute, Bethesda, Maryland 20205

The genomes of the acute retroviruses contain transforming genes (v-onc genes) that are derived from a set of chromosomal sequences (c-onc genes). V-onc genes are required for the induction and maintenance of transformation by these viruses (1). More than 15 different v-onc genes have been identified thus far. Recently, v-sis, an oncogene originally identified in simian sarcoma virus (2), has been shown to be closely related to the gene coding for human platelet-derived growth factor (PDGF) (3). In order to study the structure and regulation of the human c-sis/PDGF gene, a bacteriophage library of human placenta DNA (4) was screened with a v-sis specific probe. Three overlapping clones which contained segments homologous to v-sis were identified. A total of six v-sis related sequences were found to be distributed over a 15 kbp region. A single 4.2 kb sis-related transcript can be detected in certain human tumor cells (5), while v-sis is only 1.0 kbp in length. In order to precisely determine the structure of the human c-sis locus, we have undertaken nucleotide sequence analysis of the gene as well as construction of cDNA clones of a sis-related transcript expressed in a human glioblastoma cell line. A comparison of the organization of the genomic c-sis locus with its cDNA will be presented.

References.
(1) "Viral Oncogenes," Cold Spring Harbor Symp. Quant. Biol. 44 (1979).
(2) Robbins, K.C., Devare, S.G., Aaronson, S.A., Proc. Natl. Acad. Sci. 78, 2918 (1981).
(3) Doolittle, R.F., Hunkapiller, M.W., Hood, L.E., Devare, S.G., Robbins, K.C., Aaronson, S.A., Antoniades, H.N., Science 221, 275 (1983); Waterfield, M.D. et al., Nature 304, 35 (1983).
(4) Maniatis, T., Hardison, R.C., Lacy, E., Lauer, J., O'Connell, C., Quon, D., Sim, G.K., Efstratiadis, A., Cell 15, 687 (1978).
(5) Eva, A. et al., Nature 295, 116 (1982).

ENHANCED EXPRESSION AND SUPPRESSION OF c-ras^H ONCOGENE DURING
GROWTH AND REGRESSION OF HORMONE-DEPENDENT MAMMARY TUMORS

Y.S. Cho-Chung and F.L. Huang,
National Cancer Institute, N.I.H.,
Bethesda, Maryland 20205

The growth of 7,12-dimethylbenz(α) anthracene (DMBA)-induced
mammary carcinoma in rats is hormone-dependent and the tumors
regress following either hormone-withdrawal (ovariectomy) or
$N^6,0^{2'}$-dibutyryl cyclic adenosine $3'5'$-monophosphate (DBcAMP)
treatment (1).

In this report we present data showing that expression of a cellular oncogene ras, which is homologous to the ras gene of Harvey sarcoma virus (2), is enhanced during growth of hormone-dependent mammary tumors and that suppression of this oncogene precedes tumor
regression.

The 22 K M.W. protein is one of the two prominent in vitro translated proteins of the growing DMBA tumors as compared to the regressing tumors (3). We tested whether the 22 K protein represents the
21,000-dalton transforming gene product (p21) of a cellular ras
(c-ras) oncogene (4). The [^{35}S]methionine-labeled in vitro translation products from growing DMBA tumors were analyzed for p21
expression by immunoprecipitation with a broadly reactive rat monoclonal antibody (5) against Harvey sarcoma virus - encoded p21. A
representative analysis is shown in Fig. 1. A substantial amount of
the 22 K translated protein [lane 2] was specifically immunoprecipitated by the antibody [lane 4] and the immunoprecipitated band co-
migrated with the 22 K translated protein. The antibody also immunoprecipitated two other proteins with M.W. of 30 K and 35 K [lane 4].
The 22 K, 30 K, and 35 K proteins were absent when immunoprecipitations were carried out with the control serum, indicating that
these proteins are probably the specific products of the ras gene.

The 22 K translated protein decreases markedly in the regressing tumors within 6 hr post ovariectomy or DBcAMP treatment
[lane 3 (3)]. The antibody detected no significant amount of
p21 from the translation products of the regressing tumors [lane 5].

We next examined whether the p21 expressed in the growing DMBA
mammary tumors is the product of genes more closely related to
v-ras^H or v-ras^K. The data of the immunoprecipitation using the
monoclonal antibody (5) that reacts only with Harvey-related p21,
but not with Kirsten-related p21 species suggested that the tumor
p21 is the product of the c-ras^H gene. Hybridization studies of
the tumor mRNAs with the cloned p21 DNA probes are underway to further document this result.

Our study presents the first evidence that the in vivo growth
of a primary, hormone-dependent mammary tumor is associated with
an enhanced expression of a cellular oncogene, ras. The results
provide a possible link between the cellular counterparts of the

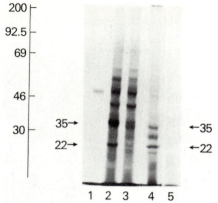

FIG. 1. Immunoprecipitation of p21 from the in vitro translation products of DMBA mammary tumor. Immunoprecipitation of p21 was carried out by the method of Furth et al. (5). (1), no messenger (2) and (3), in vitro translation products from mRNAs of growing and regressing (3 days post-ovariectomy) tumors, respectively; (4) and (5), p21 immunoprecipitates of (2) and (3) respectively.

transforming genes of viruses and hormone-stimulated growth of neoplasms. That hormone-withdrawal (ovariectomy) induces regression of tumors (1) and the decrease in the c-ras gene expression precedes the tumor regression suggests a causal role for this oncogene in the hormone-dependent mammary tumors. Indeed, an amplified expression of the 22 K protein, identified as the p21 in DMBA-tumors, has also been found in the other hormone-dependent mammary tumor, MTW9 (6).

An altered expression of p21 gene might result from either a structural alteration of the ras gene itself or from altered regulation of the gene at a regulatory locus. The activation of the c-ras^H gene in the bladder tumor cell line (EJ or T24) is linked to a single amino acid change (7). Demonstration of the transforming activity of a solid mouse skin carcinoma is also related to the structural alteration of the c-ras^H gene (8). In the mammary carcinoma, however, the p21 expression is enhanced during growth and becomes suppressed during regression, suggesting that these changes in the ras gene expression may represent a regulatory gene event; although we do not know whether the tumor ras gene might also have a structural alteration.

Importantly, both ovariectomy (hormone-withdrawal) and DBcAMP treatment resulted in the suppression of the ras gene in the regressing tumors. It is probable that an antagonistic interaction between estrogen and cAMP, as proposed earlier (9), might be involved in the enhancement and suppression of the ras gene expression in growth/regression of the mammary tumors. It is our hypothesis that an antagonistic interaction between a steroid hormone and cAMP may be exerted at a regulatory locus of the ras gene.

Our results suggest that an enhanced expression of the c-ras^H oncogene may be causally associated with hormone-dependent growth of mammary carcinomas in vivo and cAMP may play a role to suppress this oncogene.

References. (1) Cho-Chung,Y.S.,Gullino,P.M.(1974)Science 183, 87; (2) Ellis,R.W., DeFeo,D.,Maryak,J.M.,Young,H.A.,Shih,T.Y.,Chang,E.H., Lowy,D.R., Scolnick,E.M. (1980) J.Virol.36,408;(3) Huang,F.L., Cho-Chung,Y.S.,(1982)Biochem.Biophy. Res.Commun.107, 411;(4) Shih,T.Y.,Weeks, M.O.,Young,H.A., Scolnick,E.M.,(1979) Virology 96,64;(5) Furth, M.E.,Davis,L.J., Fleurdelys,B., Scolnick,E.M.(1982) J.Virol.43, 294;(6) Huang, F.L.,Cho-Chung,Y.S.,(1983)Cancer Res. 43,2138; (7) Taparowsky,E.,Suard,O.,Fasano K.,Shimizu,M., Goldfarb, M., Wigler,M.(1982) Nature 300,762;(8)Balmain,A., Pragnell,I.B.(1983)Nature 303,72;(9)Cho-Chung,Y.S. (1979)Life Sci.24,1231.

GENETIC RESISTANCE AND SUSCEPTIBILITY IN INSULIN-DEPENDENT
DIABETES ANALYSED BY HLA CLASS II ALLOGENOTOPES (DNA RESTRIC-
TION FRAGMENT POLYMORPHISM)

by   D. COHEN & J. DAUSSET
University Paris VII, Centre Hagen Hopital St. Louis, Paris
France 75010

Distribution of β DC class II restriction fragments
has been compared in 30 unrelated IDD patients and 50
healthy individuals. Various fragments differentiate
between HLA-DR3, HLA-DR4 and HLA-DR2 individuals. In
HLA-DR3 and/or HLA-DR4 individuals in whom susceptibility
is increased, two different fragments were found to be
less frequent in IDD ($p = 2.10^{-2}$ and 3.10^{-2}). HLA-DR2
patients are very rare. A fragment called DC 2.2, found
in 90% of HLA-DR2 healthy individuals, was not observed
in the 7 HLA-DR2 patients ($p = 10^{-4}$).

HLA-DR2 is increased in multiple sclerosis. 24 MS
patients were studied. DC 2.2 was found in 90% of HLA-DR2
patients (and in 90% of controls). These results suggest
that susceptibility and resistance to both MS and IDD
respectively do not depend on the same haplotypes in HLA-
DR2 individuals. Family studies are needed in order to
compare the genotypes of patients and healthy individuals.

Seventy haplotypes from healthy individuals were analysed for the presence or absence of class II β DC restriction fragments. Many correlations were noted with DC-like

specificities (DR1,2,6), others with DR specificities:

Hind III 6.9 kb with DC1-like (r = 0.85, p < 10^{-7})

Hind III 12.6 kb with DR3   (r = 1.00, p < 10^{-7})

Hind III 13.8 kb with DR7   (r = 0.91, p < 10^{-7})

Hind III 3.6 kb with DR5   (r = 0.91, p < 10^{-7})

EcoRV   "h"   with DC1-like (r = 0.68, p < 10^{-7})

EcoRV   "b"   with DR7   (r = 0.93, p < 10^{-7})

The most striking correlation was observed with DR7. Each of the three enzymes studied determined at least one fragment, found only in DR7 haplotypes. These fragments, detected by a β DC probe, gave a strong signal which remained under stringent conditions of washing. These results suggest that DR7 haplotypes carry at least one specific β DC allele. We cannot eliminate the fact that the DR7 specificity is encoded by a DC-like allele which maps either the DC or the DR region. This latter possibility could be the result of a gene conversion mechanism.

This powerful new tool permits a finer analysis to be made of the polymorphism which, according to our preliminary data, is very promising.

CHARACTERIZATION OF AN UNUSUAL ALU-RELATED FAMILY IN THE PROSIMIAN GALACO CRASSICAUDATUS

Gary R. Daniels and Prescott L. Deininger
Dept. of Biochemistry, LSU Medical Center, 1901 Perdido St., New Orleans, LA 70112, USA

A search for Alu family members present in the genomic DNA of Galago crassicaudatus revealed that there are two major types of Alu sequence in this lower primate (1,2). As shown in Figure 1, the Type I consensus sequence for galago is structurally similar to the human Alu family sequence which was described by Deininger et al. (3). Both the human and prosimian Type I Alu family consensus sequences represent an evolutionary head-to-tail tandem dimer of two 130 bp monomers. The right half of each dimer also contains a 30 bp segment which is not present in the left-half sequence.

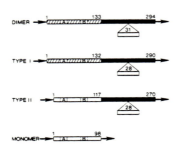

Figure 1. Structural organization of Alu families in primates. The consensus sequences for the human Alu family dimer and the galago Type I, Type II, and monomer repeats are shown schematically to demonstrate regions of homology. The crosshatched areas are clearly related to the solid regions in the diagram and thus represent a dimerization of this sequence. The A and B boxes indicate the positions of a split RNA polymerase III promoter and the arrows represent direct repeats which flank Alu family sequences.

In contrast to the dimeric structure of the Type I sequence in galago, the Type II Alu family is composed of two unrelated sequences. The right-half sequence of the Type II repeat displays strong homology to the right-half sequences of the human and galago Type I Alu families (Fig. 1). The left-half sequence, however, shows only limited homology to these sequences. A comparison of homologous sequences in the left halves of these Alu family members revealed that they are centered in regions which function as RNA polymerase III promoters and are depicted as box A and B (Fig. 1). Since the Type II Alu family is more highly conserved when comparing the base sequence of individual members than is the Type I, it may have been formed on a more recent revolutionary time scale than was the Type I dimeric sequence (2). The fact that a Type II left-half sequence probe does not hybridize to genomic DNA from other primates or mouse also suggests that this sequence was formed recently in galago.

Based on these results we propose that the structure for the prosimian Type II Alu family may have resulted from the independent integration of a new RNA polymerase III promoter adjacent to the right half of a dimeric Type I Alu family (2). In support of this idea for Type II Alu family formation, we have isolated a monomeric sequence from galago which exists as an independent repeated DNA family and corresponds to only the left half of the Type II sequence (Fig. 1).

In Fig. 2 we present the nucleotide sequence of three monomer clones, GAL 2, GAL 32, and GAL 39, which were isolated from G crassicaudatus genomic DNA and inserted into M13mp8 for DNA sequence with the galago Type II consensus sequence to indicate the relative position of transitions, transversions, and deletions within this sub-family. Overall these modifications would change the consensus sequence by 28% of its base sequence in the first 90 positions. The last 12 bases of the monomeric sequences are oligo-dA rich and precisely fit the dA-rich sequences found at the 3' end of all Alu family members. For this reason we position them 170 bp away from the left-half sequence to show their best homology to the Type II consensus sequence. The direct repeat AGTAAATGAT which flanks clone GAL 39 indicates that this monomeric sequence may be a mobile genetic element. Direct repeats flank most Alu family members indicating that they were inserted into a position in the genome which was duplicated as part of the insertion process.

```
                    10        20         30        40        50
CONS:    .........  TGCCTTGGCG  CC T GTAGCAC  AGTGGTTA G G  GCGCCAGCCA  CATACACCTA
                                   C                     T

GAL  2   GAAAAGAAAA  G..XXCA.T.  ..T..G..T.  ..A..AGTA.  ....TG...X  ....T...GG
GAL 32   GACTTTTAAA  A..XXC..T.  ..T..G..T.  .AA..AGTA.  .........C  ....TG..G.
GAL 39   AGTAAATGAT  G..XX...T.  ..T..X..T.  .AA..AGTA.  .T.......C  ....TG..AG


                    60        70         80        90 N        270        280
                                                          170
CONS:    GGGTGGTGGG  TTCGAACCCA  GCCGGGCCA  GCCAAACAAC A AAAAAAAAAA  AAAAAA....
Gal  2   AX........  ...A......  ....T.....  AXX....TG. C ..........  ..C...TATA
Gal 32   A.........  ...A......  ....T.....  AXX..C.TG. C ..........  ......AAAA
GAL 39   A.........  ...A...A..  ....C.A...  AXX....TG. A ...G......  ...GT.AATG
```

Figure 2. Nucleotide sequence of monomeric repeats isolated from G. crassicaudatus genomic DNA. The sequence of monomer clones, GAL 2, GAL 32, and GAL 39, are aligned with the Type II consensus sequence (CONS) to show regions of homology. Dotted lines in the consensus sequence indicate the position of DNA flanking the monomeric repeats. Dotted positions within a monomeric sequence indicate agreement with the Type II consensus sequence and for positions that do not agree the appropriate nucleotide is given. Deletions relative to the consensus sequence are marked with an X and inserts are placed above the line representing additions to be made at that point in the sequence. The numbering begins at the left end of the repeated DNA sequence and continues to position 90. At position 91 the Type II consensus has a region of 170 nucleotides which are not homologous to the monomeric sequences. This region has been depicted as an insert in the Type II consensus sequence to clarify the diagram.

The isolation of monomeric sequences which correspond to the left half of a newly characterized Alu family, designated Type II in galago, lends support to the proposal that the monomer may have inserted itself next to the right half of a Type I dimer to form a new type of Alu family sequence. If the Type II sequence had some selective advantage over the monomer or Type I sequence we would expect to find it in higher copy number than the other two types of sequence. This seems to be true for galago as we have found the Type II to Type I Alu family ratio to be 3:1 and the Type II to monomer ratio to be 6:1. Furthermore, all three types of sequences are expressed in vitro using a RNA polymerase III transcription system. However, the Type II Alu family sequence and monomeric sequences have the most efficient promoters. This implies that the selective advantage that Type II Alu sequences have over Type I sequences is a more efficient RNA polymerase III promoter and that the advantage that Type II has over monomer is an Alu family member right-half sequence of unknown function. The isolation of monomeric left-half sequences along with the Type II Alu family member in galago gives us two new sequences to help elucidate the function of Alu family members in mammalian species.

References: (1) Daniels, G.R., Fox, G.M., Loewensteiner, D., Schmidt, C.W., and Deininger, P.L. (1983) Nucleic Acids Res. in press. (2) Daniels, G.R. and Deininger, P.L. (1983) Nucleic Acids Res. in press. (3) Deininger, P.L., Jolly, D.J., Rubin, C.M., Friedmann, T., and Schmid, C.W. (1981) J. Mol. Biol. 151, 17-33.
Acknowledgement: This work was supported by a grant from the National Institutes of Health, GM 29848.

THE ISOLATION OF GENE SEQUENCES ON HUMAN CHROMOSOME 21

Jeffrey N. Davidson, Albert A. Davidson, and Lee A. Niswander
Eleanor Roosevelt Institute for Cancer Research and Dept. of Medicine,
University of Colorado Health Sciences Center, Denver, CO 80262

It is unclear why trisomy of 21q22 leads to Down syndrome. With the
isolation of genes located in this region, an understanding of this
genetic disease may evolve. For this reason we are searching a λ/21
library (1) for gene sequences located on chromosome 21.

Screening for recombinants without middle repetitive sequences. About
10,000 phage were mixed with E. coli LE392 and spread on agar plates.
Phage plaques were transferred to nitrocellulose (2) and hybridized to
labeled total human DNA (3). Under these conditions, phage containing
middle repetitive sequences yield a spot upon exposure to X-ray film.
The 2000 phage which failed to hybridize the probe were transferred to
new plates and rescreened twice more. The resulting set of 127 phage
appears to contain no human middle repetitive sequences.

Screening for recombinants with gene sequences. RNA purified (4) from
human tissue culture cells was reverse transcribed in the presence of
labeled dCTP and oligo dT (5). When filter transfers of phage were
probed with the labeled cDNA, twelve phage showed significant hybridization. DNA prepared from each phage was cut with EcoR1 and the fragments separated on agarose gel. Insert DNA was observed in each case.

Test for location of cloned genes on chromosome 21. DNA from human (HT
1080 fibrosarcoma), rodent (CHO-K1 or mouse A9), rodent/human hybrids

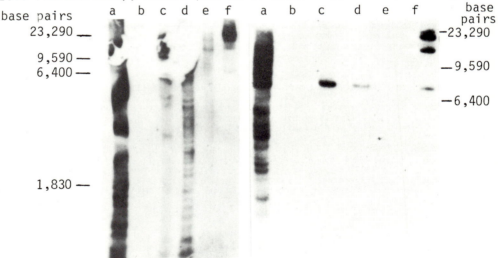

Fig.1. EcoR1 digested cellular DNA probed with 5×10^5 cpm/ml labeled CP5 DNA. 10 ug of each DNA applied per lane: (a)HT; (b)K1; (c)2FUr1; (d)WAV; (e)A9; (f)10 pg of CP5.

Fig. 2. EcoR1 digested cellular DNA probed with 5×10^5 cpm/ml labeled CP113 DNA. 10 ug of each DNA applied per lane: (a)HT; (b)K1; (c)2FUr1; (d)WAV; (e)A9; (f)10 pg of CP113.

with only a human chromosome 21 (153E9a or WAV), or hamster/human hybrid with only the long arm of human chromosome 21 (2FUr1) were cut with EcoR1 and the fragments separated by agarose gel electrophoresis and transferred to nitrocellulose (6). Filters were hybridized with labeled phage DNA. Phage CP5 (Fig. 1) gave a multiple band pattern in human and a similar pattern in somatic cell hybrids with a complete chromosome 21. Because few bands were seen in a hybrid missing the short arm, this phage must contain a low repeat sequence mainly found on the short arm of chromosome 21 and on other human chromosomes. Phage CP113 (Fig. 2) clearly hybridizes to a single band (similar in size to the phage insert), correlating with the long arm of chromosome 21. However, this phage contains a low repeat element present on other human chromosomes. Phage CP2 (Fig. 3) gives an unique band even when hybridized to EcoR1 digested total human DNA. Its human insert clearly maps only to the long arm of human chromosome 21 as do the inserts from phage CP8 and CP21G1.

Expression of a cloned gene in various human cell lines. RNA dot blots (Fig. 4) were hybridized to labeled DNA from CP8. Although it is expressed in all cells tested, the degree varies with cell-type (neuroblastoma > T-cells > B-cells > fibroblast and myeloid).

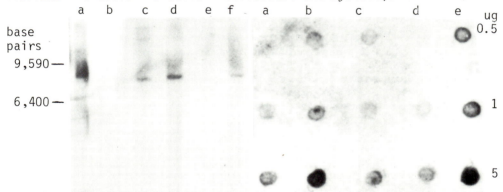

Fig. 3. EcoR1 digested cellular DNA probed with 5×10^5 cpm/ml labeled CP2 DNA. 10 ug of each DNA applied per lane: (a)HT; (b)K1; (c)153E9a; (d)2FUr1; (e)A9; (f)WAV.

Fig. 4. Total RNA from various cells probed with 5×10^5 cpm/ml labeled CP8 DNA. Varying concentrations of each cellular RNA was spotted on nitrocellulose: (a)HT; (b)HSB-2, T-cell; (c)NG37, B-cell; (d)K562, myeloblast; (e)BE2, neuroblastoma.

References: (1) Krumlauf, R., Jeanpierre, M., and Young, B.D. (1982) Proc. Natl. Acad. Sci. 79, 2971-2975; (2) Benton, W.D. and Davis, R.W. (1977) Science 196, 180-182; (3) Wahl, G.M., Stern, M. and Stark, G.R. (1979) Proc. Natl. Acad. Sci. 76, 3683-3687; (4) Chirgwin, J.M., Prazybyla, A.E., MacDonald, R.J., and Rutter, W.J. (1979) Biochemistry 18,5294-5299; (5) St. John, T.P. and Davis, R.W. (1979) Cell 16,443-452; (6) Southern, E.M. (1975) J. Mol. Biol. 98, 503-517.
Acknowledgements: Supported by grant 5-276 from the March of Dimes. ERICR publication #476.

HUMAN FACTOR IX CLONES ISOLATED WITH SYNTHETIC
OLIGOMER PROBES

L.M. Davis, R.A. McGraw, D.W. Stafford
Dept. of Biology, University of North Carolina, Chapel Hill, N.C.

Recombinant clones containing human Factor IX coding sequences
have been selected from both cDNA banks and genomic libraries using
a series of synthetic oligonucleotides as probes. The four oligomers
were synthesized manually by the solid phase phosphotriester method
(1). Their lengths and sequences were chosen according to a
published report of a Factor IX cDNA (2) in order to hybridize
specifically to the four regions of the gene shown in Figure 1.

A human liver cDNA bank was constructed in the phage vector
lambda gt-10, and, upon hybridization with the 18-mer, a partial
Factor IX cDNA of 200 bp was found. This 200 bp cDNA was in turn
used to probe a second cDNA bank (kindly provided by S. Orkin),
from which two Factor IX cDNAs were found, of approximately
550 and 3000 bases in length. The 550 base insert corresponds to the
3' most coding sequences, including the stop codon, while the 3 kb
insert contains an initiation codon at its 5' terminus and a poly A
tract at its 3' terminus. The primary sequence of this cDNA
(as well as all sequences mentioned in this report) has been
partially determined by the Sanger di-deoxy method. The templates
are either ds linear DNA or ss M13 phage DNA subclones, and the
primers are either the oligomers referred to above or Biolabs'
universal pentadecamer. In either case, the primers are end-labelled.

Two genomic libraries representing the DNA from two individuals
carrying the Factor IX Alabama variant of Hemophilia B (3) have
been constructed by ligating partial Eco RI digests of leukocyte DNA
to the phage vector lambda gt-lambda B(4). Clones containing
Factor IX DNA have been selected by hybridization with either the
oligonucleotides or one of the cDNA clones. The first genomic
clone was selected initially by hybridization to the 18-mer.
This clone contains four Eco RI fragments of 10, 7.5, 5.5, and
1.5 kb. The latter two fragments hybridize to the 3 kb cDNA.
Approximately half the sequence of the 5.5 kb fragment has been
determined by first subcloning a Sau 3A digest of the purified
fragment into the Bam HI site of the mp8 derivative of M13.
Sequencing templates were prepared from isolated plaques
according to Zinder (5); the plaques were selected either
at random or by the 3 kb cDNA. Preliminary results are shown
in Fig. 1.

Approximately half the gene (the 3' half) is found in a stretch
of 650 bases of uninterrupted coding sequence. The 5' terminus
of this exon contains a consensus splice sequence, but the junction
of divergence between this genomic clone and the published
3' non-translated cDNA(6), 100 bases beyond the stop codon,
is not a consensus splice sequence. This divergent sequence
continues for at least 60 bases. Six bases beyond the point

of divergence (in the cDNA) the genomic sequence can be realigned
for an additional 100 bases. There are 8 base pair differences
between the genomic DNA and the cDNA in these 200 bases of
3' nontranslated sequence. The nature of the insertion
is being investigated by further sequence analysis and by
Southern blots of genomic DNAs with selected probes. Other
work in progress includes an analysis of the sequence of the 1.5 kb
Eco RI fragment found in this clone, as well as a characterization of
other genomic clones selected by the 3 kb cDNA probe.

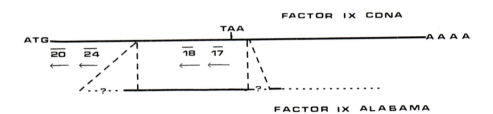

Fig. 1 Normal Factor IX cDNA and partial Factor IX Alabama
Genomic DNA.
The top solid line represents the 3 kb cDNA upon linearization by
Pst I digestion from the vector pTK218. The positions of the four
oligomers are indicated by the solid bars, and their lengths in
base pairs by the numbers below the bars. The direction and extent
of DNA sequence obtained by priming ds linear DNA with each of the
oligomers is represented schematically by the arrows.
      The lower solid line represents the portion of the Factor IX
Alabama clone which is transcribed and has been sequenced. The
dashed lines indicate the positions at which the genomic sequence
diverges from the cDNA sequence. The question marks indicate
uncertainty in the length of these insertion sequences. The dotted
lines indicate sequences which have been cloned but not analyzed.
Not shown are approximately 2000 bases of sequence which have
been determined but are not found in the cDNA.

      References - (1) R.A. McGraw, manuscript in preparation;
(2)K. Kurachi and E.W. Davie (1982) Proc. Natl. Acad. Sci.
79:6461-6464; (3)H.R. Roberts, M.J. Griffith, K.M. Braunstein, and
R.L. Lundblad (1981),in Hemophilia and Hemostasis, pgs. 85-102;
(4)M. Thomas, J.R. Cameron, and R.W. Davis, (1974), Proc.
Natl. Acad. Sci. 71:4579-4583; (5)N.D. Zinder and J.D. Boeke
(1982), Gene 10:1-10; (6)M. Jaye, H. de la Salle, F. Schamber,
A. Balland, V. Kohli, A. Findelli, P. Tolstoshev, and J. Lecocq,
(1983), Nucleic Acids Research 11:2325.

GENE TRANSFER AND AMPLIFICATION OF THE HUMAN GENE(S) ASSOCIATED WITH OROTICACIDURIA

Davis, R.E., J. Bleskan and D. Patterson
Eleanor Roosevelt Institute for Cancer Research, Denver, CO
University of Colorado Health Sciences Center, Denver, CO 80262

Oroticaciduria is a relatively rare autosomal recessive disorder associated with reduced levels of one or both of the last two enzymes of UMP (pyrimidine) biosynthesis, orotate phosphoribosyltransferase (OPRTase) and orotidine-5'-phosphate decarboxylase (ODCase)(1). The nature of possible nucleic acid alterations which lead to the enzyme deficiency are not known. In an attempt to begin studying the regulation and expression of the gene(s) associated with oroticaciduria, we initiated gene transfer experiments to isolate an expressible genomic clone and probes for the human OPRTase-ODCase.

Chinese hamster cell ovary mutants deficient in OPRTase-ODCase (2), Urd$^-$C cells, were used as recipients in DNA-mediated gene transfer using pSV2-NEO DNA and total cellular human HT1080 DNA as a co-transferable gene (3,4). Initially, cells exposed to both types of DNA were selected for neomycin resistance. Clones resistant to neomycin G-418 were then replated in media selecting for pyrimidine prototrophy, i.e., growth without uridine and hence complementation of the Urd$^-$C defect. Clones that grew under this selection were named primary transformants for human OPRTase-ODCase if after isozyme analysis these cells contained ODCase of human electrophoretic mobility (5). DNA isolated from five of these primary human transformants was then used in secondary rounds of gene transfer to reduce the total amount of human DNA in the transfected cells. A secondary human transformant for OPRTase-ODCase was isolated from these experiments using only the pyrimidine prototrophy selection procedure (additional pSV2-NEO was transferred into these cells in this experiment, but no neomycin resistance selection was done). To date we have been able to isolate one secondary transformant for human OPRTase-ODCase. This cell contains multiple copies of the neomycin gene, is neomycin resistant, contains human DNA, and expresses ODCase with human electrophoretic mobility.

A significant reduction in the total amount of human DNA present in the transfected cells occurred during the second round of gene transfer. Only a few distinct bands of human DNA were retained in the secondary human transformant for OPRTase-ODCase (Figure 1A). To aid us in making a preliminary identification of this human DNA in the Urd-C cells as human DNA coding for the human OPRTase-ODCase and to aid in cloning this material, we attempted to amplify the human OPRTase-ODCase enzyme activity, and thus the human gene(s), by exposing the secondary transformants to azauridine and selecting for increasing levels of azauridine resistance (6,7). The monophosphate of azauridine is a competitive inhibitor of the ODCase. Cells were isolated resistant to 1 mM azauridine which have 35-fold increased levels of ODCase enzyme activity compared to control cells, secondary transformants not selected for azauridine resistance. Aspartate transcarbamylase activity, an earlier step in the pyrimidine pathway, is not elevated in the azauridine resistant cells.

The azauridine resistant secondary transformant for human OPRTase-ODCase also appears to exhibit gene amplification as demonstrated by Southern blots (Figure 1B). The multiple copies of pSV2-NEO in this cell were apparently not associated with the amplification unit (Figure 1C) since similar amounts of DNA were present in amplified and unamplified cells. Additional experiments suggest that the level of amplification of the human bands is about 15-fold.

We have transferred the human OPRTase-ODCase gene(s) into CHO cells and have succeeded in amplifying the human OPRTase-ODCase gene. We are presently trying to increase the level of amplification in these cells and are attempting to isolate an expressible genomic clone of the human OPRTase-ODCase from the amplified human transformant for OPRTase-ODCase.

References -- (1) Kelley, W.N. (1983) In: Stanbury, J.B., J.B. Wyngaarden, D.S. Frederickson, J.L. Goldstein and M.S. Brown, eds. The Metabolic Basis of Inherited Disease. 5th ed. McGraw-Hill New York, p. 1202; (2) Patterson, D. (1980) Somat.Cell Genet. 6:101; (3) Wigler, M., R. Sweet, G.K. Sim, B. Wold, A. Pellicer, E. Lacy T. Maniatis, S. Silverstein and R. Axel (1979) Cell 16:777; (4) Southern, P.J. and P. Berg (1982) J. Mol.Appl. Genet. 1:327; (5) Patterson, D., C. Jones, H. Morse, P. Rumsby, Y. Miller and R. Davis (1983) Somat. Cell Genet. 9:359; (6) Suttle, P.D. and G.R. Stark (1979) J.Biol. Chem. 254:4602; (7) Suttle, P.D. (1983) J.Biol. Chem. 258:7713.

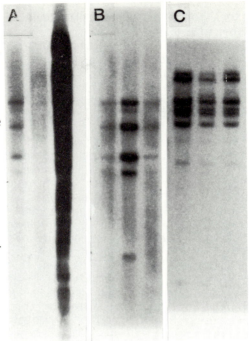

1 2 3   4 5 6   7 8 9

Figure 1. Reduction of human DNA in successive rounds of gene transfer (A) and amplification of human DNA in secondary transformant (B,C). All lanes are complete Eco R1 digests of total cellular DNA. A, 20 ug DNA per lane hybridized with nick-translated total HT1080 cellular DNA. B, 15ug DNA per lane hybridized as in A. C, Same as B except DNA hybridized to nick-translated pSV2-NEO DNA. Lanes 1,4,6,7, and 9 contain secondary transformant DNA. Lanes 5 and 8 contain azauridine resistant secondary transformant DNA. Lane 2 Urd⁻C DNA and Lane 3 primary transformant DNA.

Acknowledgements -- This work was supported in part by grants from NIH (1 F32 7086-1) and the March of Dimes (1-744).

154

ISOLATION AND PRELIMINARY CHARACTERIZATION OF A cDNA CLONE FOR HUMAN THYMIDINE KINASE

Prescott Deininger[1], Harvey Bradshaw[1], and Salvatore Carradona[2]
Dept. of Biochemistry[1], Dept. of Pharmacology[2], L.S.U. Medical Center,
1901 Perdido St., New Orleans, LA 70112, USA.

We have recently published the isolation of a lambda clone containing a functional copy of the human thymidine kinase gene (1). In addition to the full coding sequence, this gene was shown to undergo cell-cycle regulation when introduced into mouse ltk-cells. This demonstrated a remarkable conservation of the cell-cycle regulatory elements for this gene. In order to further characterize this gene and its regulatory elements, we have now cloned a full-length, functional cDNA clone for the human thymidine kinase gene.

Cloning the thymidine kinase cDNA

We chose to isolate the cDNA from a pre-existing cDNA library (2). This library had numeorus advantages for this particular isolation. First of all, it was created from a human cell line that was SV40 transformed. SV40 is known to induce the thymidine kinase gene, increasing the probability of its presence in the library. The library was also prepared in a manner which produces a high proportion of full-length copies and in a vector that puts the cloned cDNA under control of the SV40 early region promoter, allowing expression in eukaryotic cells.

We screened approximately 300,000 cDNA clones using high density plasmid screening techniques (3). Eight colonies hybridized to a fragment isolated from our genomic thymidine kinase clone and five were amplified and plasmid DNA prepared. All five DNA samples were transfected (4) onto mouse ltk-cells, and two of these clones transformed the cells to tk+ phenotype at the rate of about 10 transformants per nanogram. These two clones had a cDNA insert size of about 1550 bases, while the other three clones had somewhat shorter inserts. These results are consistent with the two transformation positive clones carrying essentially full-length cDNA inserts. One of these clones was chosen for the analyses that follow.

DNA sequence analysis of the cDNA clone

We are using a modified shotgun sequencing protocol (5,6) to sequence the cDNA insert using the dideoxy procedure (7). The sequence is not yet complete so that the reading frames cannot be determined unambiguously, but some interesting discoveries have been made. One is that there is no consensus polyadenylation sequence anywhere within 500 bases of the 3' end of the sequence, or anything even closely related to it. There are very few examples of a polyadenylated message without such a consensus sequence.

Studies on tk control

We are interested in the cell-cycle regulation of the thymidine kinase gene. Because of the low level of expression of this gene little is known about which point in the expression or by what mechanism the regulation occurs. We have shown that when ltk-cells are transformed with our genomic lambda clone containing the tk gene, that

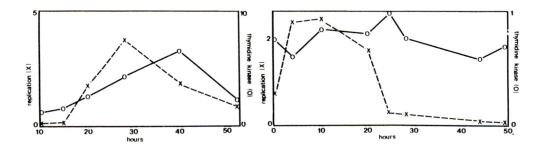

Figure 1. a. Cell synchrony on the cloned thymidine kinase gene.
Mouse ltk- cells transformed to tk+ with the genomic tk clone were
synchronized by serum starvation. After being refed, both DNA
replication and thymidine kinase activities were measured as the
cells moved through S phase. The units for the replication axis
are cpm/100000 of thymidine incorporation and the kinase activity
is in nmol of thymidine phosphorylated/min/mg of protein x 10. b.
In this experiment the mouse ltk- cells were transformed with the
cDNA clone. The replication axis is cpm/10000 and the kinase
activity is the same units as in panel a.

the resulting thymidine kinase activity is cell-cycle regulated (1,
Figure 1a). This experiment was whether the cell-cycle regulation
observed was transcriptional or occurred by an activation of the
thymidine kinase protein. We carried out the same experiment on a
mouse ltk-cell line transformed by our tk cDNA clone. This clone uses
the SV40 transcriptional signals, splice junctions and
polyadenylation, so that none of the original tk transcriptional
signals is needed. If this cDNA is regulated it would strongly suggest
a regulation based only on the protein coding sequences. The results
in Figure 1b demonstrate that this is not the case. There is no
regulation of the cDNA sequences. This suggests that the regulation of
the thymidine kinase acts at the transcriptional level, either through
transcription itself, or some form of processing.
This work was supported by NIH GM29848.

1) H. Bradshaw (1983) Proc. Natl. Acad. Sci. USA 80, 5588.
2) H. Okayama and P. Berg (1983) Mol. and Cell. Biol. 3, 280.
3) D. Hanahan and M. Meselson (1980) Gene 10, 63
4) M. Wigler, A. Pellicer, S. Silverstein, and R. Axel (1978) Cell 14,
   725.
5) P. Deininger (1983) Anal. Biochem. 129, 216.
6) P. Deininger (1983) Anal. Biochem. 135, in press.
7) F. Sanger, A. Coulson, B. Barrell, A. Smith and B. Roe (1980) J.
Mol. Biol. 143, 161.

CHARACTERIZATION OF A MUTATION IN THE PROα2(I)COLLAGEN C-PROPEPTIDE IN A CHILD WITH AN AUTOSOMAL RECESSIVE FORM OF OSTEOGENESIS IMPERFECTA.

L.A.Dickson[*], T.Pihlajaniemi[+], S.Deak[+], F.M.Pope[§], A.Nicholls[§], D.J.Prockop[+] and J.C.Myers[¶], Dpt. Biochem., U.Med.&Dent.N.J.-Rutgers Med. Sch.[+] and Sch. of Ost. Med.[*], Piscataway, NJ, Dpt. Med., U. Penn., Conn.Tis.Res. Inst.[¶], Phila., PA, and Clin.Res.Ctr.[§], Harrow, U.K.

INTRODUCTION: Osteogenesis imperfecta (OI) represents a heterogeneous group of connective tissue disorders (reviews 1,2). Phenotypic characterization of patients includes in most cases varying degrees of bone fragility, osteoporosis, blue sclerae, thin skin, and deafness. Severity ranges from very mild to death in utero. The defects in several affected people have been attributed to alterations in the structure of the major protein in the body, type I collagen, a heterotrimer consisting of two proα1(I) and one proα2(I) chains. The chains are synthesized as precursor molecules which include a central domain of about 1000 a.a. and small N- and C- terminal propeptides that are cleaved after secretion from the cell. We have characterized the defect in a patient having a moderately severe form of OI(3). The type I procollagen secreted by his fibroblasts was found to be a homotrimer consisting of only proα1(I) chains although proα2(I) chains were localized intracellularly(4). Nuclease-S1 mapping revealed a homozygous mutation in the C-propeptide of the patient's proα2(I) gene. The third cousin parents show the same defect in one of their alleles and as a result synthesize both the abnormal α1(I) trimers and normal type 1 collagen.

RESULTS: The procollagen synthesized by the fibroblasts of the patient and his parents were analyzed by DEAE chromatography and SDS-PAGE. In the child, no protein was found eluting from the column in the position of type I collagen. However, the protein eluting in the normal position of type III collagen consisted not only of type III, but contained the homotrimer of proα1(I) chains. The DEAE profile of the parents' protein showed both normal type I collagen and α1(I) trimers, again co-eluting with type III. Determination of the ratio of proα1(I)/proα2(I) mRNA in the child and his parents was within the range found in controls, and Northern blot hybridization showed a proα2(I) mRNA pattern indistinguishable from normal fibroblasts. Since assembly of the different procollagen chains has been reported to initiate in the C-propeptide(5,6), analysis of this portion of the gene for small mutations was investigated by nuclease-S1 mapping. A single stranded, 687n, DNA probe (Fig.1) coding for 80% of the C-propeptide(7) was 3' end-labeled and hybridized to mRNA isolated from the patient's and his parents' fibroblasts. Nuclease-S1 digestion revealed a 480n end-labeled fragment which appeared in a 1:1 ratio with the fully protected DNA in the hybridization with the parent's mRNA, but was the prominent band in the experiment with the child's mRNA (Fig.2). When the ionic strength of the DNA/RNA hybridization was lowered and the pH of the S1 reaction decreased, the remaining 687n band protected by the patient's mRNA gradually disappeared leaving only the 480n band (Fig.2). These results indicated that the region of mismatch must be very small and similar experiments carried out using the same DNA probe but labeled at its 5' end verified this hypothesis.

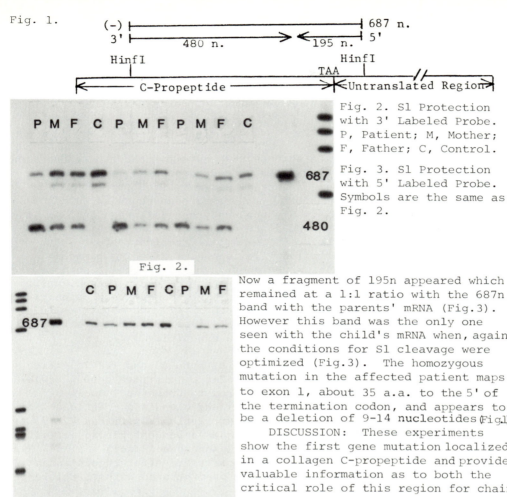

Fig. 1.

Fig. 2.

Fig. 3.

Fig. 2. S1 Protection with 3' Labeled Probe. P, Patient; M, Mother; F, Father; C, Control.

Fig. 3. S1 Protection with 5' Labeled Probe. Symbols are the same as Fig. 2.

Now a fragment of 195n appeared which remained at a 1:1 ratio with the 687n band with the parents' mRNA (Fig.3). However this band was the only one seen with the child's mRNA when, again, the conditions for S1 cleavage were optimized (Fig.3). The homozygous mutation in the affected patient maps to exon 1, about 35 a.a. to the 5' of the termination codon, and appears to be a deletion of 9-14 nucleotides(Fig.1)

DISCUSSION: These experiments show the first gene mutation localized in a collagen C-propeptide and provide valuable information as to both the critical role of this region for chain assembly and the importance of the proα2(I) chain in the normal type I heterotrimer. The heterozygous parents are phenotypically normal even though their fibroblasts secrete both α1(I) homotrimers and normal type I collagen. However, the homozygous defect is manifested phenotypically in the affected child by poor calcification of brittle bones, multiple fractures, osteoporetic limbs, and blue sclera(8). Genomic cloning of the patients DNA is currently in progress to determine which decisive a.a. have been deleted or, alternately, to show whether a frameshift mutation has occurred instigating the use of a different termination codon. REFERENCES: (1)Hollister et al.1982. Adv.Hum.Gen. 12:1.(2)Prockop & Kivirikko, N.Eng.J.Med., in press.(3)Nicholls et al. 1979. Lancet (1), 1193.(4)Deak et al. J.Biol.Chem., in press.(5) Bachinger et al. 1980. Eur.J.Biochem. 106:619.(6)Williams & Prockop 1983. J.Biol.Chem. 258:5915.(7)Myers et al.1983. J.Biol.Chem.258:10135. (8)Pope & Nicholls 1981, in Chem.&Biol. of Mineralized Conn.Tiss.(A. Veis, ed., Elsevier), p.223.

IN VITRO PHOSPHORYLATION AND INACTIVATION OF DNA TOPOISOMERASES BY VIRAL AND CELLULAR TYROSINE SPECIFIC PROTEIN KINASES

Yuk-Ching Tse Dinh[1], Tai Wai Wong[2], and Allan R. Goldberg[2],

[1]Central Research & Development Department, E. I. du Pont de Nemours & Company, Experimental Station, Wilmington, Delaware 19898

[2]The Rockefeller University, New York, New York 10021

DNA topoisomerases are enzymes that catalyze the interconversion of topological isomers of DNA via concerted breaking and rejoining of DNA backbone bonds (1-3). Bacterial and rat liver type I DNA topoisomerases, as well as DNA gyrase have been shown to form a covalent complex with DNA via a phosphotyrosine linkage (4,5). This is postulated to be an intermediate step in the DNA nicking and closing catalytic activity. An essential tyrosine residue in the active site acting as a nucleophile is thus implied. Chemical modification of the tyrosine residues in M. luteus DNA topoisomerase I and DNA gyrase with tetranitromethane leads to enzyme inactivation (6). Here we investigate if DNA topoisomerases can be phosphorylated in vitro by tyrosine specific viral pp60^{src} (7) and normal cellular TPK 75 protein kinase purified from rat liver (8) and the effect of the phosphorylation on the topoisomerase activity.

Phosphorylation of the Topoisomerases by pp60^{src} and TPK 75 – Each reaction mixture (10-25 µl) contained 2-5 µl purified pp60^{src} (0.01 unit in 10 µl, 1 unit is amount required to transfer 1 pmole of phosphate per min. at 30°C into [Val^5] angiotensin II peptide) from RSV-transformed rat fibroblast cells or partially purified TPK 75 from rat liver (both preparations free of cAMP-dependent kinase activity), 10 mM Tris pH 6.8, 3 mM MnCl$_2$, 0.05% 2-mercaptoethanol, 1 µl γ-^{32}P-ATP (3000 Ci/mmol) and 1 µg of DNA topoisomerase. After incubation at 30°C for 30 minutes the proteins were precipitated with trichloro-acetic acid and analyzed by NaDoSO$_4$/polyacrylamide gel electrophoresis. As indicated by the autoradiogram of the gel (Figure 1), E. coli type I DNA topoisomerase (gift of Dr. J. C. Wang), M. luteus DNA gyrase (purchased from BRL), calf thymus type I and type II DNA topoisomerases (gifts of Dr. L. F. Liu) can all be phosphorylated in vitro by the tyrosine specific protein kinases. None of the topoisomerase preparation has endogeneous protein kinase activity. The calf thymus topoisomerases used are partially degraded. The major polypep-

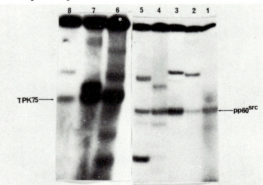

Figure 1 Autoradiogram of NaDoSO$_4$/polyacrylamide gel showing the in vitro phosphorylation of DNA topoisomerases by tyrosine specific protein kinases. (1) pp60^{src} (2) pp60^{src} + E. coli type I DNA topoisomerase (3) pp60^{src} + M. luteus DNA gyrase (4) pp60^{src} + calf thymus type I DNA topoisomerase (5) pp60^{src} + calf thymus type II DNA topoisomerase (6) TPK75 + calf thymus type II DNA topoisomerase (7) TPK75 + calf thymus type I DNA topoisomerase (8) TPK75 + E. coli type I DNA topoisomerase.

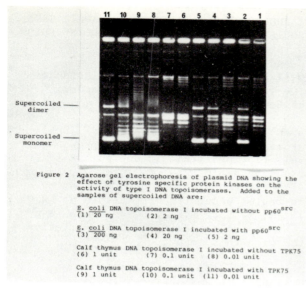

Supercoiled ―――
dimer

Supercoiled ―――
monomer

Figure 2 Agarose gel electrophoresis of plasmid DNA showing the
effect of tyrosine specific protein kinases on the
activity of type I DNA topoisomerases. Added to the
samples of supercoiled DNA are:

E. coli DNA topoisomerase I incubated without pp60src
(1) 20 ng   (2) 2 ng

E. coli DNA topoisomerase I incubated with pp60src
(3) 200 ng   (4) 20 ng   (5) 2 ng

Calf thymus DNA topoisomerase I incubated without TPK75
(6) 1 unit   (7) 0.1 unit   (8) 0.01 unit

Calf thymus DNA topoisomerase I incubated with TPK75
(9) 1 unit   (10) 0.1 unit   (11) 0.01 unit

tides, as shown by coomassie staining, were phosphorylated by the kinases along with the minor ones. For DNA gyrase, subunit A is phosphorylated to a much greater extent than subunit B. The amino acids being phosphorylated were confirmed by thin layer electrophoresis and chromatography of the acid hydrolysates of the eluted topoisomerases to be tyrosine residues.

Reduction in Type I DNA Topoisomerase Activity after Kinase Reaction – E. coli type I DNA topoisomerase was incubated with pp60src as described but with 1 mM ATP for 60 minutes. Diluted aliquots of the reaction mixture were then assayed for topoisomerase activity using supercoiled plasmid DNA as substrate. A similar experiment was performed on calf thymus type I DNA topoisomerase and TPK 75 protein kinase. As shown in Figure 2, the relaxation activity of the topoisomerases examined were reduced approximately ten-fold after incubation with the protein kinases. The protein kinases used do not affect DNA superhelicity on their own. In separate experiments, incubation of these topoisomerases with cAMP dependent protein kinases resulted in no loss of activity.

Although the tyrosine specific protein kinases can modulate in vitro DNA topoisomerase activity, the biological significance of such a reaction is presently unknown. pp60src and TPK 75 are only two of many tyrosine specific protein kinases that can be found in rat tissues. It is not certain if any of them interact in vivo with topoisomerases and thus affect DNA tanscription and replication processes. Nonetheless, it is the first instance in which phosphorylation at tyrosine residues has been shown to have an effect on enzyme activity.

References – (1) Cozzarrelli, N. R. (1980) Science 207, 953–960; (2) Gellert, M. (1981) Ann. Review Biochem. 50, 879–910; (3) Wang, J. C. (1981) The Enzymes 14, 332–344; (4) Tse, Y.-C., Kirkegaard K., and Wang, J. C. (1980) J. Biol. Chem. 255, 5560–5565; (5) Champoux, J. J. (1981) J. Biol. Chem. 256, 4805–4809; (6) Klevan, L. and Tse, Y.-C. (1983) Biochim. Biophy. Acta 745, 175–180; (7) Wong, T. W. and Goldberg, A. R. (1983) J. Biol. Chem. 258, 1022–1025; (8) Wong, T. W. and Goldberg, A. R. (1983) Proc. Natl. Acad. Sci. USA 80, 2529–2533.

ISOLATION OF A HUMAN ADENINE PHOSPHORIBOSYLTRANSFERASE (APRT) GENE, AND IDENTIFICATION OF AN ASSOCIATED RESTRICTION ENZYME POLYMORPHISM.

M.K. Dush,[*] P.J. Stambrook,[*] J.C. Clark,[*]
J. Trill[+] and J.A. Tischfield[+]
[*]Department of Anatomy and Cell Biology, University of Cincinnati
Medical Center, Cincinnati, OH 45267. [+]Department of Anatomy,
Medical College of Georgia, Augusta, GA 30912

Deficiency of adenine phosphoribosyltransferase (APRT) activity is an inherited disorder of purine metabolism which may present as elevated urinary adenine levels (1), urolithiasis due to 2,8 dihydroxyadenine stones (2), and possible renal failure (3). Individuals homozygous for APRT deficiency have been reported by several laboratories (4). To better understand the nature of mutation at the human APRT locus, we have isolated the human gene that encodes APRT activity. We have also identified a restriction enzyme polymorphism associated with this locus.

We have isolated the human APRT gene, which resides on the long arm of chromosome 16, from a lambda human genomic library, using a mouse APRT gene as a probe. Both hamster and mouse APRT genes have previously been cloned; however, they exhibit insufficient homology with their human counterpart to allow unambiguous detection of the human gene in genomic Southern blots. They display sufficient homology for identifying and isolating recombinant clones that contain human APRT DNA from a human genomic library, if screening is performed under non-stringent conditions. To facilitate such non-stringent screening, a BamHl fragment containing most of a rodent APRT coding region was sub-cloned from pBR328 into M13 phage. The resultant recombinant phage DNA was used as a probe to screen a lambda human genomic library at 57°C in 3X SSC and 10X Denhardt's solution. The DNA from one of the positive plaques (clone λHuap12) was competent in a transfection assay, in which the aprt⁻ mouse L cell line, LS24b, was used as a recipient. Starch gel electrophoretic analysis, which localizes APRT activity within the gel, demonstrates that the mouse cell aprt[+] transferents produce APRT of human origin (Figure 1). Hybridization of the mouse APRT

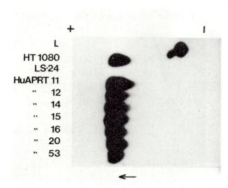

Figure 1. Starch gel electrophoresis of cell lysates that specifically localize APRT activity. Detection of APRT activity is as previously described (5). Lane L defines position of mouse APRT activity. Lane HT1080 defines position of human APRT activity. Lane LS24b depicts lack of APRT activity in a mouse aprt⁻ recipient. Lanes HuAPRT 11, 12, 14, 15, 16, 20 and 53 represent APRT activity of individual aprt⁻ mouse L cell clones transfected with λHuap12. The arrow indicates direction of migration.

gene to restriction fragments of λHuap12 DNA indicated that the
enzymes Eco R1, Hind III, Bgl II, and Sal 1 do not cut within the
gene. Each of these enzymes produces a fragment larger than 13 kb
that hybridizes with the mouse probe. Digestion with Bam H1
produces a 2.1 kb fragment which is the only Bam H1 fragment to
hybridize with the mouse APRT gene. This 2.1 kb Bam H1 fragment has
been subcloned into M13 phage. Genomic Southern blot analysis
indicates that this fragment contains only single copy genomic DNA.
Although it is the only λHuap12 Bam H1 fragment to hybridize with
the mouse gene, it contains insufficient information to transfect
aprt⁻ recipient cells to the Aprt⁺ phenotype.

The 2.1 kb Bam H1 fragment has been used as a probe to search
for restriction enzyme polymorphisms that may be associated with the
human APRT locus. Genomic DNA from 30 individuals was digested with
Bam H1, Pst1 or Taq 1 and subjected to Southern blot analysis. All
individuals produced the expected 2.1 kb Bam H1 fragment. Digestion
with Pst1 consistently produced 2 bands at 0.9 and 1.4 kb. In about
70 percent of DNA samples, digestion with Taq 1 produced 2 bands at
2.2 and 0.5 kb. In the remaining samples, Taq 1 digestion produced
an additional band at 3.0 kb (Figure 2).
Appearance of the additional 3.0 kb band is
consistent with the pattern expected for
individuals heterozygous for the loss of a
Taq 1 restriction site within or close to the
APRT gene. Additional polymorphisms associated
with the human APRT locus are being sought.

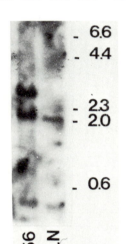

Figure 2. Southern blot analysis of a Taq 1
digest of DNAs of 2 unrelated individuals.
The size markers indicate the position of
Hind III fragments of lambda DNA.

References: 1) Van Acker, K.J., Simmonds, H.A., Potter, C. and
Camerson, J.S. (1977) New Eng. J. Med. 297:127-132 2) Gault, M.H.,
Simmonds, H.A., Snedden, W., Dow, D., Churchill, D.N. and Penney, H.
(1981) New Engl. J. Med. 305:1570-1572 3) Greenwood, M.C., Dillon,
M.J., Simmonds, H.A., Barrat, T.M., Pincott, J.R.L. and Metrewelli,
C. (1982) Eur. J. Pediatr. 138:346-349 4) Simmonds, A.H. and
Van Acker, K.J. in: The metabolic basis of inherited disease. ed.
J.B. Stanbury, J.B. Wyngaarden, D.S. Frederickson, J.L. Goldstein
and M.S. Brown. McGraw-Hill. N.Y. pp. 1144-1183 (1983)
5) Tischfield, J.A., Bernhard, H.P. and Ruddle, F.H. (1973) Anal.
Biochem. 53:545-554.

ISOLATION OF A MOUSE-LIVER ALCOHOL DEHYDROGENASE cDNA

Howard J. EDENBERG and Ke ZHANG

Department of Biochemistry, Indiana University School of Medicine
635 Barnhill Drive, Indianapolis, IN 46223.

Differences between individuals in the rate of alcohol metabolism, physiological responses to alcohol consumption, and susceptibility to alcoholism may in part be genetically based (1). Since alcohol dehydrogenase (ADH) catalyzes the rate limiting step in the oxidative metabolism of ethanol (2), it is reasonable to propose that variation in the structure and expression of the alcohol dehydrogenase genes is one of the genetic factors influencing these differences. To examine this hypothesis in a model system, we have begun a study of the structure and regulation of mouse alcohol dehydrogenase genes. The mouse alcohol dehydrogenase system has many parallels with the human. As in humans, mice have 3 classes of ADHs, and a genetic model for their formation has been proposed (3).

To begin our study, we have isolated a cDNA encoding a portion of an alcohol dehydrogenase from a mouse-liver cDNA library.

METHODS: A cDNA library was obtained from Dr. Kenneth Fong. The cDNAs were made from poly(A)$^+$ RNA extracted from the liver of a DBA/2J mouse, tailed with poly(dC), and inserted into poly(dG)-tailed, PstI-cleaved pBR322. The library was screened using a mixed oligonucleotide probe (4) synthesized by P. L. Biochemicals (see Results). Positive colonies were picked and rescreened. Covalently closed circular plasmid DNA was purified from the clone showing the strongest hybridization signal, pZK6-6. Sequencing was performed by a modification of the method of Wallace et al. (5): the mixed 14-nucleotide probe was annealed to pZK6-6 and used as the primer for dideoxy sequencing (6).

RESULTS: The sequence of the mouse-liver alcohol dehydrogenase is unknown. We therefore designed a mixed oligonucleotide probe based upon the sequence of horse ADH-EE (7) and partial sequences of rat ADH (8). The probe is complementary to the mRNA:

AMINO ACIDS:	334 335 336 337 338 ASP.PHE.MET.ALA.LYS
CODONS:	$5'\text{-GA}^U_C\ \text{UU}^U_C\ \text{AUG GCN AA}^A_G\text{-3'}$
PROBE:	$3'\text{-CT}^A_G\ \text{AA}^A_G\ \text{TAC CGN TT -5'}$

Our sequencing strategy was designed to read a portion of the coding region of pZK6-6. The 105 nucleotides sequenced thus far (Figure 1) encode 35 amino acids that match horse ADH-EE (7) or, at amino acids 298 and 310, rat ADH (8), in the position and direction expected from the primer. This identifies pZK6-6 as an alcohol dehydrogenase cDNA; it is, however, too small to contain the entire gene. Partial restriction mapping and sequencing suggest that it contains sequences encoding approximately 170 amino acids from the carboxy-terminus, along with 120 bp of 3' untranslated sequence.

Figure 1: Partial Sequence of pZK6-6

```
GCC.CAG.AAC.CTC.TCC.ATG.AAC.CCC.ATG.TTG.CTG.CTG.CTG.GGA.CGC.
Ala Gln Asn Leu Ser Met Asn Pro Met Leu Leu Leu Leu Gly Arg
Ser Gln Asn Leu Ser Met Asn Pro Met Leu Leu Leu Ser Gly Arg
Ala     300                 305                   Leu


ACC.TGG.AAG.GGA.GCA.ATA.TTT.GGC.GGG.TTT.AAG.AGT.AAA.GAT.TCT.
Thr Trp Lys Gly Ala Ile Phe Gly Gly Phe Lys Ser Lys Asp Ser
Thr Trp Lys Gly Ala Ile Phe Gly Gly Phe Lys Ser Lys Asp Ser
        315                 320                 325


GTC.CCT.AAA.CTT.GTG.---.---.---.---.---.---.
Val Pro Lys Leu Val      ←-----PRIMER------5'
Val Pro Lys Leu Val Ala Asp Phe Met Ala Lys
        330                 335         338
```

Top line: complement of the sequence. Second line: translation. Third line: Horse ADH-EE (7). Fourth line: rat ADH (8).

DISCUSSION: We have isolated and partially characterized a cloned cDNA encoding part of a mouse-liver alcohol dehydrogenase. We are in the process of screening the mouse-liver library for clones containing the remainder of the gene. This provides a starting point for testing the genetic theory of mouse ADH isozyme formation and regulation, as well as for the isolation of human ADH-cDNAs.

REFERENCES: (1) Tabakoff et al. (1983) Medical and Social Aspects of Alcohol Abuse, Plenum, N.Y. (2) Li (1977) Adv. Enzymol. 46,427. (3) Holmes et al. (1983) in Isozymes: Current Topics in Biol. and Medical Res. (ed. Rattazzi et al.) v.8, 155. (4) Wallace et al. (1981) Nucl. Acids Res. 9,879. (5) Wallace et al. (1981) Gene 16,21. (6) Sanger et al. (1977) Proc. Natl. Acad. Sci. USA 74, 5463. (7) Jornvall (1977) Eur. J. Biochem. 72,443. (8) Branden et al. (1975) The Enzymes (ed. Boyer), v.9,103.

ACKNOWLEDGEMENTS: We thank R. E. Jerome for technical assistance, and Dr. Kenneth Fong for the mouse-liver cDNA library. Supported by the Project Development Program of Indiana University School of Medicine and by the Grace M. Showalter Trust.

Polymorphic Restriction Endonuclease Sites Linked to the HLA-DR α Chain Gene: Localization and Use as Genetic Markers in Control and Insulin-Dependent Diabetes Populations.

Henry A. Erlich and Deborah Stetler, Cetus Corporation, Emeryville, CA 94608

INTRODUCTION. The human major histocompatibility complex (the HLA region), located on the short arm of chromosome 6, encodes a number of different cell surface glycoproteins which mediate a variety of functions. Genetic susceptibility to a variety of diseases shows significant association with specific serologically defined HLA types. Insulin dependent diabetes mellitus (IDDM), one of the most frequent and severe of the diseases in which HLA-linked genes have been implicated, is associated with the HLA-DR types, DR3 and DR4 (1). The genetic heterogeneity of serologically defined DR types has been demonstrated by a variety of techniques. Precisely localized DNA sequence polymorphisms within or linked to HLA-DRα and/or β chain loci offer the possibility of HLA-DR typing at the DNA level.

RESULTS AND DISCUSSION. A cDNA clone for the HLA-DR α chain (pDR α-1) (2) has been used to detect restriction endonuclease site polymorphisms within and closely linked to the HLA-DR α chain gene. Hybridization of BglII-digested human genomic DNA with pDRα-1 has revealed three allelic restriction fragment lengths: 3.8 kb, 4.2 kb, and 4.5 kb. Hybridization of EcoRV-digested human genomic DNA with the same probe has revealed two allelic polymorphic restriction fragment lengths: 9.2 kb and 13.0 kb. Using double digests of genomic DNA from individuals homozygous for each of the allelic variants, the polymorphic restriction sites have been localized precisely with respect to the HLA-DR α gene and are clustered near the 3' end. Comparison of the genomic blot pattern with BglII-PstI and BglII-EcoRI double digests with the published nucleotide sequence for two DRα genomic clones (3,4) reveals that the polymorphic BglII site which defines the 3.8 kb variant is located within an intron 41 nucleotides 5' from the 3' UT exon. The polymorphic BglII site which defines the 4.2 kb variant is located 9 nucleotides 3' of the polyadenylation signal. The localization of the polymorphic BglII and EcoRV sites is shown in Figure 1. These polymorphic restriction sites can be used as precisely defined HLA-DR α genetic markers for the analysis of genetic predisposition to HLA associated diseases like IDDM.

The distribution of the HLA-DR α allelic restriction fragment variants has been determined in control and IDDM populations (Table 1). In addition, the correlation between individual restriction fragments and serologically determined DR specificities has been examined in families by segregation analysis, in homozygous typing cells, and in hemizygous deletion variants. The 3.8 kb BglII fragment appears to be associated with the HLA-DR1 specificity and the 4.2 kb BglII fragment, with the HLA-DR3 and the DR6 specificities, suggesting linkage disequilibrium between these markers and the loci determining the DR specificities, presumably the DRβ genes. The frequency of the 4.2 kb BglII fragment is increased in the IDDM probands relative to the control population. In IDDM family analyses, the 4.2 kb fragment segregated with HLA-DR3 but not with HLA-DR4 chromosomes. This fragment therefore may represent a marker for DR3 but not DR4 associated susceptibility to IDDM.

Table 1. Frequency of HLA-DRα BglII and EcoRV alleles and selected genotypes in control and IDDM populations.

	Control	IDDM Probands
A. Allele	(n=55)	(n=12)
BglII		
3.8 kb	0.164	0.083
4.2 kb	0.164	0.5
4.5 kb	0.673	0.417
EcoRV	(n=53)	(n=12)
9.2 kb	0.377	0.50
13.0 kb	0.623	0.50
B. Genotype	(n=35)	(n=6)
BglII		
4.2/-	0.29	0.83

Allele (1A) frequencies were derived from family analyses, homozygous typing cells (most of which are from consanguineous matings), hemizygous deletion variants and informative individuals. The frequency of individuals containing at least one copy of the 4.2 kb allele are designated (4.2/-).

Fig. 3. Map of polymorphic and nonpolymorphic restriction sites (EcoRI, R; PstI; EcoRV, V; BglII, B) relative to the HLA-DRα gene.

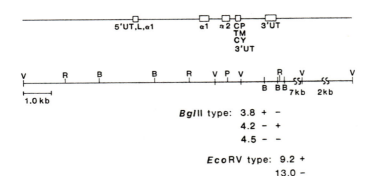

In summary, the experimental approach reported here defines precisely localized genetic markers linked to the HLA-DRα locus which will be useful in the construction of a fine structure map of the HLA region and in the genetic analysis of HLA association with disease.

REFERENCES. (1) Ryder, L.P., Svejgaavd, A. and Dausset (1981) Ann. Rev. Genet. 15, 169; (2) Stetler, D., Das. H., Nunberg, J., Saiki, R., Sheng-Dong, R., Mullis, K.B., Weissman, S.M. and Erlich, H.A. (1982) Proc. Natl. Acad. Sci. USA 78, 5966; (3) Korman, A.J., Auffray, C., Schambock, A. and Strominger, J.L. (1982) Proc. Natl. Acad. Sci. USA 79, 6013; (4) Das, H.K., Lawrance, S.K. and Weissman, S.M. (1983) Proc. Natl. Acad. Sci. USA 80, 3543.

A CELLULAR GENE HOMOLOGOUS TO v-mht IS EXPRESSED IN CHICKEN AND HUMAN CELLS.

C. S. Flordellis, N. C. Kan, M. C. Psallidopoulos, K. P. Samuel, D. K. Watson and T. S. Papas

Laboratory of Molecular Oncology, NCI, Frederick, MD 21701

We have cloned the integrated proviral genome of MH2 virus from MH2 transformed nonproducer cells (1,2). The size of the DNA provirus is 5.2 kb and its complete genetic structure is 5'-Δgag-mht-myc-noncoding cellular sequence-noncoding viral c-region. Thus, the MH2 differs from MC29, CMII and OK10 in its unique mht sequence.

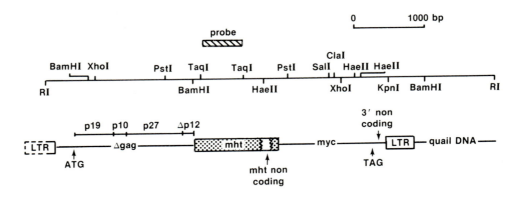

Fig. 1. Genetic map of MH2.

To investigate whether this unique sequence (mht) is part of a cellular gene we have examined whether these sequences are conserved and also if they are transcriptionally active.

Sequences Related to mht are Present in DNA of Normal Chicken and Mammalian Species Including Man. Genomic DNAs from different species were digested with restriction endonucleases which cut outside the v-mht sequence. Southern blot analysis of these digests were carried out utilizing the 800 bp Taq I/Taq I fragment which includes the v-mht coding region (Fig. 1). Distinct DNA bands can be detected in chicken, hamster and human DNA (Fig. 2). However, under our hybridization conditions no homology can be detected in the Drosophila genome. All φ restriction fragments within the species examined are different with the exception of one Pst I fragment which is shared between chicken and hamster and another between chicken and human.

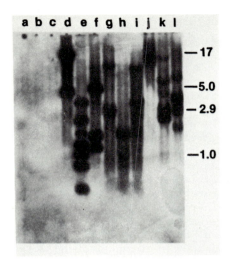

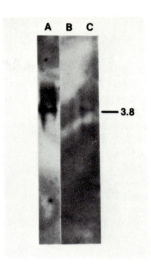

Fig. 2. Detection of mht specific sequences in genomic DNAs. 5 µgs of Drosophila mel., 10 µgs of chicken, and 20 µgs of hamster and human DNAs were digested with Bam HI (lanes a,d,g,j), Pst I (lanes b,e,h,k) and Hind III (lanes c,f,i,l). The fragments were resolved on a 0.8% agarose gel, transferred to nitrocellulose and hybridized to the nick translated probe in a hybridization buffer containing 35% formamide, 5 x SSC, 1X Denhardt's solution and 100 µg/ml denatured salmon DNA. Filters were processed as previously described (3).

Fig. 3. Expression of c-mht in chicken and human cells. Northern blot analysis was carried out utilizing 5 µgs of chicken poly RNA (lane A) and 5 µgs of poly A RNA from human cell lines, Daudi (lane B) and HL-60 (lane C).

c-mht - A Transcriptionally Active Gene. To determine whether c-mht is transcriptionally active, we have looked for presence of mht related sequences in the RNA of normal chicken cells and human cells. Poly A RNA was purified from these cell lines and subjected to Northern blot analysis utilizing mht specific probe. We have identified a common RNA species of 3.8 kb in size (Fig. 3). These results indicate that the MH2 contains only a subset of a larger, transcriptionally active cellular gene.

Refs. (1) Kan et al., 1983, PNAS, in press; (2) Papas et al., Cancer Cell, Cold Spring Harbor, 1983, in press; (3) Thomas, P. 1980, PNAS 77:5201.

LATENCY OF TUMOR INDUCTION BY METHYLCHOLANTHRENE IS H-2 LINKED

Herbert A. Freedman

Dept. Path. SUNY-Downstate Med. Ctr. B'klyn, N.Y. 11203

Influence of the H-2 locus on local tumorigenesis by the chemical carcinogen 3-methylcholanthrene (MCA) was studied in a variety of BALB congenic mouse strains. These strains differ genetically only at the H-2 locus. Thus, differences between these strains in response to tumorigenesis by MCA can most probably be attributed to this sole genetic difference. This holds true for the progeny of crosses between these strains as well.

Local tumors were induced in 21 day-old mice by injection (sc) of 100 ug MCA in 0.1 ml trioctanoin. Animals were observed three times a week for local tumor development. The resultant tumors were transplanted to and maintained in syngeneic recipients. The morphology of each tumor was checked histologically. At least five groups of mice of each genotype were used; each group consisting of 5-10 randomized mice. Although variations within groups of a given genotype were common, these variations were remarkably consistent in groups of the same genotype. Thus variations in the mean latency of tumor induction between groups of mice of the same genotype were slight. The data presented in Table I were calculated from the pooled latencies for all animals of a given genotype, not the pooled means of all groups of a given genotype.

Table I shows that although the mean latency of tumor induction in $H-2^{d/d}$ mice is not significantly different from that of $H-2^{b/b}$ animals, the mean latency of tumor induction in $H-2^{g/g}$ mice is significantly different from both ($p \leq 0.01$). Since the $H-2^g$ haplotype represents a recombination between the D end of $H-2^b$ and the K, I and S regions of $H-2^d$, this result indicates that two genes, one to the left and the other to the right of the crossover point, are involved.

The data presented in Table I also show that homozygosity for the $H-2^k$ haplotype is associated with an extremely short latency of tumor development. Since tumors in these mice are at least 0.5 cm at approximately 35 days after inoculation with MCA, it would seem as though malignant transformation must have occurred soon after exposure to the carcinogen. All of our mice are homozygous for the dominant Ah^b allele (aryl hydrocarbon hydroxylase inducible) and, as such, are all highly susceptible to local tumor induction by MCA. Thus, the effect shown is most probably at the level of tumor progression. In relatively susceptible $H-2^k$ homozygotes, the tumors progress rapidly, in relatively resistant $H-2^d$ and $H-2^b$ homozygotes they progress less rapidly.

In Table I we see that relative susceptibility associated with the $H-2^k$ haplotype is recessive with regard to d, b, and g haplotypes. All $H-2^k$ heterozygotes tested were significantly ($p \leq 0.01$) more resistant than $H-2^k$ homozygotes. However, $H-2^{k/d}$ mice are considerably more resistant than $H-2^{k/g}$ animals ($p \leq 0.01$). Since $H-2^{k/g}$ heterozygotes differ genetically from $H-2^{k/d}$ heterozygotes solely at the D region of the H-2 locus, this trait (resistance) must map to the D end of the H-2 locus. Moreover, $H-2^{k/b}$ mice are not significantly different from $H-2^{k/g}$ mice. Because the only similarity between these

TABLE I. LATENCY OF LOCAL TUMOR INDUCTION BY MCA
IN BALB CONGENIC H-2 HOMOZYGOUS, HETEROZYGOUS AND
RECOMBINANT MICE*

H-2 type	Alleles at Region K I S D				Mean (days)	Std. Dev.
k/k	k	k	k	k	35.3	(10.7)
	k	k	k	k		
d/d	d	d	d	d	91.5	(35.0)
	d	d	d	d		
b/b	b	b	b	b	88.0	(27.5)
	b	b	b	b		
b/d	b	b	b	b	67.8	(16.3)
	d	d	d	d		
g/g	d	d	d	b	62.1	(11.9)
	d	d	d	b		
k/g	k	k	k	k	62.4	(15.4)
	d	d	d	b		
k/b	k	k	k	k	72.1	(13.7)
	b	b	b	b		
k/d	k	k	k	k	121.0	(16.1)
	d	d	d	d		

*All mice are genetically identical except at the
H-2 locus. Genetic background is that of the
BALB/c strain.

genotypes lies in the D region,
the resistance conferred by b and
g haplotypes must also map to the
D region.

Lastly, homozygosity for the
H-2^b haplotype confers the same
degree of relative resistance as
does homozygosity for the H-2^d
haplotype. But, the F$_1$ progeny of
the cross between these two
strains are significantly less resistant than either parental
strain (p<0.01). Thus, although
b/d F$_1$ mice carry both D region
alleles for resistance, these
genes may interfere with each
other (interallelic interactions
and/or masking) preventing full
expression of resistance. If this
were true, then we would expect
differences in these interactions
when b and d alleles are in the
cis (on the same chromosome, g/g)
or trans (on homologous chromosomes, b/d F$_1$) configuration. However, H-2^g/g mice behave in the
same manner as b/d heterozygotes
and are significantly less re-
sistant than H-2^b homozygotes. Because, H-2^g/g and H-2^b/b mice are
genetically identical with respect to the D region of the H-2 locus,
this difference must be attributed to genes located in other regions
of the H-2 complex (K, I, etc.).

In brief, our results indicate that there are at least two
genes, one mapping to the D region, the other mapping either at the
K region, or between the K and D regions of the H-2 complex which
influence relative resistance to tumorigenesis by MCA. These genes,
or their products, interact in such a way as to either interfere with
or enhance resistance. Moreover, b and d alleles appear to influence
each other regardless of whether they are on the same chromosome
(cis), homologous chromosome (trans), or at the same or different
regions of the H-2 locus. The simplest hypothesis is that these genes
are all codominant, and that their products, the H-2 alloantigens,
interact with each other and/or with tumor antigens on the surface
of the transformed cell. These interactions influence recognition of
these tumor cells by the immune system as "self" or "non-self" which
in turn influences tumor progression (relative resistance or latency
of tumor devleopment).

Supported in part by NIH grant CA29052 and ACS grant IM-171.

ISOLATION AND CHARACTERIZATION OF HUMAN METALLOTHIONEIN-I AND II PROCESSED GENES

Lashitew Gedamu and Umesh Varshney

The Univesity Biochemistry Group, The University of Calgary, Calgary, Alberta T2N 1N4

Metallothioneins (MTs) are low molecular weight and cysteine rich polypeptides synthesized in tissues of a wide variety of organisms and in tissue cultures when induced by heavy metals (Zn, Cd, Cu) or glucocorticoids. Two major human MTs (MT-I and MT-II) polypeptides have been isolated and sequenced. In order to study the molecular mechanisms involved in the regulation of the expression of these MTs, clones containing MT gene sequences have been screened from a human library. Two processed MT genes (MT-I and MT-II) have been isolated and sequenced. They are very homologous in their coding and the 3'-untranslated regions but different in their 5'-untranslated regions. They are intronless and have a poly A sequence 3' to AATAAA, the polyadenylation signal. The MT-II processed gene unlike MT-I has no frameshift or nonsense mutations. The former codes for a protein similar to MT-II except for a single amino acid change. Both genes are flanked by homologous direct repeats and the sequences are entirely different indicating that they are located in different environments of the genome. The sequences outside the direct repeats in the MT-II processed gene are entirely different from the sequences that flank the functional MT-II gene and do not contain the concensus regulatory sequences described for most functional eukaryotic genes suggesting that these genes may not be localized in the same chromosome. Based on these observations these processed genes appear to originate by reverse transcription of mRNA to cDNA followed by insertion of the cDNA into the genome via a 5'-overhanging staggered cut in the genome. The MT-II processed gene also contains repetitive elements 5'-flanking the direct repeat. Furthermore, MT-II processed gene shows two restriction fragment length polymorphisms (RFLP's) of 4.5 and 4.8 kb when DNA from a human population of different ethnic groups is digested with EcoRI. This RFLP occurs at a high frequency and is followed in mendelian inheritance. This RFLP is likely due to a restriction site polymorphism. (Supported by AHFMR and MRC)

GENETIC LINKAGE STUDIES OF HUMAN CHROMOSOME 11

D.S.Gerhard[1], K.K.Kidd[2], J.K.Kidd[2], J.Gusella[3], & D.Housman[1]

1. Center for Cancer Research, MIT, Cambridge, MA 02139
2. Dept. of Human Genetics, Yale Univ. School of Medicine, New Haven, Conn. 06150
3. Dept. of Genetics, Mass. General Hospital, Boston, MA 02114

INTRODUCTION The use of somatic cell genetics has led to the localization of a series of genes to the short arm of chromosome 11 which include the β-globin gene cluster (1), insulin (2) and the c-Ha-ras-1 oncogene (3). The identification of restriction fragment length polymorphisms in DNA associated with these genes permits the development of a genetic linkage map of a region of the human chromosome in which these genes are located.

METHODS Lymphoblastoid cell lines have been established from two large multigenerational pedigrees which are appropriate for such linkage studies. DNA isolated from these cell lines has been used to demonstrate genetic linkage between the loci mentioned above and an additional locus defined by hybridization to a DNA probe isolated by R. WHite's lab, pADJ-762 (4). The characteristics of alleles at each locus are given to the right below:

LOCUS	PROBE	ENZYME	ALLELES	SIZE (KBP)
BETA GLOBIN CLUSTER	P×1.3[5]	HINC II	- / +	8.0 / 3.7
	PG,[6]	HIND III	- / +	8.0 / 4.5
	PA,[6]	HIND III	- / +	4.6 / 2.7
	Pψβ1-5[5]	HINC II	-- / -+ / +- / ++	7.6 / 3.0 + 4.6 / 6.0 / 3.0 + 3.0
	PHβ1[1]	BAM HI	- / +	23.0 / 9.0
pADJ-762	pADJ762[4]	BCL I	- / +	11.0 / 4.3
HRAS-1	pEJ6.6[3]	BAM HI	3 / 2 / 1	8.3 / 7.2 / 6.9
INSULIN	PHINS 321[2]	SAC I	HI / MED / LO	7.9 / 6.8 / 6.2

RESULTS Data was obtained from two pedigrees. 90 inidividuals from the first and 49 individuals from the second were typed for each marker. LOD scores were calculated for all pairwise combinations of these four loci using the computer program LIPED (7) and the results are given in the table below:

SUMMARY OF PAIR-WISE RECOMBINATION FREQUENCIES

LOCI	$\hat{\theta}$ (IN%)	TWO-SUPPORT-UNIT CONFIDENCE INTERVAL	LOD SCORE
HRAS-1 - INS	7	(2-18)	6.02
pADJ-762 - INS	15	(6-27)	3.13
pADJ-762 - HRAS-1	3	(0.8-13)	6.11
pADJ-762 - HBBC	3	(0.7-11)	8.39
INS - HBBC	18	(8-34)	1.99
HRAS-1 - HBBC	10	(2-19)	7.47

LOCI	INFORMATIVE MEIOSES (OUT OF 189)
HBBC - pADJ-762	65
HBBC - INSULIN	37
HBBC - HRAS-1	63
pADJ-762 - INSULIN	51
pADJ-762 - HRAS-1	57
INSULIN - HRAS-1	51

Statistical evidence for linkage is a function of the number of informative meioses for each marker pair. The values for each pair of markers is shown adjacent. In order for a pair of markers to be informative in a given meiosis both loci must be heterozygous. Uninformative meioses are thus the consequence of homozygosity of either marker in a given meiosis. Significant homozygosity is to be expected unless the locus has many common alleles of haplotypes.

Strong evidence for linkage is observed among all the markers tested. The most accurately estimated recombination values (i.e., those with the narrowest confidence intervals) are HRAS 1 – pADJ–762 and pADJ–762 – β'-globin gene cluster (HBBC). The obligate cross-overs observed established that pADJ–762 was located between HRAS 1 and HBBC. These obligate crossovers also established that insulin is adjacent to HRAS 1. An obligate crossover between insulin and HRAS 1 was also observed. However this crossover was not informative for the other markers tested. The pairwise linkage data presented in the table are most consistent with the gene order shown adjacent.

Predicted Gene Order

DISCUSSION The loci tested in this study span a region of chromosome 11 less than 20 map units in length. Most of the LOD scores obtained in this study are quite high by conventional criteria. However, the determination of accurate map distances and gene orders will require the assessment of additional sets of multigenerational pedigrees. Other groups have studied linkage among some or all of the markers typed in this study in other pedigrees. Our pairwise data on linkage are consistent with the data of Antonarakis and co-workers (8), Lebo et al. (9), and White and co-workers (10). A point which remains unresolved is the gene order of HRAS 1 and insulin with respect to the other markers tested. Additional examples of cross-over between HRAS 1 and insulin will be necessary to unequivocally establish gene order of these markers. The findings reported here are consistent with the assignment of the four markers tested to a DNA segment of less than 2×10^7 base pairs if we accept the rough approximation that 1 cM is equal to 10^6 base pairs. This estimate is consistent with the assignment of all four markers to the distal third of the short arm of chromosome 11 by techniques of somatic cell genetics and in situ hybridization.

(1) A. Deisseroth et al. (1978) Proc. Natl. Acad. Sci. USA 75, 1456; (2) D. Overbach et al. (1981) Diabetes 30, 267; (3) B. DeMartinville et al. (1983) Science 219, 498; (4) D. Barker et al. (1983) Int'l Human Gene Mapping Workshop VII, Abstracts p. 19; (5) B. Forget, personal communication; (6) D. Tuan et al. (1979) Nucl. Acid Res. 6, 2519; (7) J. Ott (1974) Am. J. Hum. Genet. 26, 588; (8) S. Antonarakis et al. (1983) Proc. Natl. Acad. Sci. USA in press, E. Fearon et al. (1983) Am. J. Hum. Genet. submitted; (9) R. Lebo et al. (1983) ibid 80, 4808; (10) R. White et al. personal communication; (11) R. Lawn et al. (1978) Cell 15, 1157.

ACKNOWLEDGMENT The established cell lines used to obtain DNA for the studies presented here are available from the Mutant Cell Repository, Camden, NJ.

INSERTION OF A SELECTABLE MARKER INTO VARIOUS SITES ON HUMAN CHROMOSOME #11

Tom Glaser and David Housman
Department of Biology, Massachusetts Institute of
Technology, Cambridge, Massachusetts 02139

Cell lines carrying the bacterial Neomycin Phosphotransferase gene (NPT-II) inserted in a human X-11 translocation chromosome were identified by their ability to co-segregate this marker and human Hypoxanthine-Guanine Phosphoribosyl Transferase (HPRT). This step will permit the development of hybrid cell lines in which a particular region of chromosome #11 (1000-5000 kb) has been isolated on a rodent cell background. Hybrids of this type could be created by transferring metaphase chromosomes (fragmented) from a cell line carrying the selectable marker on chromosome #11 to a rodent cell recipient (1); these hybrids could serve as resources for the construction of recombinant DNA libraries containing cloned sequences from this region (2). In particular, we are attempting to obtain sequences from the 11p13 region associated with Wilms' tumor (3). This report describes the construction and initial characterization of cell lines carrying marked X-11 chromosomes.

STABLE INSERTION OF THE NPT-II GENE IN AN X-11 CHROMOSOME

Our strategy for specifically marking a single chromosome is shown in figure 1. We have infected a mouse-human hybrid cell line with an ecotropic retroviral vector conferring resistance to G418, a neomycin analog (4). This hybrid, F2-1, is a MEL cell derivative which carries most of human chromosome #11 as an X-11 translocation involving the long arm of human X (t(11;X)(11pter>11q::Xq>Xqter)) (5). The X-11 chromosome is retained in F2-1 by HAT selection (6). Hybrid cells segregating this chromosome (less than 0.01% per doubling) can be recognized by their resistance to 6-thioguanine.

The vector, zipneoSV(X)1 (7), contains the NPT-II gene under the control of a Moloney sarcoma virus LTR promoter. Infected cells harbor a single integrated copy of this retroviral construct. Infected clones that have the construct inserted in the translocation chromosome can simultaneously lose NPT-II and human HPRT; thioguanine resistant segregants isolated from these clones should be G418 sensitive.

F2-1 cells were infected in suspension (8) using a helper-free viral stock (9), and following pretreatment with tunicamycin to block endogenous gp70 production (10). After 48 hours, infected cells were diluted into RPMI 1640 containing 15% fetal calf serum and 0.5 mg/ml G418, and distributed into 96 well culture dishes. Colonies were isolated 2-3 weeks later. As shown in Table I, 156 G418 resistant clones were recovered from three independent infections of F2-1. After passage in nonselective media, clones were split into 5 ug/ml 6-thioguanine. TG resistant segregants were isolated from 153 of the clones. Of these, 11 had lost the G418 resistant phenotype.

Genomic DNA prepared from seven of the G418 sensitive segregants was analyzed by the Southern procedure (11), and two classes were identified. Segregants in one class contain an apparently intact NPT-II sequence but do not express it phenotypically.

The second class of segregants has lost the NPT-II sequence; parental clones corresponding to these segregants presumably carry the marker on the translocation. Three out of seven clones tested which co-segregate HAT and G418 resistance belong to this class. This frequency is consistent with the relative size of the translocation chromosome, assuming random integration of the retroviral vector. Integration is thought to be essentially random although particular chromosomal regions may act as preferred target sites (12).

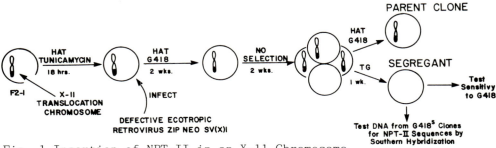

Fig. 1 Insertion of NPT-II in an X-11 Chromosome

CHARACTERIZATION OF MARKED X-11 CHROMOSOMES

We are mapping the integration sites in these clones by: [a] in situ hybridization of metaphase chromosomes (13); [b] cotransfer of G418 resistance and hybridization markers by metaphase chromosome transfer into rodent cells (14). Markers include cloned single copy and defined low order repetitive sequences (15); and [c] fusion rescue of proviral and flanking sequences. Because the retroviral construct used in this experiment contains both SV40 and ColE1 origins of replication, sequences flanking the integration site can be rescued by fusing stably infected clones with COS cells (providing SV40 early functions), and transforming competent E. coli with the resulting imprecisely excised circular molecules (16). These sequences will be used to probe genomic DNA from interspecies hybrids containing human chromosome #11s with defined deletions.

TABLE I. Analysis of 156 Infected F2-1 Clones

	Clones Co-segregating HAT & G418-resistant Phenotypes	Clones Co-segregating HAT-resistant Phenotype & NPT-II Sequence
# Screened	153	7
# Positive	11	3

REFERENCES. (1) McBride et al. (1982) Mol. Cell. Biol. 2:52; (2) Gusella et al. (1980) Proc. Natl. Acad. Sci. USA 77:2829; (3) Riccardi et al. (1978) Pediatrics 61:604; (4) Southern, P. and Berg, P. (1982) J. Molec. Appl. Genet. 1:327; (5) Zavodny, P.J., Roginski, R.S., and Skoultchi, A.I. (1983) in Hemoglobin Switching (Stamatoyanannopoulos, G. and Nienhuis, A.W., eds.) in press; (6) Littlefield, J.W. (1964) Science 145:709; (7) Cepko, C. (1983) pers. comm.; (8) Rosenberg, N. and Baltimore, D. (1976) J. Exp. Med. 143:1453; (9) Mann, R., Mulligan, R.C., and Baltimore, D. (1983) Cell 33:153; (10) Rein et al. (1982) Virology 119:185; (11) Southern, E.M. (1975) J. Mol. Biol. 98:503; (12) Varmus, H. and Swanstrom, R. (1982) in RNA Tumor Viruses (Weiss et al., eds.) p.369; (13) Harper, M.E., Ullrich, A., and Saunders, G.F. (1981) Proc. Natl. Acad. Sci. USA 78:4458; (14) Housman et al. (1983) Banbury Report No. 14: Recombinant DNA Applications to Human Disease (Cold Spring Harbor) p.197 ; (15) Gusella et al. (1982) Proc. Natl. Acad. Sci. USA 79:7804; (16) Conrad, S.E., Liu, C., and Botchan, M.R. (1982) Science 218:1225. We are grateful to Dr. C. Cepko for providing her zipneoSV(X)1 vector and to Dr. A. Skoultchi for providing the F2-1 cells. This work was supported by NIH grants GM-27882 and CA-26717.

DIFFERENTIAL EXPRESSION OF TWO CLUSTERS OF MOUSE HISTONE GENES

Reed A. Graves, Susan E. Wellman and W. F. Marzluff

Department of Chemistry, Florida State University, Tallahassee, Florida, 32306

We have isolated three clusters of mouse histone genes which are expressed in cultured mouse cells and fetal mice. The mRNAs from each of these genes can be distinguished by S1 nuclease mapping. Each gene coding for a particular histone (e.g. histone H3) has a highly conserved coding region. The untranslated regions have not been conserved among different genes coding for the same protein. Thus in an S1 nuclease mapping experiment there are two types of protected DNA fragments; the major fragment represents protection by the majority of the mRNA up to the AUG codon. The minor S1 resistant fragment extends to the end of the mRNA and represents protection by the mRNA derived from the gene. The three clones used are shown in Fig. 1. A schematic of the S1 nuclease assay is shown in Fig. 2.

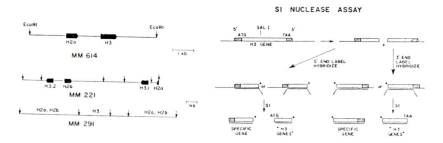

Fig. 1. The location of the histone genes in the three clones is shown. The arrows indicate the Eco R1 sites. The direction of transcription is indicated where it is known.

Fig. 2. The protected DNA fragments after hybridization and S1 nuclease digestion are analyzed by polyacrylamide gel electrophoresis and detected by authoradiography (see Fig. 3).

The proportion of the mRNA derived from each gene can be estimated by comparing the relative intensity of the two protected fragments. The three H3 genes on MM 221 and MM 291 code for a minor portion of the H3 mRNA while the other clone, MM 614, codes for a major H3 mRNA, about 40% of the H3 mRNA. Similar results were obtained with the H2a genes. The H2a gene on MM 614 codes for a major H2a mRNA, while the H2a genes from MM 221 and MM 291 code for minor H2a mRNAs. A similar pattern of differential expression was found in all mouse cells tested including teratocarcinoma cells and fetal mice.

The levels of histone mRNA are regulated in cultured mouse myeloma cells in parallel with DNA synthesis. When DNA synthesis is inhibited the levels of all the histone mRNAs decrease in parallel. This is due both to a increase in the rate of mRNA degradation and a decrease in the rate of mRNA synthesis. The effects are rapid and reversible.

Within ten minutes after inhibiting thymidine synthesis with fluoro-deoxyuridine (FUdR) histone gene transcription is reduced by a factor of four to five and the histone mRNA decays with a half-life of 12 minutes. Within ten minutes after refeeding thymidine the rate of transcription is restored to control levels (Table 1) and the steady state level of mRNA reaches control levels in 30 to 40 minutes (Fig. 3). The minor H3 mRNA derived from MM 221 and MM 291 and the major H3 mRNA derived from MM 614 recover with the same kinetics. This indicates that the higher levels of the mRNAs derived from MM 614 are due to a higher rate of transcription of these genes.

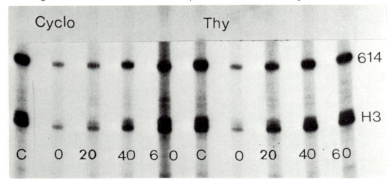

Fig. 3. Recovery of Histone mRNA levels after treatment with FUdR. Cells were treated with FUdR for 45 min (0 time) and then cycloheximide or thymidine added. RNA was prepared at the indicated times and analyzed by the S1 nuclease assay using the H3 gene from MM 614 as a probe. The H3 band represents protection to the AUG codon and the 614 band represents protection to the end of the mRNA. C are control cells.

When inhibitors of protein synthesis are added to cells which have been treated with FUdR, the levels of histone mRNA increase (Fig. 3). This increase is due to an increased rate of histone gene transcription as well as increased stability of histone mRNA (Table 1). We conclude that continued protein synthesis is necessary for decreased histone gene transcription and an increased rate of mRNA degradation. It is possible that histone mRNA metabolism and deoxynucleotide metabolism are coordinately regulated.

Table I. Effect of Fluorodeoxyuridine on Histone Gene Transcription

Treatment	CPM	H3 % of control	CPM	Actin % of control
Control	600	100	120	100
FUdR-10 min.	180	30	103	85
FUdR-45 min.	150	25	110	90
FUdR-45 min.+ Thy-25 min.	580	95	170	140
FUdR-45 min.+ Thy-25 min.	920	150	105	90
FUdR-45 min.+ cyclo-25 min.	325	55	135	110
FUdR-45 min+ puro-25 min.	360	60	120	100

Nuclei were prepared from mouse myeloma cells which had been treated with fluorodeoxyuridine for various times then thymidine (Thy), cycloheximide (cyclo) or puromycin (puro) was added for the indicated times and the nuclei were incubated with α-^{32}PO$_4$-GTP for 30 minutes and RNA prepared. The amount of histone mRNA was measured by hybridization.

HEMOGLOBINOPATHIES: DETECTION OF DEFECTIVE HUMAN β-GLOBIN GENES BY DIRECT AND INDIRECT DNA RESTRICTION ANALYSIS

Jürgen HORST[1], Renate OEHME[1], Enno KLEIHAUER[2] and Elisabeth KOHNE[2]

Abteilung Humangenetik[1] und Pädiatrie II[2], Universität Ulm, 79 Ulm FRG

INTRODUCTION. Identification of mutant genes in cellular DNA is theoretically possible because of the specificity of restriction enzymes either direct or indirect. A direct identification of the defective gene can be made if the mutation changed an enzyme's cleavage site and thus changed the normal DNA restriction pattern. The direct detection of the sickle cell gene with restriction enzyme Mst II(1-3) and the hemoglobin (Hb) M Milwaukee gene with Sst I (4) have recently been described. An indirect identification of chromosomes that carry a mutant gene relies on the presence of inherited DNA sequence polymorphisms within the cellular genome, giving rise to variations in restriction sites. Examples of this indirect diagnostic procedure are the identification of β-thalassemia-causing β-globin genes (5). In this communication we describe the direct detection of the Hb M Milwaukee β-globin gene in three generations of an afflicted family. The identification of mutant β-globin genes in a family with Hb Presbyterian has been achieved by the indirect detection method.

RESULTS. The pedigree of a family with individuals affected with Hb M Milwaukee is shown in Fig. 1. Since the parents of patient II.3 were healthy persons of 49 (I.1) and 37 (I.2) years, it can be assumed that the β-globin gene mutation occurred in one of them. Chromosomal DNA of the afflicted members and of normal controls was digested with enzyme Sst I. Blot hybridization using the β-globin probe (6) revealed three fragments of 15.5, 9.0 and 6.5 Kb (Fig.1), a pattern found to be diagnostic for the heterozygous state of Hb M Milwaukee in preliminary studies of II.3 (4). Normal controls exhibited the 15.5 Kb fragment only.

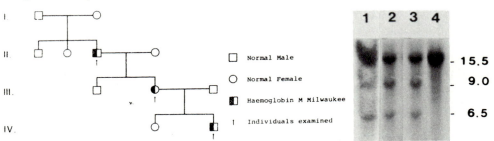

FIG.1. Pedigree of a family with Hb M Milwaukee affected members (left) and the diagnostic DNA pattern (right). II.3 (1), III.3 (2), IV.2 (3), normal control (4). Fragment sizes are in Kb.

Fig. 2 shows the pedigree of a family with individuals affected with Hb Presbyterian. To identify the mutant globin gene seven restriction sites (Hinc IIε, Hind III$^G\gamma$, Hind III$^A\gamma$, Hinc II$\psi\beta$, Hinc II 3'$\psi\beta$, Ava IIβ, Bam HIβ) of genomic DNA from all family members were analysed that have been found to be polymorphic within the β-globin gene cluster (7.9). DNA blotting and hybridization with specific probes revealed that the haplotype constellation - + - + + - + was diagnostic for the Hb Presbyterian β-globin gene carrying chromosome in the family under investigation. This haplotype - rare in mediterraneans (8.) - could also be demonstrated in normal controls.

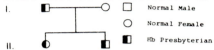

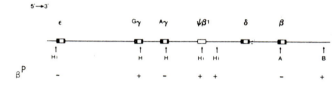

FIG.2. Chromosomal haplotype constellation of the Hb Presbyterian β-globin gene (β^P). Top: Pedigree of the family with affected members. Bottom: Human β-globin gene cluster. The arrows indicate restriction sites Hinc II (Hi), Hind III(H), Ava II(A), Bam HI(B); their presence is indicated by +, absence by - .

DISCUSSION. We have used two different approaches to identify chromosomes that carry a mutant hemoglobin gene. By means of a direct analysis of the mutant gene with Sst I it was possible to demonstrate that the β-Milwaukee globin gene DNA sequence GAGCTC of codons 67 and 68 had been transmitted over three generations. The indirect identification method of chromosomes carrying mutant β-globin genes has been used in case of Hb Presbyterian. Here linkage analysis of the mutant β-globin gene to polymorphic DNA restriction sites within the β-globin gene cluster revealed a chromosomal haplotype constellation that has so far only been found in 1% of mediterranean indiv'duals. Our results however, indicate that this haplotype constellation might be more frequent in populations of central European origin.

REFERENCES. (1) Wilson, J.T., Milner, P.F., Summer, M.E., Nallaseth, F.S., Fadel, H.E., Reindollar, R.H., Mc Donough, P.G. & Wilson, L.B. (1982), Proc. Natl. Acad. Sci. USA 79, 3628-3631; (2) Orkin, S.H., Little, P.F.R., Kazazian, H.H. Jr. and Boehm, C.D. (1982), N. Engl. J. Med., 307, 32-36; (3) Chang, J.C. & Kan, Y.W. (1982), N. Engl. J. Med. 307, 30-32; (4) Horst, J., Schäfer, R., Kleihauer, E. & Kohne, E. (1983), Brit. J. Haem. 54,, 643-648; (5) Little, P.F.R., Annison, G., Darling, S., Williamson, R., Camba, L. & Modell, B. (1980), Nature 285, 144-147; (6) Wilson, J.T., Wilson, J.B., De Riel, J.K., Villa-Komaroff, L., Efstratiadis, A., Forget, B.G. & Weissmann, S.M. (1978), Nucl. Acids Res. 5, 503-517; (7) Antonarakis, S.E., Boehm, C.D., Giardina, P.J.V. and Kazazian, H.H. Jr. (1982), Acad. Sci. USA 79, 137-141; (8) Orkin, S.H., Kazazian, H.H. Jr., Antonarakis, S.D., Goff, S.C., Boehm, C.D., Sexton, J.P., Waber, P.G. & Giardina, P.J.V. (1982), Nature 296, 627-631; (9) Kan, Y.W., Lee, K.Y., Furbetta, M., Angius, A. & Cao, A. (1980), N. Engl. J. Med. 302, 185-188.

ACKNOWLEDGEMENT. Supported by the Deutsche Forschungsgemeinschaft.

ISOLATION AND PRELIMINARY CHARACTERIZATION OF FERRITIN HEAVY CHAIN cDNA CLONE.

Swatantra K. Jain[+], Dana Boyd[+], K. Barret[+], J. Crampton[*] and Jim Drysdale[+]
[+]Tufts Medical School, Boston, and [*]University of Liverpool, Liverpool, UK.

Ferritin is the major iron storage protein in eukaryotes. Different forms of ferritin are expressed during development and in pathological states of iron overload and malignancy. Some of these forms may play different roles in iron metabolism since they differ in their intracellular distributions and in their relative rates of iron uptake and release. In addition to its role in iron metabolism, ferritin is of interest as a tumor marker and as a possible regulator of myelopoiesis (1).

The heterogeneity in tissue ferritins is largely due to differences in expression of two types of subunits, H and L, MW 21,000 and 19,000 resp. which can combine in different proportions in a 24 subunit shell to generate a series of isoferritins. The H and L subunits share extensive sequence homologies but are encoded by distinct mRNAs (2). A second isoelectric form of the H subunit is found in some tissues but the structural and metabolic relationships of the two H isosubunits are not known. Ferritin is also found to variable extents in serum in normal and pathological states. M ch of the serum ferritin is distinct from tissue ferritins in that it is glycosylated (3); it may therefore be synthesized on membrane-bound polysomes and be encoded by distinct mRNA(s).

In many cells, ferritin synthesis is regulated by iron. Much of the present evidence suggests that the apparent induction of ferritin by iron involves a cytoplasmic control. One popular hypothesis is that iron mobilizes ferritin mRNA from inactive cytoplasmic mRNP particles to functional polysomes (4).

As a first step in exploring the origins, relationships, and regulation of ferritin mRNAs we have cloned human ferritin mRNA. This paper presents an initial characterization of a ferritin cDNA clone, the organization of ferritin genomic DNA and preliminary studies of ferritin gene expresion in normal and iron-loaded HeLa cells.

Isolation of ferritin cDNA clones. A cDNA library to human lymphocyte mRNA was prepared by conventional procedures through insertion at the Pst site in pAT

153, a derivative of pBR322. This library was screened with a mixture of 32 oligo-deoxynucleotides, each containing 14 deoxynucleotides, and corresponding to all possible coding sequences of a peptide present in H but not in L subunit. The synthetic oligodeoxynucleotides were kinased and used to screen the lymphocyte library. The filters were also screened with nick-translated cDNA prepared from a preparation enriched in ferritin HmRNA by electrophoresis in acid-urea agarose gel and identified by translation followed by immunoprecipitation.

A clone reacting strongly with both probes was isolated. This clone was shown to contain human ferritin H sequences on the basis of hybrid selection and by sequence analysis. This cloned DNA is approx 550 nucleotides long and contains about 50% of the ferritin HmRNA sequence.

The H clone selected HmRNA but not LmRNA from unfractionated HeLa cell mRNA suggesting that there are substantial sequence differences in ferritin H and L mRNAs.

Southern blot analyses of human genomic DNA digested with three enzymes showed a complex pattern with approx 12 EcoRl fragments and 15 BamHl fragments. Our analysis indicates that the H chain of ferritin is composed of a family of genes containing at least 10 members that are highly homologous. Several related, but less homologous members were also detected. These may be pseudogenes or L chain genes with sequence homology to H chain genes.

In order to explore the translational model for regulation of ferritin synthesis by iron, we analyzed ferritin mRNA levels in polysomes and in mRNP particles from normal and iron-loaded HeLa cells by translation assays and by Northern blot analyses. The results show that iron does not significantly increase ferritin mRNA levels in polysomes, nor decrease ferritin mRNA levels in mRNP particles.

References: (1) Drysdale, J.W. (1982) in Advances in Red Blood Cell Biology, Weatherall, D., Fiorell, G. and Gorini, S. (eds.) Raven Press New York, p. 35. (2) Watanabe, N. and Drysdale, J.W. (1981) Biochem. Biophys. Res. Commun. 98, 507. (3) Cragg, S.J., Wagstaff, m. and Worwood, M. (1980) Clin Sci 58, 259. (4) Zahringer, J., Baliga, B.S. and Munro, H.N. (1976) Proc. Natl. Acad. Sci. 73, 857.

LOCALIZATION OF c-abl, c-sis AND c-fes ONCOGENES TO HUMAN GERMLINE CHROMOSOMES

Suresh C. Jhanwar, Benjamin G. Neel, William S. Hayward and R.S.K. Chaganti
Memorial Sloan-Kettering Cancer Center, 1275 York Avenue, New York, NY 10021

INTRODUCTION

Cellular oncogenes (c-onc genes) are highly conserved DNA sequences common to oncogenic retroviruses (v-onc genes) and vertebrate cells. Over 15 different oncogenes have been identified in acute retroviruses isolated from avian and mammalian species (1). Although their precise role in normal cell metabolism is not yet known, their high degree of evolutionary conservation indicates that they play an important role in cellular metabolism or tissue differentiation (2). Cytogenetic studies during the past 20 years on various forms of human cancer have shown that non-random chromosome abnormalities are associated with various tumors. So far, about 25 specific break sites have been identified in the human genome which are associated with specific rearrangements in tumor cells. Recent localizations of c-onc genes on chromosomes by us and others have shown that the sites of several of them correspond with the break sites. We present here germline (meiotic pachytene) chromosomal localization of the human cellular counterparts of transforming genes of three RNA tumor viruses, namely, abelson murine leukemia virus, simian sarcoma virus, and feline sarcoma virus.

MATERIALS AND METHODS

Molecular Probes. The plasmids pv-abl, pv-sis, and pv-fes contain 2.3, 1.0, and 0.4 Kb inserts, respectively. They were the generous gifts of Drs. S. Goff, S. Aaronson, and C. Sherr.

In Situ Hybridization: Chromosome preparation, hybridization, autoradiography, and grain analysis were performed according to previously described methods (3,4,5).

RESULTS

Localization of c-abl: Analysis of autoradiographic grains on 29 well spread pachytene cells revealed 49 hybridization sites. Of these, 13 occurred at a specific site on chromosome 9, namely, the chromomere region corresponding to somatic metaphase band 9q34.1 (5,6). The deviation from expected hybridization at this site was also highly significant ($p < 0.001$). Therefore, we localize the c-abl oncogene on band 9q34.1.

Localization of c-sis: Analysis of autoradiographic grains on 30 well spread pachytene cells revealed 55 hybridization sites. Of these, 17 occurred at a specific site on chromosome 22, namely, the chromomere region corresponding to the somatic metaphase band

22q13.1 (6). The deviation from expected hybridization at this site was also highly significant (p < 0.001). Therefore, we localize the c-sis, oncogene on band 22q13.1.

Localization of c-fes: Analysis of autoradiographic grains on 32 well spread pachytene cells yielded 60 hybridization sites. Of these, 19 occurred at a specific site on chromomere region corresponding to the somatic metaphase band 15q26.1 (6). In this case also the deviation from expected hybridization was highly significant (p < 0.001). Therefore, we localize the c-fes oncogene on band 15q26.1.

DISCUSSION

We confirm previous assignment by somatic cell hybridization of c-abl, c-sis, and c-fes oncogenes to chromosomes 9, 22, and 15 respectively. We also confirm the localization of c-fes to 15q26 reported recently by **in situ hybridization** on somatic chromosomes (7). We present the germ line positions of all three genes. The three chromosomes engage in specific rearrangements in leukemias. Thus, the Philadelphia (Ph^1) chromosome which characterizes chronic myelogenous leukemia (CML) is derived from the translocation t(9;22) (q34;q11) and the translocation t (15;17)(q22;q21) is seen in a proportion of acute promyelocytic leukemia patients (8). However, only one of the three oncogene sites reported here corresponds with a tumor cell associated break point, namely, c-abl at 9q34.1; in the Ph^1 translocation c-abl has been shown to move to 22q. The activation of c-myc mediated by translocation next to the Ig H gene on chromosome 14 (9) provides a model for the role of chromosome change in the development of neoplasia. The status of activation of c-abl in CML is still unknown.

REFERENCES

1. Coffin, M., Varmus, H.E., Bishop, J.M., Essex, M., Hardy, W.D., et al. (1981) J. Virol. 49, 953.
2. Bishop, J.M., (1981) Cell, 23, 5.
3. Neel, B.G., Jhanwar, S.C., Chaganti, R.S.K., and Hayward, W.S. (1982) Proc. Natl. Acad. Sci., 79, 7842.
4. Jhanwar, S.C., Prensky, W. and Chaganti, R.S.K. (1981) Cytogenet. Cell Genet. 30, 39.
5. Jhanwar, S.C., Burns, J.P., Alonso, M.L., Hew, W., and Chaganti, R.S.K. (1982) Cytogenet. Cell Genet. 33, 240-248.
6. Standing committee of Human Cytogenetic Nomenclature. (1981) Cytogenet. Cell Genet. 31, 5.
7. Harper, M.E., Franchini, G., Love, J., Simon, M.I., Gallo, R.C., and Wong-Staal, F. (1983) Nature (London) 304, 169.
8. Rowley, J.D., Golomb, H.M., and Dougherty, C. (1977) Lancet 1, 549.
9. Marcu, K.B., Harris, L.J., Erikson, J., Watt, R., and Croce, C.M. (1983) Proc. Natl. Acad. Sci., 80, 519.

REGULATION OF METALLOTHIONEIN GENES IN MENKES' DISEASE

L. Jolicoeur-Paquet, A. Zelinka, L.-C. Tsui and J.R. Riordan

The Hospital for Sick Children and University of Toronto,
Toronto, CANADA M5G 1X8

Menkes' disease is an X-linked trait characterized by severe mental retardation, neurological impairment and death usually before 3 years of age (1). Cu is redistributed in tissues (2) and, although it accumulates in some, it is effectively unavailable to copper-enzymes because of sequestering by a high affinity ligand (3). Evidence from several laboratories including this one (4) indicates that this ligand is metallothionein (MT). Since MT is inducible by copper it is not immediately evident whether Cu, which has accumulated in the cells for any reason, is responsible for the elevated level of the protein or, conversely, an enhanced inherent capacity to make more or altered MT results in copper retention. The following studies were intended to distinguish between these 2 possibilities.

Cu, Zn and Cd fluxes into and out of Menkes' lymphoblasts - If the first alternative is true then the accumulated Cu responsible for "hyperinduction" could be due either to elevated Cu influx or an inhibition of efflux. We have shown previously that Menkes' lymphoblasts accumulate greater than normal amounts not only of Cu but also of Zn and Cd (5). We have now measured the initial rates of influx of these three metals and found that these rates did not differ between normal and Menkes' cells. Furthermore, Cu did not share the same entry route with Zn and Cd, i.e. lack of competitive inhibition. That these were 2 different routes was confirmed by the finding of identical pH dependencies for Zn and Cd and a totally different one for copper. This provided evidence that it was the retention of Cu rather than the influx which was enhanced in Menkes' cells since it is the former rather than the latter which is shared by all 3 metals.

Whereas the rate but not the extent of uptake was increased by detergent permeabilizing of the cell membrane, the rate of efflux was not altered by this treatment. Therefore, metal retention was apparently due to alteration of the high affinity intracellular ligand (i.e. MT) rather than a blockage of the efflux pathway.

Metallothionein regulation - Since the above results favoured our second possibility, i.e. that increased or altered MT was responsible for Cu retention, we sought more direct evidence of this. The relative rate of MT synthesis measured by incorporation of ^{35}S-cysteine was more than twice as high in Menkes' cells as in normals indicating acceleration of synthesis rather than diminished degradation.

RNA prepared from normal and Menkes' cells (6) either with or without poly A^{+} selection was subjected to Northern blot hybridization analysis using human MT-I and MT-II probes. The increased MT mRNA levels were found to correspond to and presumably account for the overproduction of the protein in Menkes' cells. As with the steady state levels of the protein and synthetic rates, the Menkes' increments were seen when no additional metal was added to the cells and on addition of high doses of Cu, Zn or Cd. At this gross level of resolution it appears that there is "over expression" of MT genes in both the uninduced and induced states. Since Cd is the most potent inducing metal, MT mRNA levels were measured as a function of finely graded doses of the metal (0-100 μM). The results showed a cooperative response (sigmoidal dose-response curve) of normal cells to induction by Cd whereas the cooperativity was less pronounced with Menkes' cells. Furthermore, the diminution in MT mRNA levels after the peak had been reached, characteristic of normal cells (7) does not occur with Menkes' cells. The levels of these transcripts remains high and would be expected to result in greater amounts of MT protein. This behaviour may be the result of a genetic lesion in a Cd binding regulatory factor permitting it to still function but in an imperfect manner.

Discussion - Because MT genes are not located on the X-chromosome (8,9), our interpretation requires that regulation of transcription of MT-genes by metals is mediated via a trans-acting regulatory factor rather than by an autoregulatory mechanism involving only MT protein itself. To date attempts to distinguish between these possibilities have not been definitive (10-12). However, effective regulation of a mouse MT-I gene transferred to CHO cells was not dependent on the amount of MT present (12). The lack of correlation between the order of "inducing power" of the different metals (Cd >Cu and Zn) and the relative binding affinities of the metals for MT (Cu >Cd and Zn) is also inconsistent with an autoregulation model. Studies with hybrids of CHO cells and Menkes' fibroblasts also suggests that there may be an X-linked regulator of MT genes (8).

References - (1) Menkes, J.H., Alter, M., Steigleder, G.K., Weakly, D.R. and Sung, J.H. (1962) Pediatrics 29, 764; (2) Nooijen, J.L., de Groot, C.J., van den Hamer, C.J.A., Monnens, A.H., Willemse, J. and Niermeijer, M.F. (1981) Pediatr. Res. 15, 284; (3) Boyce, P.M., Camakaris, J. and Danks, D.M. (1980) Connect. Tiss. Res. 7, 205; (4) Riordan, J.R. (1983) in "Biological Aspects of Metals and Metal-Related Diseases" ed. B. Sarkar p. 159; (5) Riordan, J.R. and Jolicoeur-Paquet, L. (1982) J. Biol. Chem. 257, 4639; (6) Chirgwin, J.M., Przybyla, A.E., MacDonald, R.J. and Rutter, W.J. (1979) Biochemistry 18, 5294; (7) Enger, M.D., Roll, L.B. and Hildebrand, C.E. (1979) Nucl. Acids Res. 7, 271; (8) Hildebrand, C.E., Crawford, B.D., Enger, M.D., Griffith, B.B., Griffith, J.K., Hanners, L., Longmire, J.L. and Walters, R.A. (1982) J. Cell Biol. 95, 448a; (9) Cox, D.F. and Palmiter, R.D. (1983) Human Genet. 64, 61; (10) Searle, P., Stuart, G., Palmiter, R. and Brinster, R. (1983) J. Cell. Biochem. Suppl. 7A, 116; (11) Karin, M. and Holtgreve, H. (1983) J. Cell. Biochem. Suppl. 7A, 114; (12) Carter, A.D. and Hamer, D.H. (1983) J. Cell. Biochem. Suppl. 7A, 114

A RANDOM CHROMOSOME 6 DNA PROBE AND RFLP ANALYSIS OF HLA-TYPED FAMILIES

K.W. Klinger[1], A.W. Muir[2] and C.Gillam[3]

[1] Dept. Mol. Biol. & Microbiol. Case Western Reserve Univ.
[2] Dept. Med. Case Western Reserve Univ. Cleveland, Oh. &
[3] Dept. Biochemistry St. Mary's Hosp. Med. Sch., London

INTRODUCTION. Hereditary hemochromatosis is considered to be an autosomal recessive disorder. The causative genetic defect is unknown, but the hemochromatosis gene has been shown to be linked to the HLA region on chromosome 6 (1,2,3). We would like to identify additional cloned DNA sequences that could be used to define the hemochromatosis locus, and to provide a set of linked markers. This report describes a cloned DNA sequence localized by in situ hybridization to the short arm of chromosome 6, and the analysis of polymorphic restriction fragments generated from DNA isolated from members of HLA-typed hemochromatosis families.

RESULTS. Characterization of λ4Cll and assignment of the cloned random DNA sequence to chromosome 6. The recombinant bacteriophage λ4Cll was retrieved from a chromosome 4 library constructed by Davies and Williamson (4) from flow cytometry purified human 4 chromosomes. λ4Cll consists of EcoRl digested human DNA ligated into the vector λgt.WES-B. as diagrammed in Fig. 1, the order of EcoRl restriction fragments in the clone is: long arm of λ (21.7 kb), 3.2 kb human DNA, 2.0 kb human DNA, short arm of λ (14 kb). The human DNA insert of λ4Cll is aligned with the homologous locus in human DNA in Fig. 1. By hybridization to DNA from human/rodent hybrid cell lines, we found that 4Cll DNA hybridized to chromosome 6, rather than to chromosome 4. This clone was localized on chromosome 6 by direct hybridization in situ to metaphase spreads (5). As shown in Fig. 2, the majority of the silver grains were distributed on the short arm of chromosome 6, probably at 6p12-p22. This assignment would overlap the MHC locus,and thus the 4Cll DNA sequence might be linked to the hemochromatosis gene. Therefore we characterized the 4Cll probe for the detection of restriction fragment length polymorphisms that could be used in linkage analysis of the hemochromatosis families.

Identification of DNA sequence polymorphisms. When 4Cll DNA was hybridized to human DNAs digested with one of 10 different restriction endonucleases and transferred to filters, a restriction fragment length polymorphism was only detected when the DNA was digested with BglII. Among 9 unrelated individuals, the 4Cll probe detected a 7.3 kb BglII fragment in 6 individuals, a 6.9 kb fragment in 1 individual, and both alleles in the remaining 2 cases.

Hybridization analysis of the BglII digested DNA from
three hemochromatosis families (6, 4, and 7 members ,
respectively) did not allow us to perform linkage analysis
using the probe 4Cll. Unlike the case in the unrelated DNA
panel, only 2 individuals out of the 17 analyzed showed
the minor allele. Analysis of additional families may allow
identification of informative families.

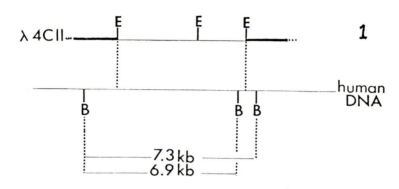

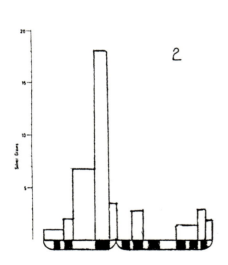

Fig. 1. Recombinant phage
4Cll. E= EcoRl restriction
sites. B=BglII restriction
sites. The heavy line
indicates lambda DNA, the
light line indicates human
insert. The human insert is
aligned with the homologous
human locus, and the lengths
of the allelic BglII
fragments are shown.

Fig 2. Localization of 4Cll DNA by in situ hybridization.
The intrachromosomal localization of 3H-labeled 4Cll DNA
over chomosome 6 from 9 cells is shown.

REFERENCES.(1) Muir, A., McLaren, G.D., Braun, W.E., and
Askari, A.D. (1978) Am. J. Hum. Genet. 30, 61A; (2)Simon, M.,
Pawlotsky, Y., Bourel, M., Fauchet, R, and Genetet, B. (1975)
Nouv. Presse Med. 4, 1432. (3) Simon, M., Bourel, M.,
Fauchet, R.,and Genetet, B. (1976) Gut 17, 332. (4) Davies,
K. and Williamson, R (1983) unpublished data. (5) Harper,
M.E. and Saunders, G.R. (1981) Chromosoma 83, 431.

STUDIES ON DRUG INDUCIBLE GENE SEQUENCES

Koch J. A.*, Fisher, C. W. *, Dilella A. G.*, Haska M.*, Steggles A. W.* and Wong J. F. †.

*Program Molecular Pathology, NEOUCOM, Rootstown, Ohio, and †Department of Chemistry, University of Oklahoma, Norman, OK.

During the screening of a recombinant DNA library derived from a phenobarbital (PB) induced rabbit liver poly (A+) mRNA population, we identified a recombinant plasmid (PB7) that corresponded to a PB inducible mRNA. The plasmid was isolated, the insert mapped using restriction enzymes, and sequenced. The sequence, which represents ca. 50% of the total mRNA, covers only a part of the N terminal region of the PB7 protein. The protein does not appear to have any homology with known cytochrome P450 sequences.

METHODS. Male rabbits were treated with PB(1), killed by cervical dislocation, the livers removed and RNA isolated from polysomes by the procedure of Palmiter (2). Poly (A+) mRNA was isolated (1), and cDNA synthesized using reverse transcriptase. Reverse transcriptase was also used for second strand synthesis. After S1 nuclease treatment and C tailing, the dsDNA was inserted into the G tailed Pst I site of PBR322. E. Coli HB101 cells were transformed and screened for antibiotic sensitivity. One recombinant plasmid (PB7) was selected for further studies. The PB7 insert was isolated by agarose gel electrophoresis and electro-elution then characterized by dot-blot hybridization using DBM paper. The PB7 mRNA was also sized by agarose gel electrophoresis followed by Southern blotting and hybridization to a nick translated [^{32}P] PB7- dsDNA probe. The PB7 insert was subcloned into M13 mp8 and M13mp9 and sequenced using the procedure of Sanger et. al (3).

RESULTS AND DISCUSSION. The dot blot experiment is shown in Fig. 1, and the DNA sequence analysis in Table 1. The data indicates that PB7 mRNA is inducible by PB treatment and represents ca 0.01% of the total rabbit liver mRNA population. On agarose gel electrophoresis, the PB7 mRNA ran with a 23s rRNA marker (data not shown). The PB7 insert was subcloned into M13mp8 and M13mp9 and both DNA strands sequenced. DNA sequence analysis shows one usable reading frame starting at nucleotide 1294, enabling the N terminal sequence of 66 amino acids to be identified. Studies are continuing on the isolation of a DNA clone that contains the 3' end of the mRNA, and on identifying the protein coded for by PB7 mRNA.

Figure 1. Dot blot assay of polysomal poly(A⁺)-
mRNA. Liver polysomal poly(A⁺)mRNA's isolated
from phenobarbital treated and untreated rabbits
were heat denatured and adjusted to 10 mM Na-
acetate, pH 4.0. Increasing amounts of mRNA were
spotted in 15 ul onto DBM-paper disks (1cm²) and
incubated at room temperature for 40 min. The
disks were washed with 0.2 M Na-acetate, pH 4.0,
and incubated at 42°C for 5 hr. in hybridization
buffer (50% formamide, 5X SSC, 25 mM Na-phosphate,
pH 6.5, 0.02% each of BSA, ficoll, and polyvinyl-
pyrrolidone) containing 1% glycine. The disks were
then hybridized to nick-translated [³²P]-pPB7 cDNA
insert (10,000 cpm/disk) in hybridization buffer
containing 200 ug/ml of denatured sonicated calf
thymus DNA for 30 hr. at 42°C. The disks were then
washed in 0.5X SSC for 3 hr. at 65°C. Hybridization was quantitated by liquid scintillation
counting. A background value of 53 cpm was
subtracted from each value. o———o , mRNA isolated
from untreated rabbits. •———• , mRNA isolated
from rabbits injected with phenobarbital. □———□ ,
mRNA isolated from rabbits administered 0.1%
phenobarbital-drinking water.

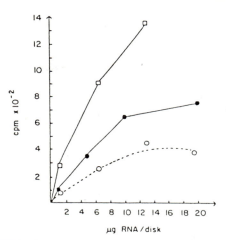

```
GGGGGGGGGG GGTGAAATGA CAAAACATTA AGGCAGTTTT ATTTCACTCC TAATGAAATG TTTATCTAAT ATATTTAGCT TAACTTCATT TTTAAAATAC
    10         20         30         40         50         60         70         80         90         100

TTAAGACGGA GGGGGCAAGA TGGCGGAATA GGAAGGGAGC ACACTGATAG TCCGGGGAGA GACAGTTTAA TAAAAGTGGA GATACTGCAG GTTCAAGGAA
    110        120        130        140        150        160        170        180        190        200

GAGTAGGGGA GGAAACAGCA GAAGAAACTC TTCCGGAACG CATGATTCAC AGTGGACCTG TGTGGAGAGC GTGGGAGCCC ACAGTTTGGG ACACCAGCGG
    210        220        230        240        250        260        270        280        290        300

CAGACTCAAC ACACCAGCGC TGGAATGCGA GGTGAGCTGA ACCTCAATAG CCCGAGACAC CAGCAGGCAA GCGGAGAGAG GAGACTAGAG GGAACGACCC
    310        320        330        340        350        360        370        380        390        400

CCCGGGCGGG GGGGAACTTC ACCAGGCTAA CTGGAAGAGA GAGAGAGAGA AAAAAAAAGG TGACTGGTGC GGACACGGGT TTCTCTCTCT CTGGTCACCT
    410        420        430        440        450        460        470        480        490        500

CTCAAGGGCG AGCAAGACAA AGAGCAGGCG CCATCTTGGA CATACGTCAT AAGCAGAGTG ACCTCAGGTC TGCACCGGCC CTGAGCCTAG CAAAAAAACC
    510        520        530        540        550        560        570        580        590        600

TGACTCTGGG TGGGGCAAAT TAACAGGAGA TTAGGACCTA GTAAATTTGT GGTGCTACTG AACTGAGACT GTGAAAAAAA GAGACGGTGG GGGAGAGAAC
    610        620        630        640        650        660        670        680        690        700

TCACAGAATT CACCTGAGTA CTCTCCAGAG ACGCTACAAT TCCGTAACTT TGGCAACCCA GTGGAGACTG AAGGAGAATT TGAGCCCACT CTGAGAGCAG
    710        720        730        740        750        760        770        780        790        800

AACAGATTCC CTGTGTGGTC CTTGGGAAAG AGCTTCTGAT CTCTGGCTCC TGTGGGTATA TAATTTGCCT GCTAACTACC TCCAACTTCA TTCAGCTGTG
    810        820        830        840        850        860        870        880        890        900

CGAATTACTT CCCTTTTGAA TCAAAAAAAT AGAGAGAGAG AGAGAGAGAG AGATCTACCA CGCCTAACCT GGGAGTGTCA CCTTTGGCAC ACCAAACAGA
    910        920        930        940        950        960        970        980        990        1000

GCTCTCAGGC CACACCCATC TCAAGCCTCT AAGCGTCCAT CAAAAACAGA CAGTCCACTT AATTTAGAGT CATAGTATAA CAAGAAAAAG CACCACAGTG
    1010       1020       1030       1040       1050       1060       1070       1080       1090       1100

AAGAAACCAA ATATCTCCAA TATGCCAAAT AACAAAGTCA AAAACCGAGG TAATAAAAAC AAGGAAGTCA CCATGACGCC CCCAAATGAA AAAAGACACC
    1110       1120       1130       1140       1150       1160       1170       1180       1190       1200

CAATTCAAGA TTATGAAGAT GATGAGATAG AAGAAATGCA AGAAGCAAGT CTCAAAAAAT TGATAAGAAC ATTAAGAAGT CTCAAAAACA
    1210       1220       1230       1240       1250       1260       1270       1280       1290
```

```
    M   L   E   L   Q   K   S   L   M   V   K   I   E   N   L   S   R   E   N   E   I   L   K   R   N   Q
AAA ATG CTT GAA CTA CAG AAA TCC TTA ATG GTC AAG ATA GAA AAT CTC TCT CGT GAA AAT GAA ATA TTA AAG AGG AAT CAA
        1300           1310           1320           1330           1340           1350           1360           1370

    N   E   T   K   Q   L   V   Q   Q   E   T   V   I   V   T   R   N   H   N   E   V   K   N   S   Y   R   S
AAT GAA ACG AAA CAA CTA GTA CAA CAG GAA ACT GTG ATA GTG ACG AGA AAT CAT AAT GAA GTG AAG AAT TCA TAT AGA TCA
        1380           1390           1400           1410           1420           1430           1440           1450

    N   E   K   H   N   R   E   P   Y   K   Q   N   G
AAT GAA AAA CAC AAT AGA GAG CCT TAC AAA CAG AAT GGG TCC CCC CCC CCC CCT GCA G
        1460           1470           1480           1490           1500           1510
```

REFERENCES. (1) DiLella A., Chiang J. and Steggles A. (1981)
Biochem. Biophys. Res. Commun. 100 155-161. (2) Palmiter R. (1974)
Biochemistry 13 3605-3615. (3) Sanger F., Nicklen S. and Coulson A.
(1977) Proc. Natl. Acad. Sci. 74 5463-5467.

ACKNOWLEDGEMENTS. Support was provided by NIH grant no. GM-
27675, and the NEOUCOM Office of Geriatrics and Gerontology.

CLONING OF cDNA ENCODING ORNITHINE DECARBOXYLASE (ODC): STUDIES
ON ODC-mRNA INDUCTION BY ANDROGENS IN NORMAL AND ANDROGEN-INSENSITIVE
(Tfm/Y) MICE

K. Kontula, C.W. Bardin and O.A. Jänne

The Population Council and The Rockefeller University, 1230 York
Avenue, New York, NY 10021

INTRODUCTION

Polyamines are thought to play an essential role in the control
of cellular metabolism and proliferation. Ornithine decarboxylase
(ODC) which catalyzes the conversion of ornithine to putrescine is
the first and rate-controlling enzyme in polyamine biosynthesis (1).
ODC activity fluctuates rapidly in response to a variety of stimuli
such as hormones, drugs and tissue regeneration, and displays a very
high turnover rate. For example, androgens increase ODC activity in
mouse kidney about 500-fold with a lag period of a few hours (2). In
order to determine in more detail how ODC activity is regulated we
prepared a cDNA clone to purified ODC-mRNA and used this cDNA as a
probe for initial studies on the regulation of ODC-mRNA by androgens
in kidneys of normal and androgen-insensitive (Tfm/Y) mice.

MATERIALS AND METHODS

ODC-mRNA was purified from kidneys of androgen-treated mice by
immunoadsorption of renal polysomes to a protein A-Sepharose column
and enriched for poly(A)-containing RNA by oligo(dT)-cellulose.
Double-stranded cDNA synthesized from this mRNA was inserted into the
Pst I site of plasmid pBR322 and propagated in E. coli. Plasmids
containing cDNA sequences coding for ODC were identified by differential colony hybridization, by radioimmunological detection (3) of
ODC-like antigens from bacterial culture media and by cell-free
translation of hybrid-selected mRNA followed by immunoprecipitation
with specific ODC antiserum. A 330-bp restriction endonuclease fragment of the selected plasmid pODC54 was labeled by nick-translation
and used to study changes in ODC-mRNA concentration in response to
androgen administration (4).

RESULTS AND DISCUSSION

After a single injection of testosterone to intact female mice,
renal ODC-mRNA concentration increased as soon as 6 hr and peaked
24 hr after steroid injection (Fig. 1). Continuous androgen treatment
for 4 days resulted in 10- to 20-fold increase in ODC-mRNA concentration in kidneys of castrated male mice whereas no induction of
this mRNA was detected in kidneys of Tfm/Y animals which have an inherent defect of the androgen receptor (Fig. 2). There was a clear
sex difference (male > female) in the level of renal ODC-mRNA indicating that even physiological concentrations of androgens are able
to regulate ODC-mRNA concentration. Regardless of the pretreatment

type and sex of the animals, Northern blots always revealed two hybridizable RNA species (Fig. 1, Fig. 2): a major band of 2.15 kb in length and a minor one of 2.7 kb. Cycloheximide given in vivo was found to block most of the androgen-induced ODC-mRNA accumulation indicating the importance of ongoing protein synthesis for the induction process and/or for normal rate of transcription.

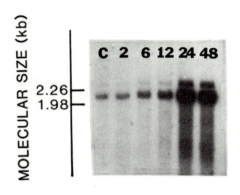

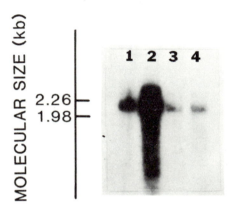

Fig. 1. Northern blot analysis of poly(A)-containing RNA from kidneys of female mice for ODC-mRNA sequences. C: control mice; other lanes: mice killed 2, 6, 12, 24 and 48 hr after injection with 10 mg testosterone.

Fig. 2. Northern blot analysis of poly(A)-containing RNA from kidneys of castrated male mice (1), castrated male mice treated for 4 days with testosterone (2), untreated Tfm/Y mice (3) and Tfm/Y mice treated for 4 days with testosterone (4).

CONCLUSIONS

1) Cloning of cDNA encoding ODC was accomplished; 2) androgens regulate ODC synthesis, at least in part, via increasing ODC-mRNA accumulation; 3) induction of ODC-mRNA by androgens does not occur in androgen-insensitive Tfm/Y animals indicating that the presence of functional androgen receptors is necessary for this process. In summary, this system should provide a very useful model for detailed studies on molecular mechanisms of androgen action and on factors that regulate polyamine synthesis by altering the transcription rate of the ODC gene.

REFERENCES

(1) Pegg, A.E. and McCann, P.P. (1982) Am. J. Physiol. 243, C212-C221. (2) Pajunen, A.E.I., Isomaa, V.V., Jänne, O.A. and Bardin, C.W. (1982) J. Biol. Chem. 257, 8190-8198. (3) Isomaa, V.V., Pajunen, A.E.I., Bardin, C.W. and Jänne, O.A. (1983) J. Biol. Chem. 258, 6735-6740. (4) Kontula, K.K., Torkkeli, T.K., Bardin, C.W. and Jänne, O.A. (1983) Proc. Natl. Acad. Sci. USA (in press).

MOLECULAR AND CYTOGENETIC CHARACTERIZATION OF FLOW SORTED MAMMALIAN CHROMOSOMES

G. Langer, K.J. Hutter, J. Barths and N. Blin

German Cancer Research Center, D-69 Heidelberg, F.R.G.

Flow analysis and sorting of fluorescence stained metaphase chromosomes constitute a new and powerful tool that complements cytogenetic analysis. Although this technique is quite complex--involving metaphase chromosomes preparation, quantitative fluorometry, computer data analysis, and statistical evaluation of results--it provides genetic material not obtainable otherwise. The use of sorted chromosomes as material for establishing chromosome specific libraries was reported for both, mouse and human species (Disteche et al., 1982; Davies et al., 1981). We have studied the flow karyotypes and sorted chromosomes of Chinese hamster cell lines and of rat and mouse tumors applying molecular and cytogenetical analyses.

1) Because of genomic shifts observed in cultured cell lines each line under investigation needs a careful examination of the karyotype. Flow karyotyping of a Chinese hamster cell line (CHV79) cultivated separately in two different laboratories showed each a distinct flow karyogram (Fig.1). Banding analysis, however, indicated that a basic set of (mainly large) chromosomes remained conserved.

FIG.1: FLOW KARYOTYPES OF CHINESE HAMSTER CELLS

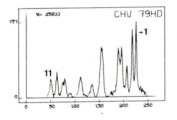
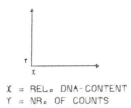
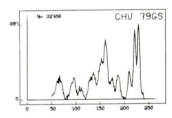

X = REL. DNA-CONTENT
Y = NR. OF COUNTS

2) In order to correlate correctly the peaks of a flow karyogram with particular chromosomes we have applied banding methods (GTG, QFD) to flow sorted chromosomes of CHV 79HD cells, thus obtaining a reference list for this karyotype (Table 1).

3) Sorted chromosomes have been used for gene mapping (e.g. Lebo et al., 1979). We have located U1snRNA sequences on peaks No.1 and 2 (Blin et al., 1982) and 5SRNA genes on chromosome No.5 in the CHV79HD karyotype, along with other gene sequences listed in Table 2.

Table 1: Distribution of CHV79HD Chromosomes in
the Flow Karyotype; Nomenclature According to the
Baltimore Conference 1975 (Ray and Mohandas, 1976)

PEAK NUMBER	PEAK SIDE	CHROMOSOME NUMBER	ORIGIN	HETEROCHROMATIN	NOR	COMMENTS
		I 45%	1	==	=	==
1	==	II 38%	3Q TER>3Q CEN::1Q26>1P22 ::7Q21>7Q TER	TWO INTERCALARY BANDS ON ONE ARM	=	==
		III 11%	2P TER>2Q TER::4P27>4P TER	==	=	RARE CHROMOSOME
2	==	IV	2	==	=	TWO HOMOLOGUES
3	==	V	4Q TER>4Q1::7Q CEN>7Q TER	CENTROMERE	P TER	==
4	RIGHT	VI 60%	5Q TER>5Q CEN::1Q25>XQ TER	==	=	==
		VII 25%	3	==	Q TER	==
4	LEFT	VIII 22%	3P TER>3P1::4Q1>4Q TER	==	Q TER	==
		IX 61%	XQ-	Q	=	==
5	==	X	5	P	=	==
	==	XI 5%	8?	P	=	RARE CHROMOSOME
6	==	XII 25%	7Q?	P	Q TER	==
	==	XIII 70%	6P-	==	P TER	TWO HOMOLOGUES
7	==	XIV	I 9Q	P AND Q	P AND Q TER	==
8	RIGHT	XV 78%	?	P	=	==
8	LEFT	XVI 82%	8P-Q- OR 9Q-	==	=	RARE CHROMOSOME
9-12	==	XVII-XXI	?	TOTAL	=	==

Table 2: Assignment of DNA Sequences to Peaks in a CHV79HD Flow Karyogram

Karyogram Peak No.	DNA Sequence
1,2	U1snRNA
3	5SRNA
4	Histone H3
1-11	AluI family
1,2	Albumin

4) For a detailed analysis of tumor genomes we have enriched by flow sorting cell line specific marker chromosomes. Marker peaks indicated by arrows were located in flow karyograms of Ehrlich ascites (EAT), Walker (W256) and Yoshida (RY HE) sarcomas (Fig.2). These markers are now being used for mapping specific sequences and as material for DNA cloning.

FIG.2: FLOW KARYOTYPES OF EXPERIMENTAL TUMOR CELLS

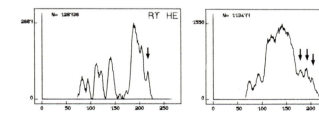
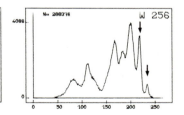

References: Blin,N., Stoehr,M., Hutter,K., Alonso,A., Goerttler,K. (1982) Chromosoma 85:723-733. Davies,K.E., Young,B.D., Elles,R.G., Hill,M.E., Williamson,R. (1981) Nature 293:374-376. Disteche,C.M., Kunkel,L.M., Lojewski,A., Orkin,S.H., Eisenhard,M., Sahar,E., Travis,B., Latt,S.A. (1982) Cytometry 2:282-286. Lebo,R.V., Carrano,A.V., Burkhart Schultz,K., Dozy,A.M., Yu,L.C., Kan,Y.W. (1979) Proc.Natl.Acad.Sci.USA 76:5804-5808.

MOLECULAR CLONING OF THE FACTOR IX GENE

Don E. Lavelle and Pudur Jagadeeswaran
Center for Genetics, University of Illinois at Chicago,
808 S. Wood Street, Chicago, Illinois 60612

Introduction:

We have been interested in hereditary disorders associated with the hematopoitic system. (1) Other than the hemoglobin mutants one of the most well known mutations in human hereditary disorders is hemophilia. There are two types of hemophilia, hemophilia A and hemophilia B. Hemophilia B is a sex linked disorder which results in production of no or defective Factor IX (zymogen of a serine protease which participates in the middle phase of the intrinsic pathway of blood coagulation). We have been interested in cloning the genes for Factor IX from both normal and defective individuals to understand the molecular basis for hemophilia B.

Results and Discussion:

As a first step in our attempts to understand the molecular basis for hemophilia B we began by cloning Factor IX cDNA. We chose an amino acid sequence in the bovine Factor IX molecule, namely glu-cys-trp-cys-gln-ala. From this we deduced possible 17 nucleotide long mixed probes, which we have synthesized. We have screened the human liver cDNA library with the kinased oligonucleotide probes by the Hanahan and Meselson high density colony screening method. The cDNA library was obtained from Dr. Savio. L. Woo. One of the clones out of this library showed a strong positive signal. From this clone, DNA was isolated and the nucleotide sequence was determined by the Maxam and Gilbert method. The amino acid sequence was predicted from the nucleotide sequence. Comparison of the predicted amino acid sequence with the already known partial amino acid sequence of human Factor IX has confirmed that we have Factor IX cDNA. During this analysis three separate papers have appeared on molecular cloning of Factor IX cDNA (2-4).

Our cDNA clone is not a complete cDNA clone. Both 5' and 3' end sequences are truncated. We have learned from S.L. Woo that Earl Davie had screened the same liver cDNA library as we had in order to isolate his cDNA clone. Our cDNA sequence differs from that of Earl Davie. The sequences differ by one amino acid codon. The cDNA that we have isolated has one internal codon less than that of Davie, ours lacking a codon for alanine. The Maxam Gilbert nucleotide sequence autoradiograph showing the alanine codon difference is given in Figure 1.

Since two different clones (ours and Davie's) were obtained from the same library, either there must be more than one copy of the Factor IX gene present in the cells, or alternatively there is only a single gene which must exhibit differential splicing. However, the lack of splicing concensus sequences in the region containing the additional codon in Davie's clone argues against the latter possibility. We have conducted Southern blot analysis of the restriction digests of human genomic DNA. Since our blots of cellular DNA show that there is only one copy of the Factor IX gene per haploid genome, we conclude that the library must have been obtained from a female. Therefore the difference of one codon is due to a polymorphism. Another group has also observed this variation (4). Therefore, it seems like a common polymorphism. We

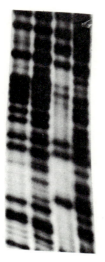

C G G A
   T G G

5'ATTCGAΔATTATTCCT3'

Fig 1: Maxam and Gilbert pattern showing the missing codon. The nuc-
cleotide sequence is given on the right side of the pattern.
The triangle within the sequence indicates the position of
the missing codon.

have also screened the genomic phage library and obtained a positive
clone. This was plaque purified. The DNA was isolated and was
transfered to nitrocllulose filter by Southern blotting. The filter was
hybridized with the nick translated Factor IX cDNA. The results
indicate that the phage DNA has Factor IX gene. Further
characterization of this clone will be presented.

Summary:

We have cloned a cDNA for Factor IX and identified a deletion
polymorphism. We have also isolated a genomic clone for Factor IX. The
characterization of the gene is underway.

References:

1. Jagadeeswaran, P., Tuan, D., Forget, B.G., and Weissman, S.M.,
Nature 296:469, 1982.
2. Kurachi, K., and Davie, E.W., Proc. Natl. Acad. Sci. USA 79:6461,
1982.
3. Choo, K.H., Gould, K.G., Rees, D.J.G., and Brownlee, G.G., Nature
299:178, 1982.
4. Jaye, M., De La Salle, H., Schamber, F., Balland, A., Kohli, V.,
Findeli, A., Tolstoshev, P., and Lecocq, J., Nuc. Acids Res. 11:2325,
1983.

ANALYSIS OF SINGLE BASE SUBSTITUTIONS IN HUMAN DNA. by N. Lumelsky, L.S. Lerman and S.G. Fischer, Dept. of Biological Sciences, State University of NY, 1400 Washington Ave., Albany, NY 12222.

Although the presence of a base substitution in DNA can sometimes be detected by the loss of the restriction site, a multiplicity of tests with a large number of endonucleases provides only a modest probability of recognition.

We have shown (1) that base substitutions in a segment of λ DNA can be detected from the positions of DNA fragments in a denaturing gradient gel, and partial identification of the particular exchange can be inferred. We have applied the same procedure to the detection of base substitutions in the human β-globin gene with respect to changes responsible for β-thalassemia. Again, substantial inference can be drawn as to the type of substitution.

The Denaturing Gradient System. The procedure and equipment for the denaturing gel electrophoresis was described previously (2). In our system, DNA molecules migrate into a polyacrylamide gel containing an ascending concentration of denaturants (urea, formamide). As DNA molecules move into the gel, they are exposed to a gradual denaturation-promoting change in the medium which is linearly equivalent (3) to a gradual increase in temperature. DNA molecules undergo an abrupt decline in mobility at a characteristic depth, resulting in positions and patterns that change little if the application of the field is continued. The strong retardation as the helix unravels provides the basis for sequence-determined separation.

Detection of Single-Base Substitutions in the Recombinant Plasmids Carrying Mutant β-globin Genes. We have analyzed five recombinant plasmids which carry five different mutant human β-globin genes(Table I).(All plasmids were gifts of T. Maniatis, Harvard University.) Plasmids were digested with the appropriate restriction enzyme and then either electrophoresed directly into a denaturing gradient gel, or first separated by size in a standard polyacrylamide gel and then run into a denaturing gradient gel to make a two-dimensional pattern.

Plasmid carrying mutation	Site of the mutation	Nature of the mutation	Separation in denaturing gel
πβ° VII	IVS1, pos 6	T→C	+(6mm)
πβ° P29	IVS1, pos 1	G→A	+(8mm)
πβ° G15	IVS2,pos745	G→C	−
πβ° K	IVS1, pos 5	G→C	+(1mm)
#39 β°	exon 2,pos25	C→T	−
IVS1β+	IVS1, pos110	G→A	+(2mm)

TABLE I

We will achieve the maximum separation in a denaturing gel if the substitution occurs in the most easily melted part of the DNA molecule. The statistical-mechanical melting theory has enabled us to make a direct theoretical calculation of the melting progression as the temperature is raised for any fragment of DNA for which the sequence of bases is known. The calculated melting pattern of a given DNA molecule guides the choice of restriction endonuclease, such that the test region will be adjacent on one or both sides to more stable regions, and less stable regions are excluded. If a substitution occurs in a

very GC-dense region and is surrounded by AT-dense regions, it is
difficult to choose useful fragment boundaries the desirable way. Our
present system is not sensitive to substitutions outside the most-
easily-melted part of a DNA molecule at present, but work now in progress will circumvent this limitation.

The result of a typical two-dimensional separation is represented in
Figure 1. We mixed the DNA of two recombinant plasmids carrying human β-
globin genes, one with a mutant β-globin gene (πβ°P29, IVS1,pos.1,G→A tran-
sition) and another one with a normal
β-globin gene(πSVWT2). The mixture was
digested to completion with Hae III.
The control sample, the plasmid containing the normal β-globin gene, was
digested alone. Hae III digestion
produces a 272 bp fragment carrying
the substitution in the least stable
region. After the separation according

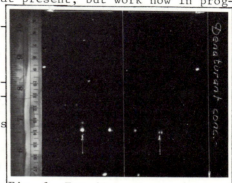

Fig. 1. Two-dimensional separation of DNA restriction fragments in a denaturing gel.

to length by conventional electrophoresis in a polyacrylamide gel, the
strip containing the broad spectrum of DNA fragments was sealed over
the top of the denaturing gradient gel perpendicular to the gradient
direction, and electrophoresis was carried out to give a two-dimensional pattern. The left and right sides of Fig. 1 are mirror images,
in that the length of the fragments increases from right to left in
the mixed pattern, and from left to right in the control, as shown.
The 272 bp fragments in the mixed sample are seen as two distinct
spots. At the same time, only one spot appears on the right side. All
other fragments form tight individual spots. The results show that a
single base substitution in the 272 bp DNA fragment produces sufficient change in retardation properties for the fragment to travel several mm less deep into the gel than wild type,and agrees with the lower
melting stability of an AT vs. a GC pair.

Detection of Point Mutations Directly in Human Genomic DNA.Simi-
lar mutations were identified in human genomic DNA. The samples were
extracted from human leukocytes as described(4). After digestion with
Hae III, two-dimensional separation was carried out as with plasmid
fragments. The DNA from the denaturing gel was transferred to the
hybridization membrane(GeneScreenPlus)(5)and then hybridized with a
[32]P-labeled probe. The hybridization conditions were similar to those
described (6). We could discriminate a single bp substitution in a 272
bp Hae III fragment in human genomic DNA. These substitutions are not
detected by any known restriction enzyme. Our theoretical analysis
shows that we should be able to detect and characterize all possible
substitutions in this 272 bp restriction fragment.

Refs. 1.Fischer,SG,Lerman,LS,PNAS 80:1579-83(1983);2.Fischer,SG,Ler-
man,LS Meth Enzym 68:183-91(1979);3.Lerman,LS,Fischer,SG,Bregman,DB,
Silverstein,KJ in:Biomolecular Stereodynamics(ed.R.Sarma)Adenine Press
1981,459-70;4.Wilson,JT et al PNAS 79:3628-31(1981);5.Levinger,L, J
Molec Biol 146:287-304(1981);6.Wahl,GM, Stern,M, Stark,GR PNAS 76:
3683-87(1979).

POSSIBILITY OF PRENATAL DIAGNOSIS OF CLASSICAL PKU BY RESTRICTION
FRAGMENT LENGTH POLYMORPHISM ANALYSIS OF THE PHENYLALANINE HYDROXY-
LASE GENE

Alan Lidsky, Fred Ledley, Anthony DiLella, Kathryn Robson, and
Savio L. C. Woo
Howard Hughes Medical Institute, Dept. of Cell Biology, Baylor
College of Medicine, Houston, Texas 77030

Classical phenylketonuria (PKU) is a typical example of inborn
errors in metabolism and is characterized by a deficiency of the
hepatic enzyme phenylalanine hydroxylase (PH) which normally converts
phenylalanine to tyrosine. The genetic disorder causes impairment of
post-natal brain development, resulting in severe mental retardation
in untreated children. The disease is transmitted as an autosomal
recessive trait and has a collective prevalence of about 1 in 10,000
among Caucasians so that 2% of the population are carriers of the
PKU trait.

In order to characterize the inherited disease at the molecular
level, we have recently reported the purification of messenger RNA
coding for PH, the synthesis of its complementary DNA and the isolation of its structural gene by molecular cloning. To develop an
analytical procedure for diagnosis of PKU at the gene level, we have
taken advantage of the existence of many benign nucleotide polymorphisms throughout the human genome some of which alter the recognition sequence of restriction endonucleases. To search for restriction site polymorphisms in the PH gene, we isolated genomic DNA from
a panel of random, but otherwise normal Caucasians and analyzed the
DNAs with a number of restriction enzymes followed by Southern blotting using the PH cDNAs as a hybridization probe. Three of the
enzymes used have revealed polymorphic fragment sizes in the PH gene
locus, Msp I, Sph I, and Hind III. The Msp I restriction site polymorphism reveals two variant fragments of 23 kb and 19 kb in length,
with frequencies of .45 and .55 respectively. Upon digestion with
Sph I, some individuals are homozygous for either a 7.0 kb band or
for a 9.7 kb band. The frequencies are .94 and .06 for the 7.0 and
9.7 kb fragments respectively. A third restriction fragment length
polymorphism is detected with Hind III. Among a number of DNA fragments common to all individuals, some are homozygous for either a
4.2 kb, a 4.0 kb , or a 4.4 kb band, and others are heterozygous for
2 of the 3 fragments. The frequencies of the Hind III fragments are
.70, .24, and .06 for the 4.2, 4.0, and 4.4 kb fragments respectively. Although the polymorphisms in the human PH locus bear no direct
relationship to the PKU trait per se, they can nevertheless be used
as a tightly linked marker, to tract the mutant PH genes in PKU
families.

The analysis of a PKU family by Hind III polymorphism is shown in
Figure I. In this family, both parents are heterozygous for the 4.2
and 4.0 kb bands as shown in lanes 1 and 2. There are 2 affected
children in this family and both are homozygous for the 4.2 kb band
as shown in lanes 3 and 4, indicating that the PKU genes in this
family are associated with the 4.2 kb fragments. An unaffected

sibling who is homo-
zygous for the 4.0 kb
band as shown in lane
5 must be free of the
PKU trait, and a sec-
ond unaffected sib-
ling who is hetero-
zygous for the 2 bands
as shown in lane 6 must
have inherited 1 copy
of the mutant gene and
1 copy of the normal
gene from either parent,
and must therefore be a
carrier of the PKU trait.

Figure I.

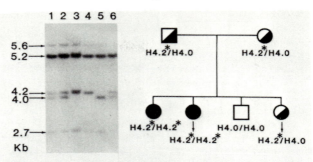

Thus, should there be a hypothetical pregnancy in this family in the
future, prenatal diagnosis of the genetic disorder can be achieved
by amniocentesis followed by analysis of chromosomal DNA isolated
from the cultured amniotic cells or chorionic villi. The polymorphism
analysis is dependent on the heterozygosity of the restriction sites
in the PH genes in the parents, so that one may distinguish the PKU
allele from the normal. Therefore, it is important to estimate the
probability of any given individual in the population to be heterozygous with respect to any of the 3 restriction site polymorphisms.
Using the frequencies of the individual fragments in a panel of 20
normal Caucasians, it has been calculated that approximately 75% of
Caucasians in the general population would be heterozygous for at
least one of these polymorphisms.

In all families studied thus far, complete segregation concordance
between the mutant PH gene, as detected with the RFLP's, and the disease
phenotype has been observed. These results strongly suggest that PKU
is the result of mutational events in the PH gene itself and is not
caused by some other trans-regulatory mechanisms. We have also used
the human PH cDNA to map the PKU locus in man. A panel of human/mouse
somatic cell hybrids containing different assortments of human chromosomes was used to localize the PH gene in the human genome. Genomic
DNA from 17 hybrid cell lines was digested with Bam HI and subjected
to Southern blot analysis using the human PH DNA as a hybridization
probe. The presence of a 20.5 kb fragment indicated the presence of
the chromosome containing the PH gene. Complete segregation concordance was observed between the presence of the PH 20.5 kb fragment and
human chromosome 12. Since the PH gene has been assigned to chromosome 12, the PKU locus is also on chromosome 12. The existence of
multiple RFLPs in the PH locus would also mean that the human cDNA
clone can serve as a polymorphic marker for chromosome 12.

We have recently isolated longer PH cDNA clones and are presently
searching for additional RFLPs in this locus. These will be useful in
increasing the percent heterozygosity observed in the population. This
would mean that we could increase the number of families for which we
could do prenatal diagnosis and heterozygote determination of classical PKU.

ISOLATION, PARTIAL CHARACTERIZATION AND CELL CYCLE REGULATION OF
HUMAN H1 HISTONE GENE IN A CLUSTER WITH CORE HISTONE CODING

SEQUENCES. F. Marashi†, M. Plumb†, L. Green†, J. Stein*, and
G. Stein†. †Department of Biochemistry and Molecular Biology and
*Department of Immunology and Medical Microbiology, College of
Medicine, University of Florida, Gainesville, Florida 32610, USA.

Summary — We describe the isolation and characterization of a human
histone gene cluster which contains at least one of each of the
five histone genes (H1, H2A, H2B, H3 and H4). Furthermore, the
cloned H1 gene is used to establish that the cellular abundance of
hybridizable H1 and core histone mRNAs is coordinately regulated
during the HeLa cell cycle and exhibits a temporal and functional
relationship to the rate of DNA synthesis.

Introduction — More than nine distinct genomic histone clusters
have been previously characterized, all conspicuously lacking H1
coding sequences (1-4). The heteromorphic organization of these
clusters indicates that the genes are not organized as simple
tandem repeats. The absence of H1 coding sequences suggests
functional and regulatory differences in human core and H1 histone
gene expression which is supported by evidence that although H1 and
core histone proteins are synthesized predominantly in S phase
(5-8), a higher basal level of histone H1 synthesis is detected in
G1 and quiescent cells than for core histones (6,7).

Results — A recombinant phage, λHHG415, containing a human H1
histone gene (Fig. 1A) was isolated using a chicken H1 histone
sequence (9) as a probe. Histone coding regions were identified by
hybridization with homologous and heterologous probes and by hybrid
selection/in vitro translation. Based on DNA sequence analysis
(Fig. 1B) the amino terminus of the encoded H1 protein shares
extensive homology with corresponding regions of H1 histones from
rabbit (93.7%), X. laevis (83.4%) and trout (83.4%). Using this H1
gene and several core human histone genes (2,10) as hybridization
probes, we have examined the levels of hybridizable histone mRNAs
throughout the cell cycle in continuously dividing HeLa cells and
following stimulation of quiescent human diploid fibroblasts to
proliferate. In both types of cell populations the representation
of core and H1 mRNAs paralleled the rates of DNA synthesis.
Moreover, inhibition of DNA replication resulted in a rapid and
coordinate reduction of core and H1 histone transcripts.

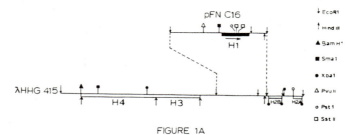

FIGURE 1A

```
-80        -70       -60       -50       -40       -30       -20       -10
CCCGGGCCCGAGCATAGCAGCAACGCAAAACCTGCTCTTTAGATTTCGAGCTTATTCTCTTCTAGCAGTTTCTTGCCACC ATG TCG GAA ACC
                                                                              Met Ser Glu Thr


GCT CCT GCC GAG ACA GCC ACC CCA GCG CCG GTG GAG AAA TCC CCG GCT AAG AAG AAG GCA ACT AAG AAG GCT
Ala Pro Ala Glu Thr Ala Thr Pro Ala Pro Val Glu Lys Ser Pro Ala Lys Lys Lys Ala Thr Lys Lys Ala
                    (10)                              (20)


GCC GGC GCC GGC GCT GCT AAG CGC ATA GCG GCG GGG CCC CCA GTC TCA GAG CTG ATC ACC AAG GCT GTG CCT
Ala Gly Ala Gly Ala Ala Lys Arg Ile Ala Ala Gly Pro Pro Val Ser Glu Leu Ile Thr Lys Ala Val Pro
                    (30)                              (40)                              (50)


GCT TCT AAG GAG CGC AAT GCC C
Ala Ser Lys Glu Arg Asn Ala                                        H1
```

FIGURE 1B

Discussion – We have isolated the first human H1 histone gene.
This H1 gene is located in a cluster with one each of core histone
coding sequences. Using this H1 gene and several core histone
genes as hybridization probes we have obtained evidence that
expression of both H1 and core histone genes is largely restricted
to the S phase of the cell cycle and that there appears to be a
temporal as well as functional relationship between DNA replication
and histone gene expression. It is interesting to note that
maximal cellular levels of core histone mRNAs appear to precede
those of H1 mRNAs, suggesting that this may be related to the
assembly of core particles which precedes H1 mediated nucleosome
condensation and the associated formation of higher ordered
chromatin structures. Tissue specificity and fluctuations in the
abundance of H1 histone protein subtypes at various stages of
development have been observed in mouse cells (11,12). The
availability of this human H1 histone gene will enable us to
examine the expression of H1 histone mRNA variants during the cell
cycle of HeLa cells.

Literature Cited

1. Hentschel, C.C. and Birnstiel, M.L. (1981) Cell 25, 301-13.
2. Sierra, F., Lichtler, A., Marashi, F., Rickles, R., Van Dyke,
    T., Clark, S., Wells, J., Stein, G., and Stein, J. (1982)
    Proc. Natl. Acad. Sci. USA 79, 1795-9.
3. Heintz, M., Zernik, M. and Roeder, R.G. (1981) Cell 24, 661-8.
4. Brusch, S. and Wells, J.R.E. (1981) Nucl. Acid Res. 9,
    1591-7.
5. Delegeane, A.M. and Lee, A.D. (1982) Science 215, 79-81.
6. Wu, R. and Bonner, W.M. (1981) Cell 27, 321-30.
7. Tarnowka, M.A. and Gablioni, C. (1978) Cell 15, 163-71.
8. Waith, W.I., Renaud, J., Nadeau, P., and Pallotta, D. (1983)
    Biochemistry 22, 1778-83.
9. Clark, S.J., Krieg, P.A., Wells, J.R.E. (1981) Nucl. Acid Res.
    9, 1583-90.
10. Plumb, M., Stein, J., and Stein, G. (1983) Nucl. Acid Res. 11,
    2391-410.
11. Pehrson, J.R. and Cole, R.D. (1982) Biochemistry 21, 456-60.
12. Lennox, R.W. and Cohen, L.H. (1983) Biol. Chem. 258, 262-8.

202

Restriction enzyme fragment length polymorphism (RFLP) of human pre-pro-parathyroid gene in isolated clones and in a population survey.

Hubert Mayer, Georg Widera, Erich Breyel
GBF -Gesellschaft für Biotechn. Forschung mbH, Mascheroder Weg 1,
3300 Braunschweig

Jörg Schmidtke
Inst. für Humangenetik, Univ. Göttingen, Nikolausbergerweg 5a,
3400 Göttingen

Parathyroid hormone (PTH) is the principal homeostatic regulator of blood calcium. The organisation of the human PTH gene is known (1). Here we describe restriction enzyme fragment length polymorphism in two genomic DNA-clones encoding human Prepro-PTH and the results of a population survey.

A pyhsical map of two   phages encoding human Prepro-PTH isolated from a human foetal liver genomic DNA library constructed in phage Charon 4 A by Lawn et al. (2) is summarized in Fig. 1. All EcoRI-fragments of the two clones cross-hybridize except the EcoRI 3'-endfragments. The two clones were furthermore distinguished in their XbaI and EcoRI cleavage sites and in the PTH-coding-EcoRI-fragments in their PstI, Sau 3A, TaqI, HaeIII, AluI cleavage sites. p2.24 has a deletion of ca. 200bp in the 3' noncoding region in comparison with the other clone. By DNA-sequenz analysis of p20.36 we can deduce the location of two intervening sequences (IVS) interrupting the PTH gene. The first IVS interrupting the 5' noncoding region of the mRNA is only partially present in the clones. The DNA-sequence of p20.36 confirms the previously determined PTH-genomic DNA-sequence (1). The results of a population survey for genomic DNA-polymorphism detectable with p20.36 are summarized in Fig. 2   While no polymorphism was found with BamHI, EcoRI, HindIII and MspI, one rare polymorphism was observed with XbaI, and two frequent polymorphisms with PstI and TaqI, respectively. The interpretation of the PstI polymorphism is outlined schematically in Fig. 2.

p20.36 detects RFLP's with a high frequency. The overall heterozygosity observed with this probe is 0.012, which is approximately three times higher than the genomic average in man (Cooper and Schmidtke, in press).

On genomic blots p20.36 cross-hybridizes with a sequence of unknown location and function. This sequence hybridizes much fainter. In the different digests it is probably represented by: EcoRI - 2kb, HindIII- 4.8kb, MspI - 2.3 and 3.3kb, TaqI - 1kb, XbaI - 5.8kb, BamHI and PstI- not detected.

References. (1) Lawn, R.M., Fritsch, E.F., Parker, R.C., Blake, G. and Maniatis, T. (1981) Cell 15, 1157-1174; (2) Vasicek, T.J., McDevitt, B.E., Freeman, M.W., Fennick, B.J., Hendy, G.N., Potts, J.T.jr., Rich, A. and Kronenberg, (1983) Proc. Natl. Acad. Sci. USA 80, 2127-2131

203

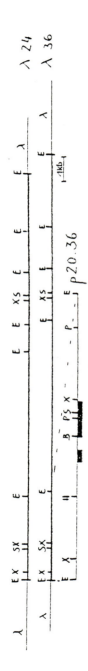

Fig.1
Restriction map of two human prepro-PTH clones.

Fig.2
Southern blotts of
chromosomal DNAs
from a population
survey.

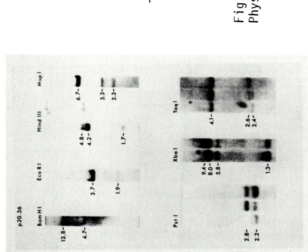

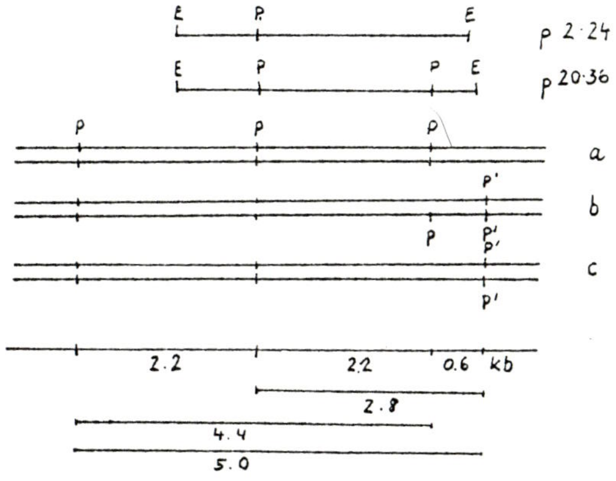

Fig.3
Physical map of Pst-polymorphism.

RESTRICTION ENZYME SITE POLYMORPHISMS OF CLASS II
HISTOCOMPATIBILITY GENE SEQUENCES IN WILD MICE

Thomas J. McConnell and Edward K. Wakeland
Dept. of Pathology, Univ. of Florida, Gainesville, Florida 32610

Genes controlling immune responsiveness in mice are located within the $\underline{I}$ region of the murine $\underline{H-2}$ complex (1). A molecular map of the $\underline{I}$ region has been obtained recently through the analysis of a genomic cosmid library (2). Four genes controlling immune responsiveness, denoted $\underline{A}_\alpha$, $\underline{A}_\beta$, $\underline{E}_\alpha$, and $\underline{E}_\beta$, have been identified and DNA probes specific for these genes have been made available. Serologic and biochemical analysis of $\underline{I}$ region gene products have demonstrated extensive genetic polymorphisms among standard laboratory mice (3) and in wild mouse populations (4,5).

We have been studying the polymorphism of these genes in wild mouse populations of $\underline{Mus\ m.\ domesticus}$, $\underline{Mus\ m.\ musculus}$, and $\underline{Mus\ castaneus}$ with the intent of determining how these genes diversify (4-6). A collection of mouse strains carrying 30 independently derived $\underline{H-2}$ haplotypes from laboratory and wild mice has been produced and the expressed I region gene products of these strains have been serologically and structurally compared (7).

In this report, we have used a DNA probe specific for $\underline{A}_\beta$ to assess the genetic variability of $\underline{A}_\beta$ in 30 $\underline{H-2}$ haplotypes. Our results reveal extensive variability in restriction enzyme sites within and flanking $\underline{A}_\beta$, indicating that the analysis of restriction enzyme site polymorphisms will be a valuable tool for the analysis of I region gene diversity in wild mice.

MATERIALS AND METHODS.   Genomic DNA was prepared by standard methods from livers (8). 20 μg of DNA from each strain was digested with 20 units of restriction enzyme for 16 hrs. under conditions described by the supplier (BRL, Bethesda, Maryland). Restriction fragments were electrophoresed through 0.7% agarose gels for 40 hours at 1.5 V/cm and transferred to nylon filters (Pall, Glen Cove, New York) by the method of Southern (9). $\underline{A}_\beta$ related sequences were detected by hybridization with a $^{32}P-$ labeled 5.8 kb genomic EcoRI fragment containing $\underline{A}_\beta^d$. This plasmid was kindly supplied by Dr. Lee Hood, California Institute of Technology. Hybridization conditions were as described (2).

RESULTS AND DISCUSSION.   Genomic DNAs from 30 mouse strains, including 11 $\underline{H-2}$ haplotypes of standard laboratory mice and 19 $\underline{H-2}$ haplotypes extracted from $\underline{Mus\ m.\ domesticus}$, $\underline{Mus\ m.\ musculus}$, and $\underline{Mus\ castaneus}$ were digested with Kpn I, Hind III, EcoRI, BamHI, Pvu II, or Pst I, and analyzed by Southern blot hybridization with a $^{32}P-$labeled $\underline{A}_\beta$ specific DNA probe derived from the genome of Balb/c ($\underline{H-2}^d$). Polymorphisms in restriction enzyme (RE) cleavage sites were detected by pair-wise comparisons between samples electrophoresed on the same gel. The results of these comparisons were tabulated as the total number of $\underline{A}_\beta$-related fragments shared by two DNAs divided by the total number of $\underline{A}_\beta$-related fragments detected in both DNAs.

Previous studies of the $\underline{A}_\beta$ polypeptides expressed by these strains have indicated that A$_\beta$ alleles can be organized into "families" of related alleles based on the structures of their A$_\beta$ polypeptides. A$_\beta$ alleles within the same family encode similar A$_\beta$ polypeptides which are identical in more than 90% of their tryptic peptides, while A$_\beta$ polypeptides encoded by alleles in separate families are identical in less than 70% of their tryptic peptides (8,9).

Our analysis of the RE site polymorphisms of A$_\beta$ in these strains is consistent with results obtained by analysis of A$_\beta$ polypeptides. Alleles in separate families generally share less than 30% of A$_\beta$-related fragments, while A$_\beta$ alleles within the same family generally share more than 50% of their A$_\beta$-related fragments.

Table 1. Matrix comparison of RE polymorphisms distinguishing A$_\beta$ alleles in separate A$_\beta$ families.

Strain	B10	B10.WB	B10.PL	B10.BUA16	B10.F	B10.S
B10	–	21[1]	11	6	15	32
B10.WB	8/38[2]	–	17	0	14	23
B10.PL	4/36	4/24	–	10	8	16
B10.BUA16	2/34	0/22	2/20	–	8	0
B10.F	6/40	4/28	2/26	2/24	–	21
B10.S	12/38	6/26	4/25	0/22	6/28	–

[1] Percentage of A$_\beta$-related restriction fragments shared in a paired comparison of the two strains listed.

[2] The numerator is the total number of shared A$_\beta$-related RE fragments and the denominator is the total number A$_\beta$-related RE fragments detected in all six digests.

The results in Table 1 are representative of comparisons between any of the 19 A$_\beta$ "families" identified among the 30 H-2 haplotypes surveyed. An example of results obtained when alleles within the same family are compared is presented in Table 2.

Table 2. Matrix comparison of RE polymorphisms distinguishing A$_\beta$ alleles within the "pq" family.

Geographical Origin of Wild Mouse Ancestor	Strain	B10.Q	B10.CAA2	B10.STC77	B10.CAS2	B10.SAA48
Laboratory inbred	B10.Q	–	100[1]	80	67	19
California	B10.CAA2	28/28[2]	–	80	67	19
Michigan	B10.STC77	24/30	24/30	–	53	17
Thailand	B10.CAS2	10/15	10/15	10/19	–	50
Michigan	B10.SAA48	4/21	4/21	4/24	6/12	–

[1],[2] See Table 1.

Most of the strains listed in Table 2 are clearly more similar than those compared in Table 1. However, B10.SAA48 is only significantly related to B10.CAS2 and does not appear closely-related to any of the other A$_\beta$ alleles in Table 2. These results demonstrate gradations in the similarity of A$_\beta$ alleles within A$_\beta$ families and indicate that a detailed analysis of these closely-related alleles may be informative about the genetic mechanisms causing the diversification of A$_\beta$ in natural mouse populations.

REFERENCES.   1) Benacerraf, B. (1981) Science 212, 1229; 2) Steinmetz, M. et al. (1982) Nature 300, 35; 3) Klein et al. (1978) Immunogenetics 9, 489; 4) Wakeland, E. & J. Klein (1979) Immunogenetics 8, 27; 5) Wakeland, E. and J. Klein (1981) J. Immunol. 126, 1734; 6) Wakeland, E. and J. Klein (1979) Immunogenetics 9, 535; 7) Wakeland & Klein (1983) J. Immunol. 130, 1280; 8) Maniatis, T., E.F. Fritsch & J. Sambrook (1982) IN: Molecular Cloning, A Laboratory Manual, p. 280; 9) Southern, E. (1979) IN: Methods in Enzymology, Volume 68, ed. R. Wu, p. 152.

THE EXPRESSION OF A PRO-OPIOMELANOCORTIN-LIKE GENE IN MURINE LEYDIG TUMOR CELLS

Michael H. Melner[1] and David Puett[1]

Dept. of Biochemistry, Vanderbilt University, Nashville, TN 37232

[1]Current Address: The Reproductive Sciences and Endocrinology
Laboratories, Dept. of Biochemistry, University
of Miami School of Medicine, Miami, FL 33101

ABSTRACT - Recent evidence has demonstrated a localization of β-endorphin (β-EP) in extra-pituitary tissues and cells, including the Leydig cells of the testis. This localization could reflect either an accumulation of the peptide or de novo synthesis within the cell in a precursor form similar to pro-opiomelanocortin (POMC) in the anterior pituitary. This study presents evidence that antibodies against β-EP and (ACTH) precipitate identical precursor molecules from total cellular mRNA translation products of M5480A Leydig tumor cells. These data demonstrate the synthesis of POMC-like mRNA in this Leydig cell tumor and implicate biosynthesis as a contributing process to the presence of these peptides in Leydig cells.

INTRODUCTION - β-EP and ACTH are derived from the POMC precursor in the pituitary following post-translational processing (1,2). Recently, immunoreactive β-endorphin has been demonstrated in the testis (3) with a specific localization in the Leydig cells (4,5). Herein, we have investigated the presence of specific immunoreactive precursor molecules in translation products from total cellular mRNA in the M5480A murine Leydig cell tumor. This tumor is a well-characterized cell line which has maintained gonadotropin-responsive steroidogenesis through multiple serial passages in vivo (6).

MATERIALS AND METHODS - Murine Leydig tumor cells were maintained by serial transplantation (6). Total RNA was prepared from Leydig tumor cells by the method of Chirgwin et al. (7) and total cellular mRNA purified on poly(U)-Sepharose 4B. Total mRNA translations were performed using a cell-free wheat germ translation system prepared by the method of Haralson et al. (8) using ^{35}S-methionine. Following translation for 90 min at 23°C, assay mixtures were centrifuged at 105,000 xg for 1 hr. Supernatants were incubated with a 1:200 dilution of antisera for 24 hr at 4°C. Normal rabbit serum was added with anti-rabbit IgG and incubated for 4 hrs at 4°C. Precipitates were centrifuged at 15,000 xg for 5 min and washed 2X. Immunoprecipitates were solubized in 7M urea, 0.125 M Tris-HCI, pH 6.8, 3% SDS, 10% β-mercaptoethanol and electrophoresed (9).

RESULTS AND DISCUSSION - Antiserum prepared against synthetic β-EP immunoprecipitated from total mRNA translation products seven distinct species as determined by SDS-polyacrylamide gel electrophoresis (Figure 1). These seven ^{35}S-methionine labeled components correspond to M_r 46 K, 44.5 K, 42.5 K, 38 K, 35.5 K, 31.5 K, and

25.5 K. Immunoprecipitations performed using antibodies directed against ACTH yielded components with identical M_r and similar relative proportions to those which utilize β-EP antisera (Figure 1). The substitution of normal rabbit serum for the primary antibody as a control demonstrated no significant non-specific immunoprecipitation (Figure 1). Multiple experiments using different mRNA preparations yielded identical results.

These data indicate the expression of a POMC-like gene in these Leydig tumor cells. Previous studies have partially characterized the POMC related peptides in rat testes. Margioris et al. (10) have determined that β-endorphin represents the major immunoreactive endorphin in the testes with no α-N-acetylated forms of β-endorphin or β-lipotropin being detected.

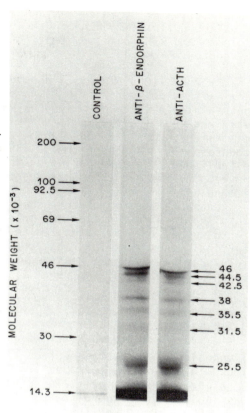

Fig. 1 Autoradiographs of antisera immunoprecipitated ^{35}S-labeled mRNA translation products following SDS-PAGE in 10% gels.

REFERENCES - Roberts, J.L., and Herbert, E. (1977) Proc. Natl. Acad. Sci. USA 74, 4826; (2) Eipper, B.A., and Mains, R.E. (1978) J. Biol. Chem. 253, 5732; (3) Sharp, B., Pekary, A.E., Meyer, N.V., and Hershman, J.M., (1980) Biochem. Biophys. Res. Comm. 95, 618; (4) Tsong, S.D., Phillips, D., Halmi, N., Liotta, A.S., Margioris, A., Bardin, C.W., and Krieger, D.T. (1982) Endocrinology 110, 2204; (5) Shu-Dong, T., Phillips, D.M., Halmi, N., Krieger, D., and Bardin, C.W. (1982) Biol. Reprod. 27, 755; (6) Ascoli, M. and Puett, D. (1978) Proc. Natl. Acad. Sci. USA 75, 99; (7) Chirgwin, J.M., Przybyla, A.E., MacDonald, R.J., and Ruter, W.J. (1979) Biochemistry 18, 5294; (8) Haralson, M.A., Sonneborn, J.H., and Mitchell, W.M. (1978) J. Biol. Chem. 253, 5536; (9) Laemmli, U.K., (1979) Nature 227, 680; (10) Margioris, A.N., Liotta, A.S., Vaudry, H., Bardin, C.W., and Krieger, D.T. (1983) Endocrinology 113, 663.

ACKNOWLEDGEMENTS - Supported in part by NIH CA09313 and AM15838. We thank Drs. Ray Zelinski, Colin Dykes, and Michael Haralson for helpful discussions. We are grateful to Dr. Nicholas Ling and Mr. Wendell Nicholson for gifts of antisera.

CONSTRUCTION OF HUMAN cDNA LIBRARIES FOR ISOLATION OF THE TERMINAL DEOXYNUCLEOTIDYLTRANSFERASE GENE. S.K. Moore, L.K. Riley, M.S. Coleman and R.C. Dickson. Dept. of Biochemistry, Univ. of KY Lexington, KY 40536

INTRODUCTION. Terminal deoxynucleotidyl transferase (TdT) is an enzyme that polymerizes in vitro deoxynucleoside 5' triphosphates onto a single-stranded oligodeoxynucleotide without template utilization. The enzyme is normally found only in cells from mammalian thymus and bone marrow and in their neoplastic counterparts. Although the in vivo function of TdT has not been established, the association of the enzyme with cells of the developing immune system has suggested that it may produce immunologic diversity (1,2).

Characterization of the gene coding for TdT may provide insights into the in vivo function and molecular mechanism for expression. To this end, we have attempted to isolate the gene coding for terminal transferase by first constructing a cDNA library. Because TdT is a low abundance message we chose two discrete approaches to enhance isolation of the gene: 1) cloning in the plasmid pBR322 using dG-dC tailing, and 2) cloning in the bacteriophage expression vector, λgtll, as developed by Young and Davis (3). Recombinants were screened for expression of terminal transferase using antibody directed against TdT.

MATERIALS AND METHODS. Construction of cDNA Libraries. Human lymphoblasts were obtained from a patient with acute lymphocytic leukemia undergoing therapeutic leukapheresis. Extracts contained high levels of terminal transferase activity. From these, polyA RNA was isolated. In vitro translation of the RNA in the presence of ^{35}S-methionine showed that only one protein, M_R=60,000, was competed out when cold terminal transferase was added prior to immunoprecipitation. cDNA libraries were constructed as described in Figures 1 and 2.

Preparation of Antibodies. Monospecific antibody was prepared by injecting rabbits with purified TdT from calf thymus. Because sera contain antibodies against E. coli proteins which would obscure specific TdT-antibody complexes, antibody samples were purified over an antigen affinity column prior to use.

Identification of Clones. Efficient screening of the libraries was achieved by utilizing antibody against TdT to detect antigen-producing clones. Briefly, the library constructed with pBR322 was printed onto nitrocellulose in a specific array, grown overnight at 37°C and lysed (3). Plaques from the phage library were plated at high density, transferred to nitrocellulose, and the lacZ gene was induced by IPTG. In both cases, remaining protein reactive sites were blocked with BSA. Nitrocellulose filters were then incubated with primary antibody. Binding of the antibody was detected by incubation with ^{125}I-Protein A and subsequent autoradiography. Controls with authentic TdT showed that as little as 500 pg of TdT could be detected.

RESULTS AND DISCUSSION. The library constructed with pBR322 was comprised of about 30,000 transformants and contained 30-50%

recombinants. Initial screening yielded 4 positive clones. Positive clones were re-screened without primary antibody and 3 bound Protein A alone. This finding was unexpected as the cDNA was derived from T-cell lymphoblasts which normally do not produce immunoglobulins. We are currently testing these clones for their ability to bind antibody directed against the F_C portion of immunoglobulins.

The library constructed with λgt11 contained approximately 50,000 recombinant phage. Preliminary screening showed 20 positive plaques. To further confirm putative clones of the gene for terminal transferase, we are curently screening clones with monoclonal antibodies to TdT. We believe that our findings, to date, indicate that it is likely we have isolated a partial cDNA for the human gene for TdT.

REFERENCES

1. Baltimore, D. (1974) Nature 248:409-411.
2. Bollum, F.J. (1975) Karl August Forster Lectures, Vol. 14, pp. 1-47, Franz Steiner Verlag, Wiesbaden.
3. Young, R.A. and Davis, R.W. (1983) PNAS 80:1194-1198.

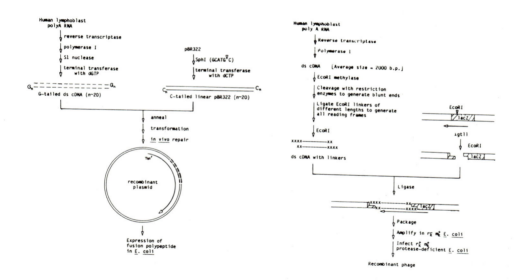

Fig 1. Construction of a cDNA library derived from human lymphoblast polyA RNA using pBR322. Expression of the cloned segment is presumably directed by the promoter for the tetracycline resistance gene of pBR322.

Fig 2. Construction of a cDNA library derived from polyA RNA from human lymphoblasts using λgt11. Expression of the cloned segment is presumably directed by the promoter for the lacZ gene of λgt11.

V-MOS EXPRESSION IN CELLS INFECTED WITH A MUTANT OF MUSV IS ACTIVATED BY A TEMPERATURE-SENSITIVE RNA SPLICING EVENT

Micheal A. Nash, Bill L. Brizzard and Edwin C. Murphy, Jr.
Dept. Tumor Biol., UTSCC M.D. Anderson Hosp., Houston, TX 77030

NRK cells infected with a ts mutant of wild-type MuSV-349, designated MuSVts110, assume a transformed phenotype at 33° but revert to a normal phenotype at 39°C. At 39°C, infected cells contain a single truncated viral gag gene polypeptide, P58^{gag} and a 4.0 kb viral RNA. At 33°C, however, a gag-gene/mos-gene fusion protein, P85$^{gag-mos}$, appears in concert with the appearance of a 3.5 kb viral RNA. Heteroduplex analysis has shown that, relative to wild-type 5.3 kb MuSV-349 RNA, the MuSVts110 4.0 kb RNA has suffered an approximately 1.5 kb deletion (Δ_1) resulting in a fusion of the middle of the gag gene p30 coding region to a downstream point near the first mos gene initiation codon. The MuSVts110 3.5 kb RNA deletion (Δ_2) includes the 1.5 kb deleted in the 4.0 kb RNA plus an additional 0.5 kb of p30 coding sequence (refer to Fig. 3).

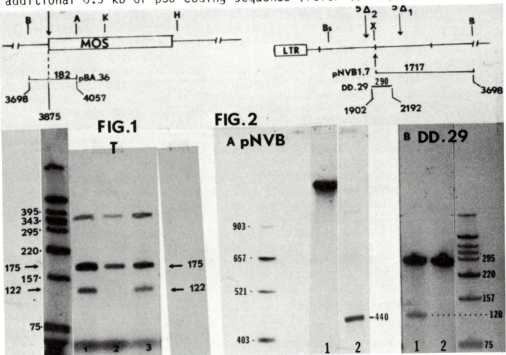

Fig. 1. Structure of the v-mos gene in MuSVts110 RNA. The 5' end labeled probe was hybridized to MuSVts110-RNA. S-1 digested and analyzed on a 4% gel in 8 M urea. pBA.36 DNA protected from S-1 digestion by RNA from cells (Lane 1), grown at 33°C; (Lane 2), shifted to 39°C; (Lane 3), shifted to 39°C, and reshifted to 33°C.

Fig. 2. Structure of the gag gene in MuSVts110 RNA. The 3' end labeled, probes were hybridized to MuSV-349 or MuSVts110 viral RNA, analyzed as in Fig. 1. Panel A: Protection of pNVB1.7 by (Lane 1) MuSV-349 RNA; (Lane 2) MuSVts110 RNA. Panel B: Protection of DD.29 by (Lane 1) MuSV ts110 RNA; (Lane 2) MuSV-349 RNA.

S-1 nuclease mapping of the mos gene end of the MuSVts110 RNA deletions, shown in Fig. 1, revealed the presence of two viral RNAs each with a distinct deletion in the MuSVts110 mos gene. As shown in Fig. 1, lane 1, RNA from infected cells grown at 33°C contains two different-sized mos genes, as evidenced by the protection of 175 and 122 bases of 5' end-labeled mos gene DNA. The second deletion mapped at an excellent splice-acceptor consensus sequence, raising the possibility that one of the RNAs was a splice product of the other. The S-1 nuclease data was correlated with the 4.0 kb and 3.5 kb MuSVts110 RNAs by temperature shift experiments combined with S-1 analysis. In contrast to RNA from cells grown at 33°C, RNA from cells grown at 39°C protects only the 175 base fragment (Fig. 1, lane 2), suggesting that it correlates with the 4.0 kb RNA. In cells reshifted to 33°C, both DNA fragments are again present (Fig. 1, lane 3). Thus, protection of the 122 base fragment correlates with the appearance and disappearance of the 3.5 kb RNA and P85gag-mos. Further S-1 analysis shows that the gag gene deletion in the 4.0 kb RNA maps at nucleotide 2104, (Fig. 2A) and in the 3.5 kb RNA at nucleotide 2017 (Fig. 2B). Of interest is the fact that near nucleotide 2017 is a splice donor site which would produce an in-frame splice with the acceptor within the mos gene.

Our data support a model in which a MuSVts110 4.0 kb RNA, containing an out of frame fusion of the gag and mos genes, is the primary transcript of the MuSVts110 viral DNA at both 39°C and 33°C. However, at 33°C a 443 base 'intron' can be spliced out of the 4.0 kb RNA, producing an in frame fusion of the gag and mos genes, and allowing the translation of the transforming protein, P85gag-mos.

FIG.3

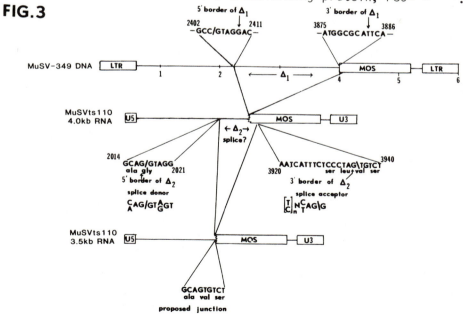

Fig. 3. Summary figure showing the deletion and splice points in MuSVts110 RNA relative to wild-type MuSV-349 RNA.

METAPHASE CHROMOSOME TRANSFER OF INSERTED SELECTABLE MARKERS:
A TOOL FOR GENE MAPPING AND ISOLATION

David L. Nelson and David E. Housman

Center for Cancer Research MIT Cambridge, MA 02138

Precise localization of mouse and human genes is limited by the resolution of currently available techniques. In particular, systematic methods for mapping mammalian chromosomal segments 10^6-10^7 base pairs in length are not currently available. To address this deficiency, we are developing an approach for mapping segments of mammalian chromosomes of this length. The method makes use of dominant selectable genetic markers introduced by retroviral vectors as selective agents for the transfer of chromosomal segments. Once isolated in a new background, these chromosome segments can be characterized and mapped using species specific repeat sequences. In order to develop this technique, we have initiated experiments in which mouse chromosome segments have been transferred to CV-1 monkey cells through the use of an inserted retroviral vector carrying the E. coli Xanthine-Guanosine Phospho-ribosyl transferase (gpt) gene (1).

INSERTION OF A SINGLE VECTOR GENOME INTO CAK CELLS. In the experiment illustrated, the pseudo-diploid mouse cell line CAK (2) was infected with ecotropic gpt virus (3) after tunicamycin (4) treatment. Selection was applied and yielded gpt[+] colonies. Three colonies (CAKgpt1, CAKgpt2 and CAKgpt5) were cloned and DNA was prepared from each. In Figure 1, DNA from each of these clones as well as from CAK cells, was digested with Eco RI, electrophoresed through a 1% agarose gel, transferred to nitrocellulose and hybridized to a probe specific for gpt sequences (5). Since Eco RI does not cut within the introduced gpt vector, viruses inserted into different genomic regions give different sized bands. Since each of the clones exhibits a gpt positive band of a different size, it is clear that the inserted gene is in a different location in each. The presence of only one band in each gpt[+] clone indicates that only a single gpt gene has been introduced into each cell clone. CAK DNA shows no hybridization.

METAPHASE CHROMOSOME TRANSFER TO MONKEY CELLS. Metaphase chromosomes were prepared (6) from CAKgpt5 cells and were applied to CV-1 monkey cells. Colonies positive for the gpt gene were selected and cloned. Transferrants containing mouse chromosomal segments should contain mouse repeat DNA which hybridizes to a total mouse DNA probe (7). We used DNA dot blotting (8) as a technique to determine the presence and quantity of mouse DNA in the transferrants. In Figure 2, DNA prepared from two transferrant cell lines, CVC5 2.1 and CVC5 2.3 was filtered onto a nitrocellulose membrane using a filtration manifold, along with standard DNAs prepared by mixing mouse and monkey DNAs at various percentages of mouse DNA to total 100 ng. The filter was hybridized to ^{32}P labeled total mouse DNA. The two transferrants

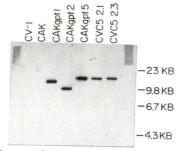

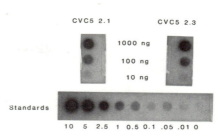

FIGURE 1. DETECTION OF INTEGRATED gpt CARRYING RETROVIRAL VECTORS. DNAs WERE ECO RI CLEAVED AND ELECTROPHORESED ON A 1% AGAROSE GEL. SOUTHREN TRANSFER WAS FOLLOWED BY HYBRIDIZATION TO ^{32}P-LABELED pBRgpt, A PLASMID CONTAINING THE E. COLI GPT GENE. THE FINAL WASH WAS 0.1x SSC, 0.1% SDS AT 55° C.

FIGURE 2. DETECTION OF CO-TRANSFERRED MOUSE REPEAT DNA SEQUENCES. DNAs WERE APPLIED TO NITROCELLULOSE THROUGH A MANIFOLD (S&S MINIFOLD). STANDARDS WERE CONSTRUCTED BY MIXING MOUSE DNA WITH MONKEY DNA TO TOTAL 100 NG AT THE PERCENTAGES GIVEN. THE FILTER WAS HYBRIDIZED TO ^{32}P-LABELED TOTAL MOUSE DNA. FINAL WASH: 0.1x SSC, 0.1% SDS AT 55° C.

gave clear hybridization, while negative control CV-1 DNA did not. This technique allows an estimation of the amount of mouse DNA co-transferred with the gpt gene. 100 ng of DNA from both transferrants when compared to the DNA standards, shows roughly the same hybridization as the 1 or 0.5% standards. By this method, we estimate that 10 to 20% of the gpt containing chromosome has been transferred. This agrees well with published estimates of the size of chromosome transferred as measured by cytogenetic methods (9).

TRANSFER OF AN INTEGRATED COPY OF THE gpt VECTOR WITH METAPHASE CHROMOSOMES. Figure 1 also shows DNA prepared from the two chromosome transferrants. If the gpt+ transferrants were derived from the transfer of an intact chromosomal segment surrounding the gpt gene, then Eco RI sites flanking the vector would be preserved, and the gpt+ bands in the transferrants would be the same as that in their parent. This is the case. CVC5 2.1 and CVC5 2.3 both have a gpt hybridizing band of the same size as their parent, CAKgpt5. Control CV-1 DNA shows no hybridization.

DISCUSSION. We have demonstrated introduction of a selectable gene into a mouse chromosome and use of that marker to transfer the adjacent chromosomal segment to a monkey cell. Using cloned low-order repeat DNAs (10), we have begun to map this and other segments of the mouse genome transferred to monkey cells. We have also extended the technique to human chromosomes employing hamster cells as recipients. This technique should prove very valuable in the fine resolution mapping of mammalian genomes, and in the isolation and cloning of large chromosomal regions.

References (1) Mulligan, R.C. and Berg, P. (1981) Mol. Cell. Biol. 1, 449; (2) Farber, R. and Liskay, R. (1979) Cytogenet. Cell Genet. 23, 3; (3) Mann, R., Mulligan, R.C. and Baltimore, D. (1983) Cell 33, 153; (4) Rein, A., Schultz, A.M., Bader, J.P., and Bassin, R.H. (1982) Virol 119, 185; (5) Southern, E.M. (1975) J. Mol. Biol. 98, 503; (6) Lewis, W.J., Srinivasin, P.R., Stohoe, N. and Siminovitch, L. (1980) Som. Cell Genet. 6, 337; (7) Gusella, J.F., Keys, C., Varsanyi-Breiner, A., Kao, F-T, Jones, C., Puck, T.T. and Housman, D. (1980) PNAS 77, 2829; (8) Kafatos, F.C., Jones, W.C. and Efstratiadis, A. (1979) Nucl. Acid Res. 7, 1541; (9) Olsen, A.S., McBride, O.W., and Moore, D.E. (1981) Mol. Cell Biol. 1, 439; (10) Gusella, J.F., Jones, C., Kao, F-T., Housman, D. and Puck, T.T. (1982) PNAS 79, 7804.

LOCATION OF MURINE LEUKEMIA VIRUS SEQUENCES WITHIN THE MURINE MAJOR HISTOCOMPATIBILITY COMPLEX, H-2

Christine Pampeno[1], Ruth Kornreich[1], Anthony Rossomando[1], Andrew L. Mellor[2], Elizabeth Weiss[2], Richard Flavell[2], Angel Pellicer[1] and Daniel Meruelo[1].

[1]Dept. of Pathology, New York Univ. Med. Center, NY, USA
[2]Biogen Research Corp., Cambridge, MA, USA

Studies in our laboratory investigating the H-2 linked resistance to Radiation leukemia virus-induced thymomas have evoked the possibility that viral DNA sequences may be located within the murine major histocompatibility complex (MHC) (1-4). To test this possibility, a viral probe, derived from a cloned ecotropic AKR provirus (5), was used to screen 38 overlapping cosmids encompassing 25 class I related H-2 gene sequences of the C57BL/10 mouse genome (6). Four of the 38 cosmids hybridized with the viral probe under stringent conditions. These four cosmids, H6, Bl.19, H43, and Bl.15, belong to a group of 10 overlapping cosmid clones defining four class I gene related sequences in a region of 90 kilobases of DNA. This cluster has been mapped to the T1 region of the MHC (manuscript in preparation).

Figure 1 shows a schematic diagram of the four over-lapping cosmids. Bam H1 digests of the cosmid clones were electrophoresed and transferred to nitrocellulose filters (7). The DNA blots were hybridized, under stringent conditions, with one of several probes. Regions hybridizing to the 5' or 3' end of the H-2 genes were detected with probes pH2111 and pH211 (8), respectively, and are indicated by dark boxes. Two viral probes, derived from the envelope protein gene sequences of the ecotropic AKR virus, were used. The pEco probe is a 2.7 kb SalI/Bam H1 fragment which includes the gp70 sequences of the cloned provirus, AKR 623 (5). The p15E probe is a 700 bp Xba I/ Pst I fragment located distal to the 3' end of the region of AKR encoding gp70 (9). Viral hybridizing fragments were positioned by 1) aligning the size of the hybridized fragment to the Bam H1 map 2) noting the presence of viral sequences in overlapping cosmids or their absence in non-overlapping cosmids 3) comparing the cohybridization of viral and H-2 gene probes.

Two regions within the H-2 cosmid cluster appear to be associated with retroviral sequences (Fig. 1). One region, hybridizing with both pEco and p15E probes, is located at the rightmost regions of cosmids H6 and H43. This region is not present in the Bl.19 cosmid. A Bam H1 fragment of Bl.19 which hybridizes with pEco, overlaps with the leftmost regions of cosmids H6 and H43. Cosmid Bl.19

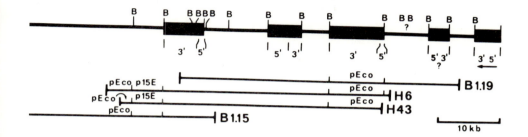

Figure 1.

lacks a p15E sequence, suggesting the presence of a defective viral genome. Preliminary experiments also indicate that neither of the two viral sequences is associated with LTRs.

The existance of Bam H1 fragments which only hybridize with viral probes suggests that virus sequences are linked to H-2 genes in this cosmid cluster as opposed to a homologous interaction between H-2 and viral DNA sequences as has been reported for HTLV (10). A linkage between minor histocompatibility antigens and retroviral DNA sequences has also been observed (11).

The viral sequences within this H-2 cluster are currently being subcloned and their expression and effect on class I gene expression will be studied. It is hoped that their study will lead to a better understanding of the association between retroviruses and the H-2 gene family.

References: (1) Meruelo et al. (1978) J. Exp. Med. 147, 470; (2) Meruelo, D. (1980) J. Immunogenet. 7,81; (3) Meruelo, D. and Kramer, J. (1981) J. Transplant. Proc. 13, 1858; (4) Meruelo, D. (1979) J. Exp. Med. 149,898; (5) Chan et al. (1980) Proc. Nat'l Acad. Sci. 77,5779; (6) Mellor, A.L. et al. (1982) Nature 298,529; Golden,L. et al. (in preparation); (7) Southern, E. (1975) J. Mol. Biol. 98,503; (8) Steinmetz, M. et al. (1981) Cell 24,125; (9) Chattopadhyay,S.K. et al. (1982) Nature 295,25; (10) Clark,M.F., Gelmann,E.P. and Reitz, M.S. (1983) Nature 305,60; (11) Meruelo, D. et al. (1983) Proc. Nat'l Acad. Sci. 80, 5032; Blatt, C. et al. (1983) Proc. Nat'l Acad. Sci. in press.

Acknowledgements: Supported by grants CA22247, CA31346 from the N.I.H. and grant IM-163 from the American Cancer Society. DM is a Leukemia Society of America Scholar. CP is a fellow of the Cancer Res. Institute/F.M. Kirby Found.

CARRIER DETECTION BY GENE ANALYSIS IN A FAMILY WITH HAEMOPHILIA
B (FACTOR IX DEFICIENCY). [1]I.R. Peake, [1]B.L. Davies,[1] A.L. Bloom and
[2]G.G. Brownlee. [1]Department of Haematology, Welsh National School of
Medicine, Cardiff, U.K.,[2]Sir William Dunn School of Pathology, Oxford, U.K.

Introduction   Factor IX deficiency (Haemophilia B),although less common than
factor VIII deficiency (Haemophilia A) occurs in approximately 1 in 30,000 males,
and, in its severest form, results in severe bleeding into muscles and joints.
Carrier detection in such families by assay of plasma factor IX levels (IXC) can,
however, be unsatisfactory because of extremes of lyonisation and the large range
seen in normal individuals (50-200 u/dl). Levels of factor IX antigen (IXAg) can
also be unhelpful since up to 30% of affected males have detectable antigen levels
Several laboratories have now reported the successful cloning of the human factor
IX gene (1,2,3). The use of genomic and c-DNA probes to study the defective
gene in five patients with factor IX deficiency who developed inhibitors to
factor IX following treatment has also been reported (4). We have examined the
use of specific gene probes in order to study the inheritance of the affected
factor IX gene in a similar family in which the affected individual appears to
show a partial gene deletion.

Results   Patient TC is a ten year old boy with severe factor IX deficiency who,
at the age of 7 years developed an inhibitor (IgG) to factor IX. Although
his family can be traced back through almost 100 years, no history of excessive
bleeding could be found. Eight female relatives covering four generations were
available for study, and the IXC and IXAg levels are given in table 1 (normal
range 50-200 u/dl). Reduced levels were recorded on this occasion in the sister
and mother. Specific gene probes have been produced in Oxford, the details of
which have been reported (1). Although the exact extent of the gene deletion in
TC is not at present clear, four genomic probes (which cover a large area in the
middle of the gene including the exon coding for part of the factor IX linking
peptide, and all the exon coding for the factor IX activation peptide), failed to
hybridise with restriction enzyme digests of the patient's DNA following agarose
gel electrophoresis and Southern blotting. Specifically using ECoRI and one of
these probes (probe II) a 4.8 Kb fragment was detected in normal DNA (and DNA
from haemophilia B patients without inhibitors) but this band was missing in TC.
Since factor IX deficiency is an X-linked disease, it would be expected that the
gene level (as measured by darkening of the band on the autoradiograph) would
be twice as much in normal females (XX) than in normal males (XY). This was
clearly shown with the probe II/ECoRI combination. When this analysis was
performed in the eight female relatives of TC, six gave signal strengths similar to
that obtained with normal female DNA (table 1). However the patient's sister
and mother gave signals similar or less than the normal male signal, indicating
that they carried the affected gene (XX[1]). These results were confirmed by
scanning the autoadiograph with a Joyce-Loebl Chromoscan[R].

Discussion   The finding of a gene deletion in TC agrees with results published
previously (4) where 4 of 5 similar patients had deletions. It would seem reasonable to suggest that the patients inability to synthesise part or all of the factor IX

Table 1 - TC Family

	FIXC (u/dl)	FIXAg[1] (u/dl)	Estimation of Autoradiograph Signal[2]
Patient TC	<1	<10	−
Sister	38	33	+
Mother	24	32	+
Grandmother	66	54	++
Great Grandmother	80	72	++
Maternal Aunt	72	77	++
[3]Female Cousin 1	76	50	++
[3]Female Cousin 2	60	55	++
[3]Female Cousin 3	51	66	++

[1]By Laurell assay   [2]Normal male = +   [3] Daughters of Maternal Aunt
                          Normal female = ++

molecule results in the recognition of the transfused normal factor IX as 'non-self', resulting in the observed immunological response. Interestingly using a sensitive monoclonal antibody based ELISA for IXAg, low levels of a IXAg were detectable in TC's plasma, although the dose response curve was not parallel to that for normal plasma IXAg. This would tend to suggest a partial deletion in this patient, and preliminary results with a c-DNA probe confirm the presence of some areas of the gene. Using the probes which fail to detect the gene, the results not only suggest that diagnosis of possible further affected members in the family may be possible (perhaps prenatally) but that carrier detection based on the strength of binding of the gene probe can be performed. These results, together with the factor IXC and antigen levels strongly suggest that the patient's sister and mother are carriers, but that the defect arose as a mutation at this level. The father was clinically normal although no data is available. However the apparent non-carrier status of the aunt would rule out his being affected. Clearly the carrier diagnosis technique requires the analysis of identical amounts of DNA. The inclusion of a second probe for a non-linked autosomal gene marker is being investigated in order to control the DNA levels analysed.

References
1. CHOO, K.H., GOULD, K.G., REES, D.J.G. and BROWNLEE, G.G. Nature 1982, 299, 178-180.
2. KURACHI, K and DAVIE, E.W. Proc. Natl. Acad. Sci., 1982,79,6461-6464.
3. JAYE, M., de la SALLE, H., SCHAMBER, F., BALLAND, A., KOHLI,V., FINDELI, A., TOLSTOSHEV, P. and LECOCQ, J.P. Nucleic Acids Research 1983,11,2325-2335.
4. GIANELLI, F., CHOO, K.H., REES, D.J.G., BOYD, Y., RIZZA, C.R.and BROWNLEE, G.G. Nature, 1983, 303, 181-182.

NONRADIOACTIVE DETECTION OF EUKARYOTIC GENES ON SOUTHERN BLOTS.

R. Pergolizzi, C. Brakel, R. Lang, M. Solanki, and S. Mowshowitz.

Enzo Biochem, Inc., 325 Hudson Street, New York, N.Y. 10013.

Biotinylated DNA probes (Langer et al., 1981) were used to analyze Southern blots of mouse and human DNA for repeated and unique genes. DNA probes containing 2'-deoxyuridine 5'-triphosphate 5-allylamine biotin (Bio 11-dUTP) were made by either nick translation or by 3'-terminal labeling with terminal deoxynucleotidyl transferase. Following transfer and hybridization, hybridized biotinylated DNA was visualized with one of three detection complexes. The complexes were composed of streptavidin, a biotin binding protein, and a multiply biotinylated enzyme, either horseradish peroxidase, acid phosphatase or alkaline phosphatase.

Blots were hybridized with pBR322 carrying either mouse or human 28S rDNA fragments. As expected, the probes were found to have extensive homology. However, the structure of the 28S DNA genes differed; we observed a low dosage 3.0 kilobase sequence in mouse but not human DNA.

When the sensitivity of the nonradioactive hybridization/detection in Southern transfers was examined, rDNA sequences were observed in as little as 40 nanograms of restricted genomic DNA.

Sensitivity enhancement techniques were applied to the analysis of single copy sequences in genomic blots. Beta globin sequences in human DNA were examined.

Langer, P.R., A. Waldrop and D. Ward (1981) Proc. Natl. Acad. Sci., U.S.A., 68, 6633.

Southern, E.M. (1975) J. Mol. Biol. 98, 503.

Organization and Expression of Endogenous MMTV Proviruses in C3Hf/He and C3Hf/Ki Mice.

Brian J. Popko and Robert J. Pauley

Dept. of Microbiology and Immunology, Univ. of Miami School of Medicine, Miami, Fl 33101

All laboratory strains of mice, in addition to most feral mice examined, contain copies of the Mouse Mammary Tumor Virus (MMTV) integrated into their genome (endogenous infection) (1). The Balb/cfC3H, C3H/He and C3H/Ki strains of mice are infected with the milk-transmitted C3H MMTV and have mammary tumor-incidences of approximately 90% at 1 year of age. Balb/c strains that lack the milk-transmitted virus have mammary tumor-incidences of less than 2% at 2 years; whereas, C3Hf/He and C3Hf/Ki mice, which also lack the milk-transmitted virus (due to foster-nursing on virus-free mothers), have tumor-incidences of approximately 80 and 30%, respectively, at 2 years (2). The relatively high tumor-incidence observed in C3Hf/He mice has been shown to be conveyed to progeny mice from either parent via the endogenous MMTV Unit V or Mtv-1 (3,4). This endogenous unit has also been shown to be capable of producing virus in milk of lactating C3Hf/He mice (4). Furthermore, some mammary tumors that arise in C3Hf/He mice contain integrated proviruses in addition to their normal endogenous MMTV content, which is presumably the result of Unit V amplification (5,6,7). We have examined the organization and expression of the endogenous MMTV units of the C3Hf/He and C3Hf/Ki mouse strains to evaluate the role of the endogenous MMTV proviruses in mammary tumorigenesis in these strains.

The various endogenous MMTV proviruses produce characteristic-sized fragments upon EcoRI digestion (8). DNA from C3Hf/He mice contained EcoRI fragments specific for the MMTV Units Ia, II, V, VII and IX; whereas, C3Hf/Ki DNA contained fragments specific for Units Ia, II, III, IV and IX. In order to determine if the endogenous MMTV proviruses of these strains are transcriptionally active, an RNA Dot-Blot assay was implemented. MMTV RNA levels were similar (approximately 0.004% of total RNA) in mammary glands from C3Hf/He and C3Hf/Ki animals. RNA sizing analysis of poly A^+ RNA isolated from C3Hf/He and C3Hf/Ki mammary glands detected a 9.0 kb RNA transcript representative of the full-length MMTV genome, a 3.8 kb spliced transcript specific for the envelope region of the genome, and a 1.7 kb RNA species that contains sequences derived predominantly from the MMTV's LTR region. Because the methylated status of a particular gene has generally provided a good indication of that genes transcriptional status (with transcriptionally active genes containing less ^{Me}CpG than inactive genes), we sought to obtain an indication which endogenous MMTV provirus is (are) the source of MMTV RNA in the mammary glands of C3Hf/He and C3Hf/Ki animals by examining DNA from these tissues for hypomethylated MMTV sequences. In order to determine which (if any) endogenous MMTV provirus contains hypomethylated sequences, double-digestions were performed with EcoRI and either the

methyl-sensitive enzyme HpaII or HhaI. These digests revealed hypomethylated sequences in the endogenous MMTV Unit Ia and V of C3Hf/He
mammary gland DNA and extensive hypomethylation of the endogenous
Unit IV in C3Hf/Ki mammary gland DNA. Finally, mammary tumors from
the C3Hf/He and C3Hf/Ki strains were examined for MMTV proviruses in
addition to the normal endogenous MMTV units of these strains using
the restriction enzyme EcoRI. EcoRI fragments containing MMTV sequences in addition to the EcoRI fragments of normal endogenous
proviruses were detected in 2 of 4 C3Hf/He and 0 of 2 C3Hf/Ki mammary
tumors.

These results indicate the following:

1) C3Hf/Ki mice, which have a moderate mammary tumor-incidence, lack
   the endogenous MMTV provirus (Unit V) that has been implicated in
   mammary tumorigenesis in C3Hf/He mice.
2) Similar levels and species of MMTV RNA are expressed in C3Hf/He
   and C3Hf/Ki mammary glands, and because milk from C3Hf/He animals
   has been shown to contain MMTV particles, it appears that, at
   least at the transcriptional level, C3Hf/Ki mammary glands have
   the potential to produce MMTV virions.
3) Hypomethylation data implicate the endogenous MMTV Units Ia and V
   of C3Hf/He mammary glands and Unit IV of C3Hf/Ki mammary glands
   in the MMTV transcriptional activity observed in these tissues.
4) Amplification of an endogenous MMTV provirus does not appear to
   be necessary for mammary tumorigenesis in either the C3Hf/He or
   C3Hf/Ki mouse strains.

References. (1) Cohen, J.C. and Varmus, H.E. (1979) Nature 278, 418-
423. (2) Bentvelzen, B. and Higlers, J. (1980) in Viral Oncology,
(ed. Klein), 311-355. (3) Van Nie, R. and Verstraeten, A. (1975)
Int. J. Cancer 16, 922-931. (4) Michalides, R., et al. (1981) Cell
23, 165-173. (5) Cohen, J.C. and Varmus, H.E. (1980) J. Virology 35,
298-305. (6) Michalides, R., et al. (1981) J. Virology 39, 367-376.
(7) Etkind, P.R. and Sarkar, N.H. (1983) J. Virology 45, 114-123. (8)
Traina, V.L., et al. (1981) J. Virology 40, 735-744.

ISOLATION AND CHARACTERIZATION OF A SINGLE-COPY PROBE
FOR A HUMAN DNA REPAIR GENE

Jaime S. Rubin, Valerie Prideaux,
Gordon F. Whitmore and Alan Bernstein

Ontario Cancer Institute, Toronto, Ontario M4X 1K9, Canada

A number of human hereditary conditions, including xeroderma pigmentosum (XP), ataxia telangiectasia and Fanconi's anemia, exhibit increased sensitivity to a variety of DNA damaging agents and a predisposition to cancer. This increased sensitivity is often ascribed to a defect in some aspect of DNA repair. Although it is evident that the human DNA repair system is determined by a number of genes, there is little detailed knowledge concerning them.

We have addressed this problem by using DNA-mediated gene transfer techniques to identify a human DNA repair gene (1). A Chinese hamster cell line, UV-20, deficient in DNA repair (2, 3) was chosen as a recipient for gene transfer studies. This cell line, like XP cells, is sensitive to a variety of DNA damaging agents and is defective in the initial incision step of excision repair. This cell line is approximately 7 times more sensitive to UV light and 70 times more sensitive to mitomycin-C (MM-C) as the parental hamster line. In addition to their repair deficient phenotype, these mutants were chosen as recipients for DNA-mediated gene transfer because they are capable of stably incorporating and expressing foreign DNA at a relatively high frequency. Also, using highly repetitive human DNA sequences (Alu sequences) as probes, human DNA can be distinguished from hamster DNA, demonstrating the presence of transferred human DNA in the transformed cell lines and allowing an initial characterization of the transfected DNA.

High molecular weight DNA from repair proficient human HeLa cells was used as a donor and selection for repair proficiency involved growth in media containing MM-C. A drug concentration was chosen that would eliminate the possibility of any surviving repair deficient cells while not reducing the survival of any generated repair proficient cells. A number of primary and secondary transformants, resistant to both MM-C and UV light, have been generated by this procedure: primary transformant, X25, and the corresponding secondary, X25-37; primary transformant, X38, and the corresponding secondary, X38-69.

Using Southern blot analysis with ^{32}P-labelled genomic human DNA as a probe, it was found that these cell lines contain multiple restriction fragments that specifically hybridize to the human DNA probe, clearly demonstrating that these transformants contain human DNA. Also, independently derived transformants contain common restriction fragments, further demonstrating the association of these human sequences to the DNA repair proficiency phenotype and thus the human DNA repair gene.

In order to isolate a single-copy subfragment of the gene that could then be used to isolate the DNA repair gene, a genomic library of one of the secondary transformants, X25-37, was constructed in the bacteriophage λgtWES. DNA from this transformant was completely digested with the restriction enzyme EcoRI, ligated to similarly digested phage, and then packaged in vitro. Approximately 1 x 10⁶ recombinants were screened by in situ hybridization with a radio-actively labelled human DNA probe.

A number of recombinants containing human inserts have been isolated and subcloned in the plasmid pBR322. The size of these human inserts corresponds to the size of restriction fragments in the secondary transformant that hybridize to the human probe. One of these inserts hlUV has been analyzed as to its restriction sensitivities (Fig. 1) with the aim of isolating a subfragment that did not hybridize to a human probe. One such restriction fragment, a 0.8 kbp PvuII-SphI fragment, has been isolated and also subcloned into pBR322. Work is currently in progress to conclusively demonstrate that this fragment is indeed a single copy fragment of a human DNA repair gene by examining the restriction fragments of human, UV-20 and DNA repair proficient transformants that hybridize to this probe. Such a probe will enable us to screen existing genomic DNA and cDNA libraries in order to clone a biologically active DNA sequence.

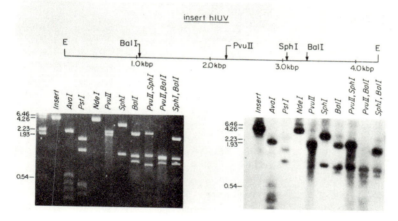

FIG. 1. Restriction Enzyme Sensitivity of Insert hlUV. Left panel: Ethidium Bromide Staining; Right panel: Hybridization Probe to ³²P-labelled Human DNA.

References — (1) Rubin, J.S. et al. Nature, in press; (2) Thompson, L.H. et al. (1980) Somat. Cell Genet. 6, 391; (3) Thompson, L.H. et al. (1982) Somat. Cell Genet. 8, 759

ACKNOWLEDGEMENTS: This work was supported by the National Cancer Institute of Canada. JSR is the recipient of a Research Studentship from the National Cancer Institute of Canada.

A POSSIBLE B CELL GROWTH FACTOR PRECURSOR

Sahasrabuddhe C.G. [1], Morgan J.W. [1], Wright D.A. [2], Adlakha R. [3], and, Maizel A. [1]. Departments of [1] Pathology, Section of Pathobiology; [2] Genetics; [3] Chemotherapy Research, UT M.D. Anderson Hospital, 6723 Bertner Ave., Houston, Texas 77030

Introduction: Recent studies show that clonal proliferation of B lymphocytes, a major aspect of the humoral response, may be mediated by soluble lymphotropic factor(s). Human B cell growth factor (BCGF) is a low mw (12KD) lymphotropic protein capable of inducing S-phase entry in population(s) of normal human activated B cells (1), and supporting the proliferation of factor dependent normal human B cell lines (2). We report here our results on the studies of mRNA for BCGF, and discuss the possible existence of a biologically active precursor of BCGF.

Results: Polysomal RNA was prepared from 24 hr. lectin activated human peripheral blood lymphocytes (PBL). This RNA was sized on a sucrose gradient (3) and the RNA from each fraction was translated in vitro using the Xenopus Laevis Oocyte system (4). The translation products were bioassayed for BCGF activity utilizing BCGF dependent long term normal human B cell lines (2). An estimated size of mRNA for BCGF was determined to be >15S (Fig 1). This raised the possibility that BCGF might be a product obtained from a large precursor protein. As we have been unable to detect a high mw protein with BCGF activity in lymphocyte conditioned media (LYCM)(1), a cytoplasmic extract (CYTO) was prepared from 72 hr. lectin activated PBLs (5), partially purified through DEAE ion exchange chromatogaphy and bioassayed for BCGF activity (2). Studies on the kinetics of appearance of intracellular (CYTO) and extracellular (LYCM) BCGF revealed; (a) The pool of CYTO-BCGF existed prior to activation (Table 1), (b) This pool apparently did not decrease at a rate corresponding to the rate of appearance of LYCM-BCGF (Fig 2). To exclude methodological artifact, similar cytoplasmic extracts (CYTO) and LYCM from a continuously growing CEM cell line were prepared and bioassayed. Neither LYCM nor CYTO preparation exhibited BCGF activity (Table 1).

Discussion: Recent studies show that mRNA for mouse epidermal growth factor (EGF) codes for a precursor protein of which less than 5% represents the biologically active 53 aa long EGF (6). Our results indicate that unlike IL-2 mRNA (7), yet similiar to EGF mRNA (6), BCGF mRNA may code for a significantly large precursor protein molecule. EGF, NGF and insulin precursors were determined through the use of antibodies against the known biologically active products. In most of these cases biological activities of precursors were not tested. Our studies suggest that BCGF may be unique in that it may exist intracellularly as a biologically active precursor(s). Elucidation of how B cell growth factor is synthesized and processed may provide new insight into B cell neoplasia.

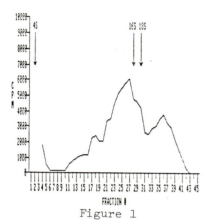

Figure 1

Table I

Samples assayed at 5%	³H-thymidine incorporation (CPM)
-	100
PBL-LYCM[A]	8771
CEM-CYTO[B]	221
CEM-LYCM	232
CEM-CYTO	286

A. LYCM AND CYTO PREPARED FROM UNSTIMU-LATED PBLs AND CEM WERE PARTIALLY PURIFIED THROUGH DEAE ION EXCHANGE CHROMATOGRAPHY AND BIOASSAYED.

B. FOR PREPARING LYCM, CELLS WERE CULTURED AT 10^6/ML; THE CYTOPLASMIC EXTRACTS WERE DILUTED TO THE SAME EXTENT AS LYCM.

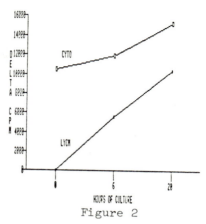

Figure 2

Figure 1: RNA from sucrose gradient fractions were translated in Xenopus laevis oocytes(4) and bioassayed(2). Smooth moving ΔCPM average of each group of six fractions is plotted against fraction number.

Figure 2: PBLs from normal donors were stimulated with lectin (1), LYCM was recovered at various times and corresponding cytoplasmic extracts (CYTO) were prepared from cells (5). Both LYCM and CYTO were partially purified through DEAE and bioassayed (2). ΔCPM is plotted against time.

1. Maizel, A., Sahasrabuddhe, C.G., Mehta, S., Morgan, J., Lachman, L., and Ford, R.: Proc. Natl. Acad. Sci. (U.S.A.) 79:5998, 1982.
2. Maizel, A., Morgan, J., Mehta, S.R., Kouttab, N.M., Bator, J.M., and, Sahasrabuddhe, C.G.: Proc. Natl. Acad. Sci. (U.S.A.) 80:5047, 1983.
3. Bleackley, R.C., Caplan, B., Havele, C., Ritzel, R.G., Mosmann, T.R., Farrar, J.J., and Paetkau V.J.: J. Immunol. 127:2432,1981.
4. Gurdon, J.B., Lane, C.D., Woodland, H.R., and Marbaix, G.: Nature (London) 233, 177, 1971.
5. Murphy Jr., E.C., and Arlinghaus, R.B.: Virology 86:329, 1978.
6. Gray, A., Dull, T.J., and Ullrich, A.: Nature 303, 722, 1983.
7. Taniguchi, T., Matsui, H., Fujita, T., Takaoka, C., Kashima, N., Yoshimoto, R., and Hamuro, J.: Nature (London) 302, 305, 1983.

SEQUENCE ANALYSIS OF ALPHA-1-ANTITRYPSIN DEFICIENCY ALLELE, PiS

Daniel Schindler, Barbara Wallner-Philipp, Richard Tizard, Russell Chan, William Kelley, and Richard Flavell, Biogen Res. Corp., 14 Cambridge Center, Cambridge,Mass. 02142

Alpha-1-antitrypsin, a protease inhibitor found in blood, is present at a concentration of 1.3 g/l, in the same range of concentration as immunoglobulin G. It can inhibit many proteases, but shows a high affinity for polymorphonuclear neutrophil elastase. It is composed of 394 amino acids and 3 carbohydrate chains(1). The most common deficiency allele is PiS which gives a mild serum deficiency of 60% of the normal value. The frequency of this allele can reach 12% in southern Europeans, about the same incidence as sickle cell anemia in blacks in the United States. The frequency of the PiS allele in the United States is 7%(2). The protein from deficient people, the S protein, has been shown to have an almost normal blood clearing time so that the defect is either in synthesis or export of the protein from the liver(3). Some thallasemia syndromes in man and a serum albumin deficiency in rats(4) have been shown to be the result of abnormal processing of the messenger RNA. In particular, the intervening sequences are incorrectly spliced. Although the mutations causing these diseases are usually found in the intervening sequences, several beta-hemoglobin deficiencies have mutations in the coding sequence which lead to altered splicing(5,6). Here we show the sequence of a PiS coding sequence around the mutation site and suggest that the major defect in S protein synthesis is the result of abnormal splicing of the messenger RNA.

Plasmids containing DNA sequences corresponding to the messenger RNA of alpha-1-antitrypsin were sequenced to give a nucleotide sequence which codes for a polypeptide chain of 418 amino acids. The first 24 amino acids comprise the signal peptide(7) and the last 394 are identical to the sequence of mature alpha-1-antitrypsin except for amino acid 264 which is valine in our sequence and glutamate in the wild type protein(Figure 1). This is the amino acid change of the PiS allele. The nucleotide change is an A in wild type becoming a T in the mutant. This changes a GA dinucleotide to a GT which is the conserved dinucleotide at the beginning of almost all introns. In fact the sequence around this dinucleotide has 7 bases of 9 the same as the consensus 5' splicing site(8) and is the same except for one nucleotide as three real splicing sites. The reduced amount of S protein synthesized may be the result of lowered amounts of correctly spliced messenger RNA as the newly formed spliced site may be used 40% of the time to reduce the amount of messenger RNA having the complete coding sequence. Further experiments are planned to test this possibility.

```
      Alpha-1-antitrypsin
        wild type       263 LEU GLU ASN 266
                            CTG GAA AAT
        PiS                 LEU VAL ASN
                            CTG GTA AAT
   Consensus 5' splice      CAG GTG AGT
        site                A̅       A̅
   Mouse mu heavy chain     CTG GTA AAC
   Xenopus alpha globin     CAG GTA AAT
   SV40 late mRNA           CTG GTA AAG
```

Figure 1. Sequence comparison of PiS mutant to wild type, the consensus sequence 5' splicing site, and other known splicing sites which differ by one nucleotide.

1) Carrell, R.W. et al., Nature 298,329-334(1982). 2) Fagerhol, M.K., Postgrad. Med. J. 52 Suppl. 2,73-83(1976). 3) Jeppsson,J.-O., Laurell,C.-B., Nosslin, B. and Cox,D.W., Clin. Sci. molec. Med. 5,103-107(1978). 4) Esumi, H. et al., Proc. Nat. Acad. Sci. USA 80,95-99(1983). 5) Orkin S.H. et al., Nature 300,768-769(1982). 6) Goldsmith M.E. et al., Proc. Natl. Acad. Sci. USA 80,2318-2322(1983). 7) Leicht, M. et al., Nature 297,655-659(1982). 8) Mount, S.M., Nucleic Acids Res. 10,459-472(1982).

Nucleotide sequence of cloned cDNA encoding rat prepro parathyroid hormone.

Hans-Jürgen Schmelzer, Gerhard Gross and Hubert Mayer
GBF - Gesellschaft für Biotechnologische Forschung mbH,
Mascheroder Weg 1, 3300 Braunschweig, FRG

Parathyroid hormone (PTH) an 84 amino acid polypeptide is the principal homeostatic regulator of blood calcium in mammals. The DNA-sequence of cDNA from bovine (1) and human (2) PTH is known. In order to study the evolution of the PTH gene we have cloned and partially sequenced rat PTH cDNA.

Using a modification of the cDNA cloning strategy of Okayama et al. (3) and starting from 1µg poly A-containing mRNA extracted from rat thyroid and parathyroid glands, we isolated 3000 hybrid cDNA colonies. One clone was identified by colony hybridisation with a bovine cDNA probe. Restriction map analysis of the clone showed that it contained a 780 bp cDNA insert. Partial sequencing of the insert showed that the clone contained ca. 350 bp 3'noncoding region and a ca. 400 bp coding region (Fig. 1) from which the amino acid sequence of the rat prepro-parathyroid hormone was deduced. Comparison of the sequences of pre-pro-PTH from four different species allows one to examine which regions have been conserved during evolution and could thus have some functional significance. An extensive amino acid (AA) homology is found between rat, human, bovine and porcine PTH in the amino and carbocyterminal region of PTH (Fig. 2). The three AAs amino terminal to the pre-hormone are identical in the four species, which could be thought to have functional importance for the conformational recognition by the enzyms that cleave the pre-peptide. In the region AAs 60-70 there is a considerable nonhomology between rat PTH and that of the three species but a consensus in the ß turn. This secondary structure could be thought to play a role for the conformational recognition by enzymes that cleave PTH into an amino terminal and c-terminal part in liver and kidney (cleavage after AA34). The extensive amino acid homology is reflected at the nucleotide level (Fig. 3). It is striking that the number of silent substitutions that have taken place is much less than that theoretically expected. Several properties of mRNA (its stability, translatability, processing from precursors) might place constraints on the primary and secondary structure of the mRNA. The identity of the nucleotides at AA-3 indicates presumably the insertion point of an intron on the chromosomal PTH rat gene in analogy to the human PTH gene.

References. (1) Kronenberg, H.M., McDevitt, B.E., Majzoub, J.A., Nathans, J., Sharp, P.A., Potts, J.T.jr. and Rich, A. (1979) Proc. Natl. Acad. Sci. USA 76, 4981-4985; (2) Hendy, G.H., Kronenberg, H.M., Potts, J.T.jr. and Rich, A. (1981), Proc. Natl. Acad. Sci. USA 78, 3765-3769; (3) Okayama, H., Berg, P. (1982) Mol. Cell. Biol. 2, 161

229

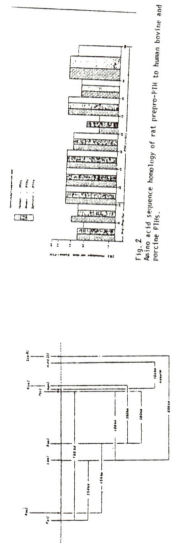

Fig. 2
Amino acid sequence homology of rat prepro-PTH to human bovine and porcine PTHs.

Fig.1
Restriction map of rat prepro-PTH cDNA clone.

```
1-  100...GATGATCCTC..ATGCTGGCAG...TTTATCTCCT..TACCCAGACG..GATGGGAAAC..CCGTTAAGAA..GAGAGCTATC..AGTGAAAATAC..AGCTTATGCA..CAACCTGGGC
                          XXXXXX   XX   XXX XXXXX          XXX X X XX X            X XXXXXXXXX     XXXX XX X     XXXXXXXXX          XXXXXXX
1-  100...TATGATTGTC..ATGTTGGCA4..TTTGTTTTCT..TACAAAATCG..GATGGGAAAT..CTGTTAAGAA..GAGATCTGTG..AGTGAAAATAC..AGCTTATGCA4..TAACCTGGGA

101- 200...AAACACCTGG..CCTCTGTGGA..GAGGATGCA4..TGGCTGAAG44..AAAAGCTGCA..AGATGGTCAC..AATTTTGTTA..GTCTTGGAGT..CCAAAATGGCT..GCCAGGAAGG
                     XXXX   XX      XXXXX X X   XXXXXXX X X   XXXX X XX X XXXXX   X X   XXXXXXX      X X XXXXX X   X XXXXXXX X
101- 200...AAACATCTGA..ACTCGATGGA..GAGAGTAGAA..TGGCTGCGTA..AGAAGCTGCAC..GGATGTGCAC..AATTTTGTTG..CCCTTGGAGC..TCCTCTAGCT..CCCAGAGATG

201- 300...GCAGTTACCA..GAGGCCCACC..AAGGAGGAGG..AAAATGTCCT..TGTTGATGGC..AATTCAAAAA..GTCTTGGCGA..GGGGGACAAA..GCTGATGTGG..ATGTATTAGT
                     XXXX   XX      XXXXXXXXX   XX  XXXXX  X         XX X XXXXX X       X X XXXXX      XX  XXXXX     XXXXXXX
201- 300...CTGGTTCCCA..GAGGCCCCGA..AAAAGGAAG..ACAATGTCTT..GGTTGAGAGC..CATGAAAAA..GTCTTGGAGA..GGCAGACAAA..GCTGATGTGA..ATGTATTAAC

301- 323...TAAGGCTAAA..TCTCAGTAAA..TGC  rat
                     XXX XXXX   XX XXXX  XX
301- 400...TAAAGCTAAA..TCCCAGTGAA..AAT  human
```

Fig. 3
Nucleotide sequence of rat prepro-PTH mRNA compared with human prepro-PTH mRNA. Identical nucleotides are indicated by*

CHARACTERIZATION OF A STEROID REGULATED GENE OF <u>DROSOPHILA</u>.

R.A.Schulz, L.Cherbas, M.M.D.Koehler, and P.Cherbas

Cellular and Developmental Biology, The Biological Laboratories, Harvard University, Cambridge, MA. 02138

The EIP 28/29 gene of <u>Drosophila melanogaster</u> is a single-copy gene located on chromosome III at 71C3.4-D1.2 (1,2). It was isolated as a gene whose protein products, the ecdysteroid-inducible polypeptides (EIPs) 28 and 29, are synthesized at an elevated rate during treatment of the Kc cell line with active ecdysones (3). The kinetics, dose-dependence, and insensitivity to cycloheximide of EIP 28/29 transcript induction suggest that the EIP 28/29 gene is a primary hormone-responsive gene in Kc cells (4). Thus EIP 28/29 gene regulation can be utilized as a model system to investigate the control of gene expression by a steroid hormone.

Interestingly, the EIP 28/29 gene, even in homozygous form, directs the synthesis of 6 polypeptides (1,2,5) (Figure 1). While as many as 4 polypeptides may be formed due to post-translational acetylation, two polypeptides – EIP 28III and EIP 29III – appear to be primary translation products of the EIP 28/29 gene (6). Since these two polypeptides are non-allelic (2), the question remained how two distinct protein products could be generated from a single-copy gene.

Figure 1. Two dimensional separations of EIPs 28 and 29 from pulse-labeled control (C) or 20-hydroxyecdysone (E) treated Kc cells. The synthesis of the 6 polypeptides is induced 8-fold by hormone and the 3 to 1 ratio of EIPs 28 to EIPs 29 remains unchanged after induction.

The transcription unit for the EIP 28/29 gene in Kc cells has been elucidated by comparing the nucleotide sequence of the complete gene and portions of several cDNA clones, by S1 nuclease analysis of RNA-DNA hybrids, and by primer extension experiments (7). It contains 4 exons (designated $\int$, α, β, and γ) of 117, 194, 261, and 410 bp separated by introns of 992, 110, and 59 bp (Figure 2). The predicted mature RNA transcript is 982N in length, with a protein coding capacity of 28,100 daltons. This analysis is consistent with the size measurements of the inducible EIP 28/29 RNA in Kc cells as determined by Northern analysis following deadenylation (1). The transcription unit is identical in both control and ecdysone-treated cells; specifically, induced transcripts initiate at the same nucleotide as the basal transcripts. Additionally, the 150 bp region immediately upstream of transcriptional initiation contains an interesting series of repeats and substantial homology to the SV40 enhancer sequences.

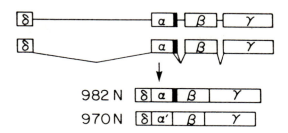

Figure 2. The EIP 28/29 transcription unit in Kc cells. Two EIP 28/29 RNAs are generated from the primary EIP 28/29 gene transcript by alternative splicing. The 982N and 970N RNAs may represent distinct EIP 28 and EIP 29 transcripts, respectively.

The availability of characterized cDNA clones, as well as a detailed understanding of the EIP 28/29 gene transcription unit, has allowed us to study the fine structure of EIP 28/29 RNAs. Whereas Northern analysis has identified a single size class of inducible RNA in Kc cells, S1 nuclease protection and primer extension experiments indicate that two forms of RNA are generated from the primary RNA transcript by alternative splicing pathways (8) (Figure 2). The longer, more abundant RNA contains the complete α exon spliced to the complete β exon. The shorter, less abundant RNA lacks 12 nucleotides from the 3' end of the α exon. Sequencing of cDNAs corresponding to the two RNAs demonstrated that different splice donor sequences separated by 12 nucleotides are utilized in the removal of intron sequences separating the α and β exons. This alternative splicing phenomenon occurs with the same efficiency in control and ecdysone-treated cells, demonstrating that the differential processing of these RNAs is not under hormonal control. Both the ratio of the two RNA forms and the predicted amino acid composition of translated polypeptides suggest that these RNAs may represent distinct EIP 28 and EIP 29 transcripts. Therefore, the alternative splicing phenomenon represents a mechanism by which to obtain two distinct polypeptides from a single-copy gene.

References - (1) Savakis,C.,Koehler,M.M.D. and Cherbas,P. (1983) submitted to EMBO J.; (2) Cherbas,L. and Cherbas,P. (1983) submitted to Nucl. Acids Res.; (3) Savakis,C.,Demitri,G. and Cherbas,P. (1980) Cell 22, 665-674; (4) Bieber,A. and Cherbes,P., unpublished observations; (5) Cherbas,P.,Cherbas,L.,Savakis,C. and Koehler,M.M.D. (1981) Amer. Zool. 21, 743-750; (6) Koehler,M.M.D.,Bieber,A. and Cherbas,P., manuscript in preparation; (7) Cherbas,L.,Schulz,R.A., Koehler,M.M.D. and Cherbas,P. (1983) submitted to Cell; (8) Schulz, R.A.,Cherbas,L. and Cherbas,P., manuscript in preparation.

Acknowledgments - This work was supported by grants from the American Cancer Society (CD107A) and the National Institutes of Health (GM29301). R.A.S. is a post-doctoral research fellow of the N.I.H.

EXCLUSION LIMITS OF DNA RESTRICTION FRAGMENTS
ON GEL FILTRATION MEDIA

Cheri Seitz
Pharmacia Fine Chemicals, Piscataway, New Jersey 08854

Gel filtration is frequently used to separate labelled nucleotides from double stranded DNA. Data reporting the exclusion limits of nucleic acids for the types of Sephadex, Sepharose, and Sephacryl gel filtration media commonly used has not been readily available. In order to ease the task of selecting the proper media, we have determined the size of DNA restriction fragments which elute in the void volume of 11 different Pharmacia gel filtration media.

METHODS: One column was packed to a volume of 10 ml for each of the following: Sephadex G-25, G-50, G-75, G-100; Sephacryl S-200, S-300, S-400, S-500; Sepharose CL-6B, CL-4B, CL-2B. The buffer used was 20mM Tris-HCl, 1mM EDTA, 0.1M NaCl, pH 7.5. Blue Dextran 2000 was applied to each column to determine the void volume.

A lambda DNA Hind III/ΦX-174 RF DNA Hae III restriction digest, containing 19 fragments ranging in size from 72-23130 base pairs, was obtained from Pharmacia P-L Biochemicals, Inc. Twenty-five micrograms were run on each column. Eluant samples corresponding to the void volumes were electrophoresed on PAA 2/16 gradient gels in a Tris-acetate buffer system. (40mM Tris, 20mM NaOAc, 1mM EDTA, pH 8.0.)

RESULTS: Eighteen of the nineteen fragments composing the digest are visible when 0.4 micrograms of the sample is electrophoresed under the conditions shown in Figure 1. Figure 2 shows the relationship between the number of base pairs and the distance migrated on the PAA 2/16 gel. A comparison of the eluent samples with the complete digest shows that all fragments of the digest are

Figures 1A-C. Electrophoresis of excluded restriction fragments on polyacrylamide 2/16 gradient gels. 1A. Sephadex. Lanes 1&10: standard; 2&3:G-25; 4&5:G-50, 6&7:G-75; 8&9:G-100. 1B. Sephacryl; 1&10:standard; 2&3:S-200; 4&5:S-300; 6&7:S-400; 8&9:S-500. 1C. Sepharose. 1&10:standard; 2&3:CL-2B; 4&5:CL-4B; 6&7:CL-6B. Pre-equilibration: 40 min., 75V; pre-electrophoresis: 40 min., 75V; electrophoresis: 70 min., 100V; staining: 1 microgram/ml ethidium bromide in distilled water, 1/2 hour.

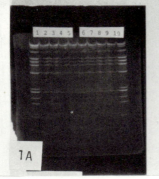
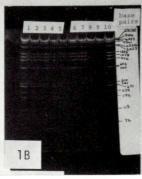
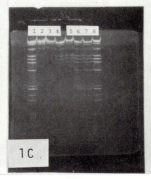

excluded from Sephadex G-25, G-50, G-75
and G-100. Sephacryl S-200 and S-300 each
excluded fragments of 118 or more base
pairs. S-400 had an exclusion limit of
271 pairs and S-500 excluded 1078 base
pairs. Sepharose CL-6B, CL-4B and CL-2B
had exclusion limits of 194, 872, and 1353
base pairs, respectively. (See Figure 3.)

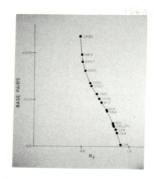

Figure 2. Base pair migration
on PAA 2/16 gel. Log-log plot.

Figure 3. Exclusion limits
in number of base pairs.

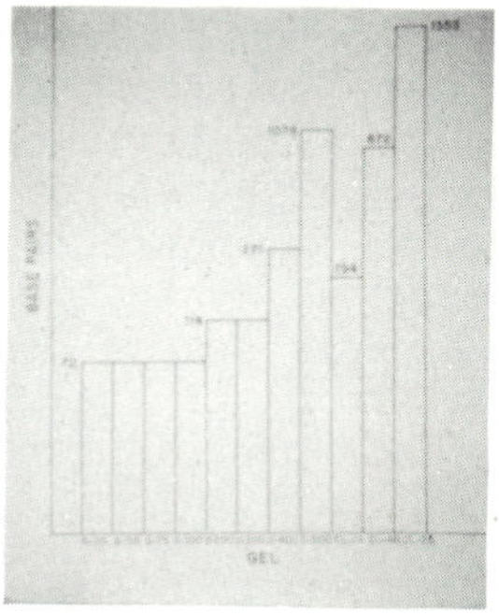

DISCUSSION: The broad size range of the
restriction digest used made it necessary to
electrophorese the eluents on gradient gels
as originally suggested by Jeppesen[1]. The
use of a 2-16% polyacrylamide concentration
made it possible to separate all the fragments
on one gel (Figs. 1A-C), and resulted in
sharper bands than found possible with single
concentration gels. We also confirmed Jeppesen's finding that if the
logarithms of the number of base pairs of the fragments are plotted
against the logarithms of the distances they have moved from the
beginning of the gradient, the points approximately fit a sigmoid-
shaped curve, with an almost linear central portion (Figure 2).
    The lack of restriction fragments smaller than 72 base pairs
prevented us from more narrowly defining the exclusion limits for
Sephadex. Also, the fact that Sephacryl S-200 and S-300 showed the
same exclusion limit probably reflects the lack of suitable markers
between 72 and 118 base pairs.
    The exclusion limits reported here for Sephacryl and Sepharose
confirm data on the exclusion limits for proteins and dextrans.
These show that the fractionation range of Sephacryl S-300
approaches that of Sepharose 6B. Sephacryl S-400 has a fractionation
range between that of Sepharose 6B and 4B, and the Sephacryl S-500
exclusion limit approximates that of Sepharose 2B. Earlier studies[2]
showed that Sephacryl S-1000 can be used for fractionating nucleic
acids up to 15 to 20 kilobase pairs.

1. Jeppesen, P.G.N. (1974) Anal. Biochem. 58. 195-207.
2. Work from Pharmacia Fine Chemicals. Data on file.

HIGH LEVEL EXPRESSION OF v-mos PROTEIN OF MOLONEY MURINE SARCOMA VIRUS IN E. COLI

Arun K. Seth and George F. Vande Woude

Laboratory of Molecular Oncology and LBI-Basic Research Program, NCI-Frederick Cancer Research Facility, P.O. Box B, Frederick, Maryland 21701

We have constructed a recombinant plasmid by inserting the v-mos gene of MSV (HT-1) at Cla I site of pJL6, a plasmid vector that contains λ phage Pl promoter and sequences coding for the first fifteen amino acids of the cII gene. Upon induction of the λ phage promoter at 42°C the bacteria harboring the recombinant plasmid (pA28) produce cII-mos fusion protein corresponding to 5-10% of the total cellular proteins. SDS-polyacrylamide gel electrophoresis of the total bacterial proteins indicates that the cII-mos fusion product is a protein of Mr 40,000. The bacterial mos protein is efficiently immunoprecipitated with the antiserum raised against the c-terminal synthetic peptide. As expected, the immunoprecipitation of E. coli mos is completely blocked by the c-terminal peptide. "Western blot" analysis with the same antiserum also reveals a distinct protein band in the range of 40,000 daltons.

Construction of cII-mos Expression Plasmid

The pJL6 (1) DNA was linearized with ClaI and repaired with dGTP and dCTP using klenow fragment. The mos gene was obtained by cleaving the pHT-10 (2) DNA with XbaI and HindIII and isolating the 1150 bp fragment from a polyacrylamide gel. Since an inframe termination codon is present upstream to the initiator ATG of mos gene, the fragment was therefore repaired with dCTP and dTTP and treated with S_1 to remove the terminator and yield flush ends. The two blunt-ended fragments were then ligated together and transformed into the E. coli strain DC646. The recombinant clones were screened by in situ colony hybridization. The DNA from one of the positive clones containing the insert in proper orientation was further transformed into the E. coli strain MZ-1, a λ lysogen that carries a temperature-sensitive mutation in the repressor gene.

Synthesis of cII-mos Fusion Protein in E. coli

The E. coli strain MZ-1 harboring the recombinant plasmid pA28 or vector pJL6 was initially grown at 32°C followed by induction at 42°C. The proteins were labeled with ^{35}S-methionine before and after the temperature shift and resolved by SDS-polyacrylamide gel electrophoresis. The gel pattern (Fig. 1) clearly showed the synsynthesis of an additional protein Mr 40,000 daltons in pA28 lysogens. No corresponding protein was synthesized in lysogens carrying the original vector pJL6, suggesting that 40 Kd bacterial product is a cII-mos fusion protein. Approximately 5-10% of the total bacterial proteins was estimated to be the 40 Kd cII-mos fusion protein.

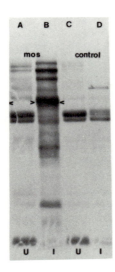

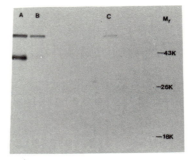

Fig. 2. Immunoprecipitation of v-mos protein synthesized in E. coli: Bacterial extracts labeled as in Fig. 1 were immunoprecipitated with the anti-C3 serum, Lanes: A, pA28 in the absence; and B, in the presence of c-terminal synthetic peptide; C, pJL6 immunoprecipitated with the same antiserum. The positions of molecular weight markers are indicated on the right.

Fig. 1. Induction of recombinant plasmid encoded protein: Bacterial extracts of pA28 cells labeled with ^{35}S methionine at 32° (A) and at 42° (B). Bacterial extracts of pJL6 cells labeled with ^{35}S methionine at 32° (C) and at 42° (D).

Immunoprecipitation of Plasmid (pA28) Encoded Protein

The ^{35}S-labeled extracts of E. coli strain MZ-1 carrying pA28 were precipitated with anti-C3 serum (3) and analyzed by SDS-polyacrylamide gel electrophoresis. The autoradiogram (Fig. 2) of the gel revealed a 40 Kd protein and as expected the 40 Kd protein disappeared when the immunoprecipitation was performed in the presence of soluble synthetic peptide. The immunoprecipitation of control cell extracts did not reveal any 40 Kd protein, further indicating that 40 Kd polypeptide is indeed a cII-mos fusion product.

References. (1) Lautenberger, J., Court, D., and Papas, T. (1983) Gene 23, 75-84; (2) Blair, D.G., McClements, W.L., Oskarsson, M.K., Fischinger, P.J., and Vande Woude, G.F. (1980) Proc. Natl. Acad. Sci. 77, 3504-3508; (3) Papkoff, J., Verma, I., and Hunter, T. (1982) Cell 29, 417-426.

TRANSFORMANTS ISOLATED FOLLOWING T24 DNA GENE TRANSFER EXPRESS A RECEPTOR BINDING Fcγ

K.D. Somers, A.E. Campbell, M.L. Beckett, M. Patten-Aardrup, and G.L. Wright, Jr.
Department of Microbiology and Immunology, Eastern Virginia Medical School, Norfolk, VA 23501

The presence of membrane receptors for the Fc portion of IgG molecules (FcγR) has been demonstrated on monocytes, macrophages, neutrophils, B and T lymphocytes, and related cell lines (1,2). FcγRs are known to be involved in phagocytosis and antibody-dependent cellular cytotoxicity and are believed to be involved in the process of transmembrane signaling leading to modulation of certain cellular functions including regulation of the immune response and differentiation. In addition to cells of the immune system, several nonlymphoid, virally transformed, and neoplastic cells have been found to express FcγR (1,3). FcγR expression on nonlymphoid tumor cells is thought to be due to the passive acquisition of FcγR shed by lymphoid cells infiltrating the tumor. The demonstrated lack of FcγR expression on most tumor cells grown in long term culture supports the hypothesis of FcγR expression by passive acquisition (4,5). We have recently determined that T24 bladder carcinoma cells express a membrane receptor that binds the Fc portion of human IgG as measured by indirect immunofluorescence and rosette formation with IgG coated erythrocytes. T24 cells are known to carry an activated c-Ha-ras-1 gene in which alteration of a single codon confers transforming activity to the encoded 21,000 dalton protein. How this or other transforming proteins mediate the process of cellular transformation and malignancy is virtually unknown. The detection of a membrane receptor for Fcγ on T24 cells raised the possibility that this membrane alteration might be a direct or indirect result of the activated oncogene. Expression of this receptor might contribute to loss of growth control and may serve as a marker of oncogene activation. We now report that focus-derived cellular transformants obtained following transfection of NIH3T3 cells with T24 cellular DNA express a membrane receptor that binds the Fc portion of human IgG as a non-selectable marker. Consistent with our hypothesis, transformants derived from transfection of NIH3T3 cells with a molecularly cloned T24 oncogene express a receptor that binds the Fc portion of mouse IgG.

RESULTS and DISCUSSION High molecular weight DNA isolated from T24 cells was used to transfect NIH3T3 cells using the calcium phosphate coprecipitation method (6). The transforming activity of the DNA preparation was 0.05 foci/µg of T24 DNA transfected. Transformed foci were isolated by the cloning cylinder trypsinization method and grown to mass culture. Evidence for the expression of a cell surface receptor for the Fc portion of human IgG on T24 cells and two T24 DNA transformants (3T3/2A and 3T3/4A) is presented in Tables 1 and 2. All assays were performed by indirect immunofluorescence using human whole IgG, F(ab')$_2$ or Fc fragments as the primary antibody and fluorescein-labeled goat antihuman IgG as the secondary antibody. T24, 3T3/2A and 3T3/4A cells express a receptor which binds whole human IgG and Fc, but not the F(ab')$_2$ portion of IgG or mouse IgG. The Fc binding to the control monocytic-like cell line U937 is reduced by pre-absorbing the Fc with 3T3/2A and 3T3/4A, but not with control NIH3T3 cells (Table 2). The ability of 3T3/2A and 3T3/4A cells to compete for the human FcγR on U937 cells demonstrates that the transformants constitutively express on their surface a receptor that binds human Fcγ. Since T24 cells contain an activated c-Ha-ras 1 oncogene, we

Table 1. Detection of a Receptor Binding to Fcγ on T24 cells and T24 DNA Transformants

Cells[2]	Human IgG[1]				Mouse IgG[1]
	whole	F(ab')$_2$	Fc	PBS	whole
T24	33	0	45	0	0
3T3/2A	51	0	33	0	0
3T3/4A	62	0	42	0	0
NIH3T3	0	0	0	0	0
U937	54	0	42	0	42[3]
44-91	6	0	1	0	42
109-3-2	7	0	0	0	41
3T3/7B	4	0	2	0	35
P3X63Ag8	NT[4]	NT	NT	0	58

% Positive Immunofluorescence with

[1] All IgG fractions were used at a concentration of 1.0 mg/ml.
[2] T24 is a human bladder carcinoma cell line. U937 is a human monocytic-like cell line known to express FcγR. Cell lines 44-91 and 109-3-2 were provided by M. Barbacid and are NIH3T3 cells transformed with the molecularly cloned T24 oncogene (8). 3T3/7B is a transformant derived from transfection of NIH3T3 cells with molecularly cloned v-mos DNA provided by M. McGeady. P3x63Ag8 is a mouse plasmacytoma cell line known to express mouse FcγR.
[3] 100% of mouse IgG binding is accounted for by the IgG2a isotype
[4] NT = not tested

Table 2. T24 DNA Transformants Block Binding to a Human Fcγ Receptor

Cells	Unabsorbed	Absorbed with[1]		
		NIH3T3	3T3/2A	3T3/4A
3T3/2A	49	49	11	8
3T34A	49	39	8	6
U937	58	53	17	17

% Positive Immunofluorescence

[1] Fc fraction of IgG (1.0 mg/ml) was absorbed with 10^7 cells of each cell line and residual binding was detected by fluorescein-labeled goat anti-human IgG.

sought to determine if NIH3T3 cells transformed with a molecularly cloned T24 oncogene would express Fc binding activity. Table 1 demonstrates that two NIH3T3 transformants containing an activated T24 oncogene (44-91 and 109-3-2, gift from M. Barbacid) express a membrane receptor that binds mouse IgG, but lack any binding activity for human IgG or derivative fragments. In addition, one transformant induced by molecularly cloned v-mos (3T3/7B) also binds mouse IgG. These results suggest that Fc membrane binding activity may serve as a marker of oncogene function.

The function of FcR on tumor cells remains speculative. FcR on malignant cells could convey a growth advantage for the tumor cell, perhaps by causing membrane purturbation leading to cell proliferation (7). FcR expression on tumor cells may play a role in escape from immune surveillance since antibodies bound to tumor cells by FcR (noncytotoxic antibodies) may serve to mask tumor cell-specific antigens and therefore function as blocking factors leading to enhancement of tumor growth.

REFERENCES (1) Unkeless, J.C., Fleit, H. and Mellman, I.S. (1981) Adv. Immunol. 31, 247-270; (2) Kerbel, R.S. and Elliott, B.E. (1983) in Methods in Enzymology (Langone, J. and VanVunakis, H. eds.) Vol. 93, 113-147; (3) Witz, I.P. (1977) Adv. Canc. Res. 25, 95-148; (4) Kerbel, R.S., Pross, H.F. and Elliott, E.V. (1975) Int. J. Canc. 15, 918-932; (5) Kerbel, R.S., Pross, H.F. and Leibovitz, A. (1977) Int. J. Canc. 20, 673-679; (6) Graham, F. and Van der Eb, A. (1973) Virology 52, 456-467; (7) Shearer, W.T., Philipott, G.W. and Parker, C.W. (1973) Science 182, 1357-1359; (8) Pulciani, S. Santos, E., Lauver, A.V., Long, L.K., Robbins, K.C. and Barbacid, M. (1982) Proc. Natl. Acad. Sci. USA 79, 2845-2849.

LINKAGE CONSERVATION AND ONCOGENE MAPPING IN THE CHINESE HAMSTER.

R.L. Stallings, A.C. Munk, J.L. Longmire, J.H. Jett, & B.D. Crawford
Life Science Div. Los Alamos Nat'l. Lab., Los Alamos, NM 87545

A panel of Chinese hamster x mouse somatic cell hybrid clones which have segregated hamster chromosomes has been used to assign 31 drug-resistance and enzyme gene loci to chromosomes in the Chinese hamster (Cricetulus griseus)(1-6). This clone panel, in conjunction with flow cytometric techniques, is being used to assign oncogene loci to chromosomes in this species. A summary of current mapping assignments and a description of our approach to oncogene mapping are described here. These studies should provide information on the evolutionary origin and rearrangement of oncogene loci in several mammalian species,and may offer insights regarding the significance of specific chromosomal alterations which are observed during the multistep neoplastic progression of cells derived from the Chinese hamster (7,8).

Mapping Approaches Using Cell Hybrids

Cell hybrids made by fusion of hamster spleen or fibroblast cells with mouse C11D (TK$^-$, Oua^R) cells were selected in medium supplemented with HAT or HAT + Ouabain. Each member of the clone panel (29 independent clones) was characterized by G-banded karyotype analysis, and starch gel electrophoresis to examine the presence of hamster isozymes. Concordant segregation of hamster isozymes and chromosomes has permitted the assignment of loci to each chromosome listed in Table 1 (1-6).

By comparing linkage relationships determined for the Chinese hamster to homologous loci assigned to mouse and human chromosomes, we have shown 8 conserved linkage groups in these three species (1-6). Published synteny of oncogenes to several of these conserved linkage groups in the mouse and human genomes allows us to predict chromosomal locations of several oncogenes in the Chinese hamster (summarized in Table 1). Additional oncogenes for which comparative mapping information is not available or not of predictive value include: myc, N-myc, mos, N-ras, fms, erb-B, sis, myb, yes, and ros.

Table 1. Comparative Synteny of Enzyme and Oncogene Loci That Have Been Mapped In Chinese Hamsters, Mice and Humans.

Loci	Hamster	Mouse	Human
PEPS		5	4
PGM2			
ADK			10
ESD	1	14	13
NP			14
PEPB		10	12
GSR		8	8
GLO		17	6
PGM1			
ENO1			
PGD	2	4	1
AK2			
DTS			5
GALT			9
APRT		8	16
GAA	3		17
IDH2			15
LDHA		7	11
HRAS1	?		11
FES	?		15
PGM3			6
ME1	4	9	
PKM2			15
MPI			
SRC	?		20
ADA			
ITPA	6	2	
AK1			9
ABL	?		
ERBA	?		17
TK		11	
GALK	7		
ACP1		12	2
TPI	8	6	12
KRAS2	?		
GPI	9	7	19
PEPD			
HRAS2	?	X	X

We are mapping oncogene loci and testing the predictions summarized above, by Southern filter hybridization analyses of hybrid cell DNAs, using cloned v-onc or homologous c-onc nucleic acid sequence probes (provided by several different laboratories).

Mapping Approaches Using Flow-Sorted Chromosomes

We also are attempting oncogene mapping by filter hybridization analyses using DNA derived from specific Chinese hamster chromosomes, resolved and purified by flow sorting methods.

Chromosomes from whole Chinese hamster embryo (WCHE) cells are isolated for flow analysis and sorting by a modified hypotonic lysis procedure, during which chromosomes are stained with the fluorescent dye, propidium iodide (8). The univariate flow karyotype (Fig. 1) is a histogram showing the number of chromosomes with a specific fluorescent intensity (DNA content). By flow techniques, the distribution of chromosome types within a population can be determined, relative frequency of occurrence of specific chromosomes measured, and relative chromosomal DNA content quantified (8). By appropriate placement of sorting windows, chromosomes can be sorted with > 80% purity. DNA purified from 10^5-10^6 sorted chromosomes can be used directly for dot-blot hybridization analyses, or cleaved with restriction endonucleases for resolution and detection of specific gene fragments by Southern hybridization methods. Flow sorting of chromosomes from euploid cells thus provides an adjunct approach to gene mapping using somatic cell hybrids.

Investigators in our laboratory have shown the utility of the Chinese hamster as a model system for the study of karyotypic changes in cancer. Euploid Chinese hamster fibroblasts exhibit a multistep evolution of phenotype, during the spontaneous process of neoplastic development (7). This neoplastic progression is accompanied by progressive changes in the karyotype (8). Mapping of oncogene loci in this species may aid in understanding the role that specific chromosome alterations play in tumorigenesis.

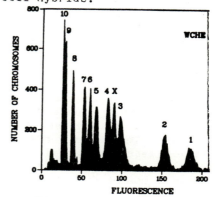

Fig. 1 Univariate flow karyotype for euploid Chinese hamster cells. (Chromosomes stained with propidium iodide)

References. (1) Stallings, R. and Siciliano, M. (1981) Somat. Cell Genet., 7:683-698; (2) Stallings, R. and Siciliano, M. (1982) J. Hered., 73:399-404; (3) Stallings, R., Siciliano, M., Adair, G., Humphrey, R. (1982) Somatic. Cell Genet., 8:413-422; (4) Siciliano, M., Stallings, R., Adair, G., Humphrey, R., and Siciliano, J. (1983) Cytogenet. Cell Genet. 35:15-20; (5) Adair, G., Stallings, R., Friend, K., and Siciliano, M. (1983) Somat. Cell Genet., 9:477-487; (6) Stallings, R., Adair, G., and Siciliano,M. (1983) Somat. Cell Genet., In press; (7) Kraemer, P., Travis,G., Ray, F. A., and Cram, L. S. (1983) Cancer Res., 43:4822-4827; (8) Cram, L. S., Bartholdi, M., Ray, F. A., Travis, G., and Kraemer, P. (1983) Cancer Res., 43:4828-4837;

(supported by the Los Alamos Natl. Lab., U.S. Dept. of Energy (O.H.E.R.), NIH Flow Cytometry National Resource (L. S. Cram, P.I., Grant RR01315).

A HUMAN-LIKE PREPROINSULIN LEADER SEQUENCE DIRECTS PROTEIN SECRETION IN YEAST

P.O. Stepien, R. Brousseau, R. Wu*, S. Narang and D.Y. Thomas
Molecular Genetics Section, Division of Biological Sciences, National Research Council of Canada, 100 Sussex Dr., Ottawa, and *Section of Biochemistry, Molecular and Cell Biology, Cornell University, Ithaca, NY 14853, USA

INTRODUCTION. We are interested in studying factors affecting stable expression of foreign genes in yeast and in E. coli. For this purpose we have investigated expression of a synthetic proinsulin gene using fusions of this gene with different leader sequences. Our previous studies (1) have shown that lack of a leader sequence gives no detectable production of proinsulin in Saccharomyces cerevisiae, while the presence of 30 amino acid long or 280 amino acid long leaders from yeast galactokinase gene leads to a low level of production of proinsulin (22 and 119 nanograms per mg of total protein) found within yeast cells. In this paper we present studies on the influence of a human secretion leader peptide on expression and export of preproinsulin by yeast.

RESULTS AND DISCUSSION. The preproinsulin leader sequence was synthesized chemically using triester methods and was ligated to the synthetic human proinsulin gene (2). The sequence is shown in Fig. 1. Differences from the natural human amino acid sequence are at amino acid positions 2, 5, 11 and 15; the sequence 25-28 connects the two genes and codes for methionine in order to enable CNBr cleavage of proinsulin from the leader.

The preproinsulin gene was fused to the yeast alcohol dehydrogenase promoter ADH1, cloned into a high copy number vector pYT 7810 and transformed into yeast. The map of this plasmid is shown in Fig. 2 (pPS4). The plasmid pPS6 containing the proinsulin gene without the leader sequence served as a control. Preproinsulin levels in cell extracts and in growth medium were measured by a radioimmunoassay for human C-peptide and radioimmunassay for human insulin.

The results indicate that the plasmid pPS4 can direct synthesis of preproinsulin in yeast. The level of production (measured by the C-peptide radioimmunoassay) is 2160 nanograms per mg of total yeast protein. In contrast to this,, transformants carrying plasmid pPS6 did not produce detectable levels of preproinsulin. The level of production in strain pPS4 is 21 times higher than that of the most effective protein fusion of proinsulin with a yeast galactokinase leader (1).

The presence of the hydrophobic pre-sequence leads also to partial secretion of the synthesized product to the yeast medium; between 10 to 25% of preproinsulin is secreted. During the secretion process the preproinsulin molecule is cleaved and the site of cleavage is adjacent to the C-peptide. The exact position of this site is being investigated.

The dramatic difference in levels of production of preproinsulin and the proinsulin fusions may be attributed to stabilizing effects of the human secretion leader sequence even within the yeast cell. Possibly it is differently compartmentalized or the hydrophobic human leader gives greater resistance against proteolysis. Both hydrophilic leaders from the yeast galactokinase or the hydrophobic leader from the cloned yeast killer toxin (results unpublished) did not have this effect.

REFERENCES

(1) P.O. Stepien, R. Brousseau, R. Wu, S. Narang and D.Y. Thomas, Gene, 24 (1983) 289–297.
(2) R. Brousseau, R. Scarpulla, W. Sung, H.M. Hsiung, S. Narang, R. Wu, Gene, 17 (1982) 279–289.

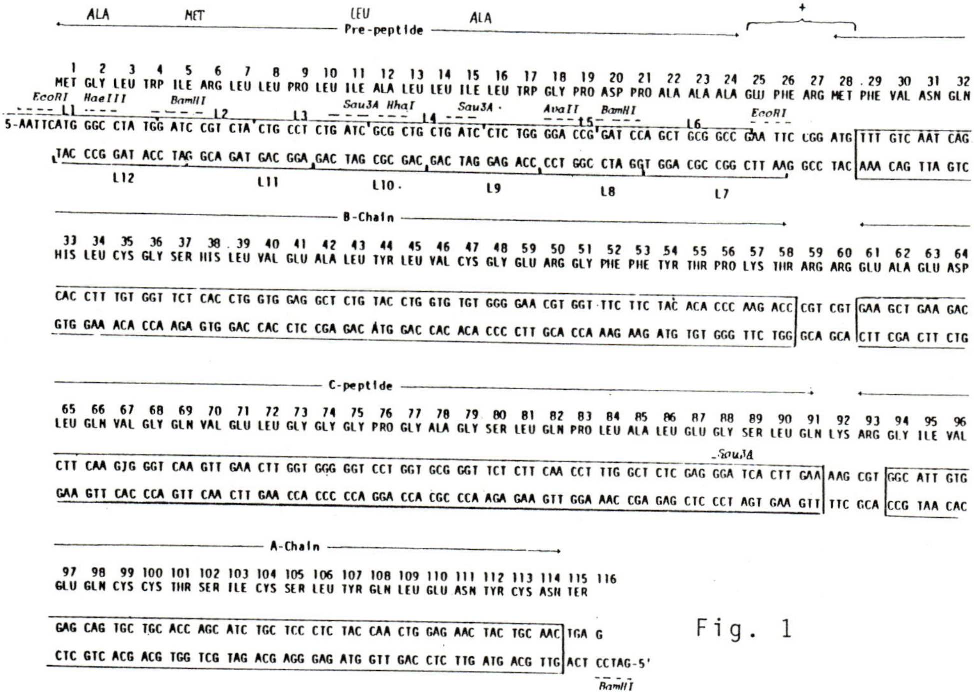

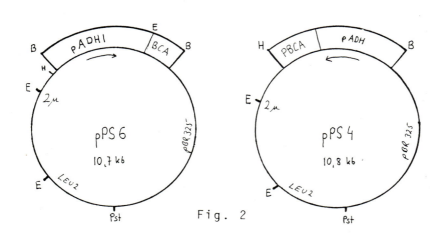

Fig. 1

Fig. 2

MECHANISMS OF DEXAMETHASONE AND BLEOMYCIN REGULATION OF PROCOLLAGEN SYNTHESIS AND TYPE I PROCOLLAGEN mRNAs. Kenneth M. Sterling and Kenneth R. Cutroneo, Department of Biochemistry, School of Medicine, University of Vermont, Burlington, Vermont 05405.

The mechanism of the glucocorticoid inhibitory effect on collagen synthesis was determined in vivo and in fibroblast cell culture using analogous neonatal chick and embryonic chick skin and lung fibroblast culture models. Dexamethasone treatment of neonatal chicks resulted in a time and dose dependent selective decrease of skin and lung collagen synthesis. Total RNA isolated from the skin of chicks receiving various doses of dexamethasone showed dose-related decreases of type I procollagen proα1(I) and proα2(I) mRNAs by dot hybridization. Dexamethasone treatment of chick skin and chick lung fibroblasts resulted in a selective decrease of procollagen synthesis. Dexamethasone-treated chick skin and chick lung fibroblasts also had decreased levels of type I procollagen proα1(I) and proα2(I) mRNAs in proportion to the decreases of cell layer procollagen synthesis.

Embryonic chick skin and chick lung fibroblasts were also used to study the effect of bleomycin, a cancer chemotherapeutic agent which causes skin and lung fibrosis, on collagen synthesis and the cellular contents of type I procollagen mRNAs. Bleomycin treatment of primary chick skin fibroblasts and chick lung fibroblasts resulted in a selective, dose dependent increase of cell layer procollagen synthesis. Solid support hybridization of total cellular RNA to ^{32}P-labeled proα1(I) and proα2(I) cloned cDNAs did not indicate an increase of total cellular type I procollagen mRNAs in bleomycin treated cells. However, bleomycin treatment of chick skin fibroblasts caused an alteration in the distribution of type I procollagen mRNAs among the nuclear, cytoplasmic and polysomal subcellular fractions. Both the nuclear and cytoplasmic type I procollagen mRNAs were significantly decreased in concentration after bleomycin administration. In contrast, the polysomal type I procollagen mRNAs were significantly increased in both chick skin and chick lung fibroblasts treated with bleomycin. These data indicate an mRNA partitioning mechanism for the bleomycin-induced increase of cell layer procollagen synthesis.

Administration of dexamethasone to bleomycin treated fibroblasts resulted in an inhibition of the bleomycin-induced increase of cell layer procollagen synthesis. The increased amounts of polysomal type I procollagen mRNAs in bleomycin treated fibroblasts were also reduced by subsequent administration of dexamethasone. The data indicate that glucocorticoids and bleomycin regulate type I procollagen mRNAs by different mechanisms, yet glucocorticoids are able to reverse the bleomycin-induced increase of polysomal type I procollagen mRNAs. Supported by Grants AM 19808 and HL 14212 from the NIH.

RESTRICTION FRAGMENT LENGTH POLYMORPHISMS IN ACHONDROPLASTIC DWARFISM AND THANATOPHORIC DWARFISM

Charles M. Strom and Charis E.L. Eng

Department of Pediatrics &
Joseph P. Kennedy, Jr.
Mental Retardation Research Center
University of Chicago
5841 South Maryland Avenue
Box 413
Chicago, IL 60637

The chondrodystrophies are a group of congenital dwarfing conditions that involve defective cartilage formation. Achondroplastic dwarfism (AC), an autosomal dominant disorder, is the most common chondrodystrophy, occurring in 1:2600 live births (1). Thanatophoric dwarfism (TD) is a lethal congenital dwarfing condition. The mode of inheritance of TD remains a matter of debate (1-5).

Type II collagen is the major collagen type found in cartilage and is comprised of 3 α1(II) collagen chains. Strom and Upholt have successfully isolated genomic clones corresponding to the α1(II) procollagen gene (unpublished results). In this study we have used the subclone pgHCol(II)al to demonstrate restriction fragment length polymorphisms (RFLP) in the α1(II) procollagen gene in a patient with TD and in a patient with AD.

Maps of the genomic clone LgHCol(II)b and the subclone pgHCol(II)al are shown in Fig. 1. The arrow is directed at the approximate position of the 3' end of the gene. The raised portion has been sequenced by Strom and Upholt and contains the fourth exon from the 3' end of the gene and codes for the last 15 amino acids of the triple helical region, the 27 amino acids of the carboxytelopeptide and the first 54 amino acids of the carboxypropeptide (unpublished results).

Fibroblasts were obtained from a skin biopsy of a patient with AC and from a patient with TD from the NIGMS Human Mutant Cell Repository (GM1422). Cells were cultured in Eagle's Medium and DNA was prepared by proteinase K digestion (6). Normal DNA was obtained from fresh placentas or peripheral blood from laboratory volunteers (6). Fifteen μg of DNA were digested to completion with the 75 units of restriction endonuclease BamHl at 37° overnight in 150mM NaCl, 6mM Tris-HCl, pH 7.9, 6mM MgCl$_2$ and 100μg/ml bovine serum albumin. Control digestions of lambda DNA were used to assure completeness of digestions. The digested DNA was electrophoresed on 1.0% agarose gels, transferred to nitrocellulose and hybridized to pgHCol(II)al which had been made radioactive by nick translation (7). The BamHl digestions of the DNA of 6 controls and the patient with TD hybridized with pgHCol(II)al are shown in Fig. 2A. This filter clearly shows that the normal DNA has a single band at the expected size of 4.2kbp but that the TD DNA has two bands, one at 4.2kbp and a second, more intense band at 6.4kbp. In Fig. 2B, a BamHl digestion of the DNA from the patient with AD is compared with those of two controls. The achondroplastic DNA has an intense 6.2kbp band in addition to the expected 4.2kbp band. The AD and TD electrophoresed contiguously on the same gel confirmed that the 6.2kbp AD band migrates slightly faster than the TD 6.4kbp band. Preliminary results using Hinfl digestions of AD and TD DNA revealed that the polymorphisms are different in these disorders.

The increased intensity of the polymorphic bands with respect to the control bands, although the same amount of DNA was applied to the gels, suggests that the RFLP's are due to an insertion of repeating sequences complimentary to pgHCol(II)al. Since the probe and the 4.2kbp normal BamH1 fragment are completely contained within the type II procollagen gene, this insertion must occur within the gene.

We have now analyzed 6 placentas and 9 peripheral blood samples of normal subjects and have found 1 placenta and 3 blood samples to contain BamH1 RFLP's. None of these, however, have the 6.4 or 6.2kbp band present in the DNA of TD or AD. Studies are underway to fully define the nature of these insertions and to analyze the inheritance pattern of these polymorphisms.

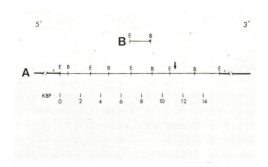

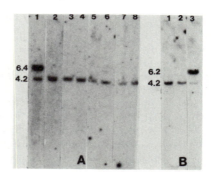

Fig. 1. Restriction maps of human type II collagen gene. A, genomic clone LgHCol(II)b; B, subclone pgHCol(II)al; E is EcoR1; B is BamH1.

Fig. 2. Southern blots of BamH1 digestions of control, TD and AD DNA with pgHCol(II)al as probe. A, lane 1 15µg of TD DNA; lanes 2-8, 15 g of DNA of 7 controls. B, lane 1-2, 15 g DNA of 2 controls; lane 3, 15 g of AC DNA.

REFERENCES. (1) Smith, D.W. (1982) in Recognizable Patterns of Malformations, (Saunders Co.); (2) McKusick, V. (1982) in Mendelian Inheritance in Man, (John Hopkins Press); (3) Harris, R. and Patton, J.T. (1971) Clin. Gen., Vol. 2, pp. 61-72; (4) Marateaux, P. and Lamy, M. (1968) Arch. Fran. Ped., Vol. 2, p. 241; (5) Sillence, D.V., Horton, M.D., and Rimoin, D.L. (1979) Am. J. Path., Vol. 3, p. 813; (6) Maniatis, T., Fristch, E.F., and Sambrook, J. (1982) in Molecular Cloning, (Cold Spring Harbor); (7) Southern, E.M. (1979) Methods Enzymol., Vol. 68, pp. 152-176

Allele Specific Hybridization Using Oligonucleotide Probes of Very High Specific Activity: Discrimination of the Human β^A and β^S-globin Genes

Anna B. Studencki and R. Bruce Wallace
Molecular Genetics Dept., City of Hope Res. Inst., Duarte, CA 91010

The repair activity of E. coli DNA polymerase I (Klenow fragment) was used to prepare nonadecanucleotide hybridization probes which were complementary either to the normal human β-globin (β^A) or to the sickle cell human β-globin (β^S) gene. Template directed polymerization of highly radiolabeled α-^{32}P-deoxyribonucleoside triphosphates (3200, 5000 and/or 7800 Ci/mmol) onto nonamer and decamer primers produced probes with specific activities ranging from 1.0-2.0 X 10^{10} dpm/μg. The extremely high specific activities of these probes made it possible to detect the β^A and β^S single copy gene sequences in as little as 1 μg of total human genomic DNA as well as to discriminate between the homozygous and heterozygous states. This means that it was possible to detect 0.5-1.0 X 10^{-18} moles of a given single copy sequence.

Hybridization of the internally ^{32}P labeled nonadecanucleotide probes 19A (5' CTCCTGAGGAGAAGTCTGC 3') and p19S' (5' pGCAGACTTCTCC-ACAGGAG 3') to human genomic DNAs is shown in the figure. 31 hr Bam H1/Eco R1 digests of 1 μg samples of $\beta^A\beta^A$, $\beta^A\beta^S$ and $\beta^S\beta^S$ genomic DNAs were resolved on a 1% Seakem HGT agarose mini-gel (0.2 X 8 X 13 cm). 85 min Bam H1 digests of 16 and 160 pg λHβG1 samples and of 3 and 30 pg pBR322-HβS samples were also included as markers on this gel. These markers contained the β^A and β^S genes, respectively. The gel membrane was hybridized for 21 hr at 53°C with a 19A probe preparation which had a specific activity of 1.4 X 10^{10} dpm/μg (Panel A). After 4.75 days of autoradiography, this probe was removed by washing the gel for 10 min at 60°C in 2X SSPE, 0.1% SDS. The gel was re-hybridized for 23 hr with a p19S' preparation which had a specific activity of 1.55 X 10^{10} dpm/μg. The re-hybridized gel was autoradiographed for 2.8 days (Panel B). Hybridization mixes contained: 2.5 X 10^6 cpm/ml ^{32}P labeled probe, 10 μg/ml sonicated, denatured E. coli carrier DNA, 0.3% SDS and 5X SSPE (1X SSPE = 10 mM sodium phosphate, pH 7.0, 0.18 M NaCl, 1 mM EDTA).

N.B. The site of the $\beta^A \rightarrow \beta^S$ point mutation is underlined in the probe sequences given above.

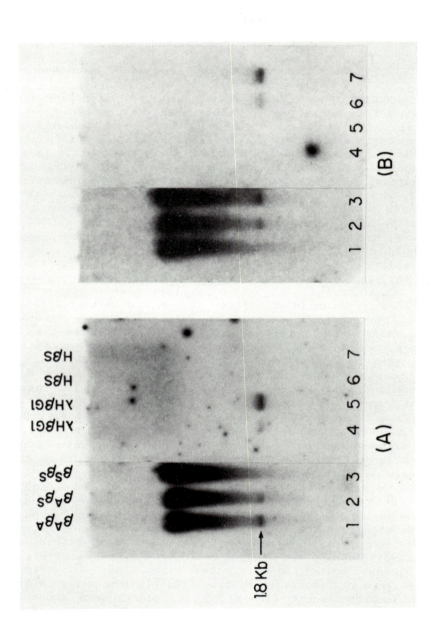

AN ENZYME-IMMUNOBINDING ASSAY
FOR FAST SCREENING OF EXPRESSION OF
TISSUE PLASMINOGEN ACTIVATOR cDNA IN E. COLI

John C.-T. TANG and Shirley H. LI

Biogen, 14 Cambridge Center, Cambridge, Massachusetts

INTRODUCTION. Tissue plasminogen activator (TPA) has been isolated from normal human tissues and certain human cell lines in culture. The enzyme is a serine protease which converts an inactive zymogen, plasminogen to plasmin, and causes lysis of fibrin clots. The high affinity of TPA for fibrin indicates that it is a potential thrombolytic agent and is superior to urokinase-like plasminogen activators. Recently, TPA has been cloned and expressed in E. coli (1, 2, and R. A. Fisher and M. D. Rosa, unpublished results). Using TPA as a model protein, we report here the development of a direct, sensitive enzyme-immunoassay for the screening of a cDNA expression library using specific antibodies and peroxidase-labeled second antibody.

MATERIALS AND METHODS. Preparation of E. coli lysates. The E. coli transformants were either replica plated onto nitrocellulose membranes or grown in microtiter plates, and harvested in exponential phase. For those colonies grown on nitrocellulose sheets, the bacteria cells were treated with chloroform vapor, and then lysed with lysozyme and DNase (3). E. coli cells grown in microtiter plates were lysed in situ with lysozyme (230 µg/ml) and EDTA (4.5 mM) for 15 min. at 20°C. Nitrocellulose membranes that contained E. coli samples were dried completely at room temperature. Microtiter plates containing E. coli lysates were incubated for 3 hours at 37°C in order to absorb protein. Enzyme-Immunobinding assay. To identify gene products in the bacterial lysates, the nitrocellulose membranes were incubated 30 min. at 20°C in blocking solution containing 3% bovine serum albumin. They were then incubated 3 hours at room temperature with anti-TPA diluted in the blocking solution. The membranes were extensively washed with PBS four times (10 min. each wash) and subsequently incubated with peroxidase conjugated-second antibody in the blocking solution. After washing with PBS as described above, the antigen-antibody complexes were assayed for the presence of peroxidase activity. The enzyme assay mixture consisted of 0.01% O-dianisidine and 0.66% H_2O_2 in 10mM Tris-HCl buffer, pH 7.5. For samples coated to microtiter plates, the enzyme-immunobinding assays were run as described for nitrocellulose membrane assays, with slight modifications. The microtiter plates were washed with 0.01% Tween 20 in PBS (PBS-Tween) before adding blocking solution. In the blocking and washing steps, 200 µl of wash were used for each well. Wells were incubated with 50 µl of first antibody and enzyme-labeled second antibody solution. The peroxidase activity bound to the antigens in the plate was assayed by using O-phenylenediamine.

RESULTS AND DISCUSSION. The procedures described here utilized both bacterial cells grown in microtiter plates in liquid media and those grown on a solid phase (nitrocellulose membranes). These assays are more sensitive and convenient than the published procedures for screening of cDNA expression libraries (3). The old method employing ^{125}I-labeled second antibody and replica plating of cells onto a nitrocellulose filter, takes 2 to 4 days to complete. Based on the application of the antigen to

Table 1. Enzyme-immunobinding assay for screening of expression cDNA.

Position	Peroxidase Activity (Absorbance 492 nm)					
	1	2	3	4	5	6
A	0.044	0.059	0.073	0.204	0.063	0.253
B	0.069	0.243	0.075	0.250	0.071	0.060
C	0.075	0.007	0.059	0.070	0.075	0.245
D	0.245	0.066	0.070	0.073		

nitrocellulose sheets, a similar enzyme-immunoassay for screening supernatants of hybridomas making monoclonal antibodies has also been described (4). However, our new procedures provide a unique way for screening various regulatory systems for a particular construct obtained from recombinant DNA technology. In addition to screening for the expression of genetic products, the recombinant molecules can be semiquantitatively determined by using a soluble substrate for peroxidase (Table 1 and Figure 1). One of the advantages of this method is that it allows a preliminary selection of high expression colonies among many positive candidates. The recombinant TPA in some of these expressed cells has been isolated and refolded for both enzymatic and immuno-chemical studies. We have been able to confirm the enzymatic activity of E. coli TPA by using coupled photometric assays (5). These TPA activities were enhanced by fibrin and fibrinogen present in the assay mixture and inhibited by specific antiserum against TPA (J. C.-T. Tang, unpublished results).

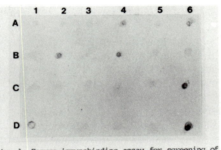

Fig. 1. Enzyme-immunobinding assay for screening of expression cDNA.

References. (1) Pennica, D., Holmes, W.E., Kohr, W.J., Harkins, R.N., Vehar, G.A., Ward, C.A., Bennett, W.F., Yelverton, E., Seeburg, P.H., Heyneka, H.L., Goeddel, D.V. and Collen, D. (1983) Nature 301, 214; (2) Edlund, T., Ny, T., Ranby, M., Heden, L.-O., Palm, G., Holygren, E. and Josephson, S. (1983) Proc. Natl. Acad. Sci. USA. 80, 349; (3) Helfman, D.M., Feramisco, J.R., Fiddes, J.C., Thomas, G.P. and Hughes, S.H. (1983) Proc. Natl. Acad. Sci. USA 80, 31; (4) Hawkes, R., Niday, E. and Gordon J. (1982) Anal. Biochem. 119, 142. (5) Tang, J. C.-T., Li, S., McGray, P. and Vecchio, A. (1984) in "Enzyme Engineering VII" ed. A.I. Laskin et al., in press.

Acknowledgments. We thank Dr. J. E. Smart for encouragement and discussion. We are grateful to Dr. R. A. Fisher and Dr. M. D. Rosa for providing us with the E. coli constructs. We also thank Miss Donna Roberto for editorial assistance.

MOLECULAR BASIS OF HEREDITARY TYROSINEMIAS: PROOF OF THE PRIMARY DEFECT BY WESTERN BLOT

R.M. Tanguay, C. Laberge, A. Lescault, J.P. Valet, J.L. Duband and Y. Quenneville

Human Genetics Unit, CHUL, Research Center and Dept. of Medicine, Univ. Laval, Ste Foy, P.Q. Canada G1V 4G2

INTRODUCTION

Hereditary tyrosinemia is an inborn error of the metabolism of the aromatic amino acid, tyrosine (1).   In the French Canadian population, the incidence varies between 1:800 livebirths in a large geographic isolate to 1:12,000 in the general Quebec population (2 and Quebec Network of Genetic Medicine registry).   In the geographic isolate, the carrier rate is 1:15.   There are at present no tests available for heterozygote detection. The great majority of patients suffer from the acute form of the disease and die of acute biochemical fulminant hepatitis or of liver failure through cirrhosis within months of birth.   A few rare patients in these families develop the chronic form of the disease with vitamin D dependent rickets and terminal hepatocarcinoma in their pre teen years.

The putative enzymatic defect in tyrosinemia seems to reside in the ultimate step of the transformation of tyrosine into fumarate or succinate by fumaryl acetoacetate hydrolase (FAAH: EC 3,7,1,2) (3). Thus FAAH activity is deficient in acute hereditary tyrosinemia while 20-30% residual activity is found in the chronic phenotype.   Organic derivatives of both natural substrates succinylacetoacetate and fumarylacetoacetate have been identified in urine of patients (3) and in the amniotic fluid permitting prenatal and neonatal diagnosis of the disease (4-5).   However the molecular nature of the enzymatic defect remains unknown.

RESULTS

The putative enzyme involved in tyrosinemia, FAAH was purified from rat liver (in preparation). The enzyme monomeric polypeptide of 40,000 dalton was further purified by preparative SDS-polyacrylamide gel before immunization in rabbits. Proteins from autopsy or biopsy liver material were separated on SDS-gels, blotted on nitrocellulose filters and probed with the rabbit FAAH antibody and with a second goat ^{125}I anti-rabbit IgG.

The antiserum against rat FAAH cross reacts with the human FAAH which is of slightly higher M.W. (Fig. 1, lane 1-4). As shown in this figure, the putative antigen is absent from livers of all tyrosinemia patients with the exception of the patients showing the chronic phenotype (lane 8). All 14 patients examined gave identical results.

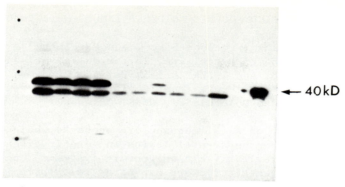

Figure 1 - Immunolot with anti rat FAAH antiserum. Livers from control (lane 2 to 5), acute (lane 6,7,9-11) and chronic tyrosinemic patients (8) and rat (12). M.W. standards (1).

CONCLUSION

This work gives for the first time the structural proof for the absence of an enzymic protein as the major defect in hereditary tyrosinemias. The acute form shows a total absence of the 40,000 dalton enzyme. On the other hand, in the less severe chronic form, the residual FAAH activity correlates well with the residual amount of the 40,000 dalton protein pattern detected by western blot analysis. Thus both forms of the disease can be easily differentiated at the enzymatic level. Work in progress in this lab on the isolation and restriction mapping of this gene should point out the molecular defect in both types of tyrosinemia. Hopefully it should lead to a restriction polymorphism based carrier test for preventive genetic medicine and help in our understanding of the dynamics of aromatic acid degradation in relation to energetic homeostasis of essential amino acids in eukaryotes.

SUMMARY

Two types of human hereditary tyrosinemia have been delineated by western blot with an anti rat FAAH antibody. The acute form is characterized by the absence of FAAH while the chronic form has a lowered content.

Supported by the Conseil de Recherche Medicale du Canada and Le Reseau de Medecine Genetique du Quebec.

BIBLIOGRAPHY

(1) Gentz, J., Jagenburg, R., Zetterstrom, R. (1965) J. Pediatr. 66, 670-696; (2) Bergeron, P., Laberge, C. and Grenier, A. (1974) Clin. Genet. 5 157-162; (3) Lindblad, B., Lindstedt, S. and Steen, G. (1977) Proc. Natl. Acad. Sci USA 79 4641-4645; (4) Gagne, R., Lescault, A., Grenier, A., Laberge, C., Melancon, S.B. and Dallaire, L. (1982) Prenat. diagn. 2 185-188; (5) Grenier, A., Lescault, A., Laberge, C., Gagne, R. and Mamer, O. (1982) Clin. Chim. Acta. 123 93-99.

USE OF CHEMICALLY MODIFIED NUCLEIC ACIDS AS IMMUNO-DETECTABLE PROBES
IN HYBRIDIZATIONS.

Paul Tchen[1], Robert Fuchs[2], Evelyne Sage[3], and Marc Leng[3]
1. Institut de Pathologie Moleculaire, 24 rue du Fg. St. Jacques,
    75014 Paris, France, and INSERM U-155, Paris, France
2. Institut de Biologie Moleculaire et Cellulaire, Strasbourg, France
3. Centre de Biophysique Moleculaire, CNRS, Orleans.

Immuno-detectable probes ("immunonucleic probes") would be
useful to search for the fundamental lesion in genetic diseases in
close linkage with a previously cloned genomic fragment, and in
the construction of a genetic linkage map using restriction fragment
length variants. Long stretches of DNA adjacent to the sequence of
a given immunonucleic probe could be immunoprecipitated after
solution hybridization and used to screen a DNA library. Starting
with a probe of known chromosomal location, it would be theoretically possible to obtain rapidly sets of clones corresponding to
defined chromosomal domains. Immunonucleic probes could also be
used to detect specific gene sequences with regular immunochemical
techniques. We are presently developing a method based on the
chemical modification of guanine residues in ribo or deoxyribo-
nucleic acids using 7-iodo-N-acetoxy-N-2-acetylaminofluorene (AAIF).

METHODS: AAIF and anti N-2 (guanosin-8 yl)-acetylaminofluorene
(anti Guo-AAF) were prepared as previously described (1,2). Probes
were prepared by reacting the nucleic acids with a 2 fold excess in
weight of AAIF (2 mM sodium citrate buffer, pH 7, 2 hours, 37°C).
Excess of reactant was removed by ethyl ether extraction. Hybridizations were performed at 65°C following standard procedures.

RESULTS: Reconstruction experiments were done to test the
feasibility of the immunopurification of gene sequences after
solution hybridization with homologous immunonucleic probes. Table
1 shows that AAIF modified DNA (DNA-AAIF) can be immunopurified.
Results of immunopurification after solution hybridization are
shown in Table 2. These results suggest that immunonucleic probes
could be used to purify gene sequences and their adjacent domains.
Immunochemical detection of genes sequences on nitrocellulose or
nylon filters were done after "in situ" hybridizations with immunonucleic probes prepared with single or double stranded DNA or RNA.
The detection sensitivity was in the picogram range. Contrary to
radioactive probes, immunonucleic probes can be used at high concentrations without significant background, and immunochemical
detection provides high resolution. Techniques accelerating the
renaturation rate plus high probe concentrations were used
successfully for rapid detection of gene sequences.

CONCLUSION: Immuno-detectable probes can be prepared with ribo
or deoxyribo, single or double-stranded nucleic acids by a simple
chemical reaction with AAIF. The modified nucleic acids can be
recognized by specific antibodies. They have a long shelf life
(more than 2 years). They can be immunoprecipitated after solution
hybridization and can potentially be used to purify gene sequences
and their adjacent genomic domains. They can also be visualized on

filters by regular immunochemical techniques after "in situ" hybridization. We believe that such probes would prove useful for rapid study of large genomic domains, gene mapping and routine diagnostic tests.

TABLE 1

Antibodies	% of immunoprecipitated DNA	
	Control	DNA-AAIF
normal serum	< 0.1	0.1
Anti Guo-AAF	0.2	81.9
anti Guo-AAF (purified)	< 0.1	71.9

Radioactive λ DNA was prepared by nick-translation and divided in two parts. One part was treated with AAIF and the other kept as a control. Each part was divided into 3 aliquots which were incubated respectively with normal serum, anti Guo-AAF antiserum and anti Guo-AAF affinity purified antibodies (1% antiserum, 1x SSC, 2% sarcosyl, 15 hours at 4°C)(SSC is 150mM NaCl and 15mM citrate). Formalin fixed Staph. a. cells were added. After 15 minutes at room temperature, the aliquots were centrifuged and the pellets were rinsed once in 1x SSC, 2% sarcosyl and once in 1x SSC, 5% sarcosyl. Supernatants of each sample were pooled. Pellets and supernatant were analyzed by Cerenkov counting. The percentage of immunoprecipitated DNA was calculated by using the formula: 100 (cpm of the pellet)/(cpm of the pellet + cpm of the supernatant).

TABLE 2

Probe:	DNA-AAIF	
Target DNA	Carrier DNA	% of reannealed immuno-precipitated molecules
λ	+	33.9
	−	33.1
pBR 322	+	0.4
	−	0.3

λ DNA and pBR 322 plasmid DNA were nick-translated to a specific activity of ~4×10^8 cpm/µg. In each experiment, 20 ng of radioactive λ DNA were mixed with 200 ng of DNA-AAIF immunonucleic probe, with or without 6 µg of sheared herring sperm DNA, in a final volume of 80 µl of hybridization solution (2x SSC, 25 mM KH_2PO_4, 2mM EDTA, 0.5% SDS, pH 7). Hybridizations were done in sealed capillary tubes at 65°C for 72 hours, after 5 minutes denaturation at 100°C. After hybridization, the content of each tube was treated as indicated in legend to Table 1. The percentage of reannealed immunoprecipitated molecules was calculated using the formula:
100 [(cpm of the pellet)/(cpm of the pellet) + 0.5 x (cpm of the supernatant)].

REFERENCES

(1) Lefevre, J.F., Fuchs, R.P.P. and Daune, M.P. (1978) Biochemistry 17, 2561-2567.
(2) Guigues, M. and Leng, M. (1979) Nucleic Acids Res. 6, 733-744.

EFFECTS OF CHEMICAL CARCINOGENS AND VIRAL ONCOGENES ON THE NEOPLASTIC PROGRESSION OF SYRIAN HAMSTER EMBRYO CELLS: EVIDENCE FOR A THREE STEP PROCESS.

David G. Thomassen, Mitsuo Oshimura, Tona Gilmer, Lois Annab, and J. Carl Barrett

National Institute of Environmental Health Sciences, Research Triangle Park, N.C. 27709

We have previously demonstrated that chemical carcinogen induced neoplastic transformation of Syrian Hamster Embryo (SHE) cells is a progressive, multistep process. To understand the nature of carcinogen-induced events and the role of oncogenes in this process, we have compared the susceptibilities of normal, diploid SHE cells and carcinogen-induced preneoplastic SHE cells to oncogene-induced neoplastic transformation by transfection with genomic clones of either Harvey murine sarcoma virus (HaSV) or Rous sarcoma virus (RSV). We present evidence that HaSV and RSV DNAs can induce neoplastic transformation of carcinogen-induced preneoplastic cells, but not of their normal parental cells. In addition, we present evidence suggesting that oncogene-induced transformation of preneoplastic cells involves 2 steps.

Normal SHE cells treated with HaSV DNA were morphologically normal, did not escape cellular senescence, but did grow in agar at a low frequency ($<10^{-5}$). DES-4 cells, a line of preneoplastic SHE cells induced with the human carcinogen diethylstilbestrol, formed progressively growing tumors in nude mice <3 weeks after HaSV DNA treatment while pBR DNA treated cells were nontumorigenic. Tumors formed with DES-4 cells treated with 50 ng of DNA, whereas SHE cells treated with 5000 ng of DNA were nontumorigenic. Co-transfection with HaSV and p-SV2-neo DNAs and selection for antibiotic resistance indicated that SHE cells were recipients for exogenous DNA but this treatment did not result in transformation of SHE cells. However, 50% of the cotransfected DES-4 cells were neoplastically transformed and expressed elevated levels of HaSV RNA. In addition, DES-4 cells transfected with RSV DNA formed tumors in nude mice while RSV DNA treated SHE cells did not. These results support the hypothesis that Ha-ras and src oncogenes can complete the neoplastic transformation of cells following carcinogen treatment but that these oncogenes alone are insufficient to cause neoplastic transformation of normal cells.

The clonal evolution of neoplastic transformation induced by HaSV DNA was examined by cotransfecting cells with pSV2-neo and HaSV DNA followed by selection for antibiotic (G418) resistance (neo^R) encoded by pSV2-neo. Fifty percent (7/14) of neo^R clones were tumorigenic and 4/4 of those clones tested expressed Ha-ras RNA. Transfection with pSV2-neo DNA alone gave 17/18 nontumorigenic, neo^R clones. There was no correlation between growth in agar and tumorigenicity by HaSV transformed cells. Some grew in agar, expressed high levels of HaSV RNA, but were nontumorigenic. Cytogenetic analyses demonstrated that DES-4 cells are aneuploid with a near diploid chromosome number. No karyotypic alterations were observed in 20 neo[R] clones regardless of their HaSV expression. In contrast, oncogene-induced tumor derived cell lines at first passage had extensive structural abnormalities and a considerable number of double minute chromosomes. We propose that Ha-ras oncogene converts DES-4 cells to a near neoplastic state and that additional karyotypic changes are required for cells to form tumors in nude mice. Thus, neoplastic progression of the cells requires carcinogen-induced immortalization, expression of Ha-ras oncogene, and karyotypic evolution.

THE HUMAN ALDOLASE B GENE: STUDIES TOWARD UNDERSTANDING HEREDITARY FRUCTOSE INTOLERANCE.

Dean R. TOLAN, William H. ROTTMANN and Edward E. PENHOET
Dept. of Biochemistry, University of California, Berkeley, CA

The widespread metabolic disorder, hereditary fructose intolerance, has been shown to be caused by a defect in the gene for the liver aldolase enzyme (1). The disease appears to be manifested in a heterogeneous fashion where both defects in the catalytic properties and/or levels of the enzyme are found. Diagnosis of the disease is commonly made in infants when illness develops due to the ingestion and failure to digest fructose. In order to understand more precisely the molecular changes which give rise to the disease, the study of the human aldolase B gene in both normal and fructose intolerant patients has been undertaken.

METHODS. The isolation of a cDNA coding for human aldolase B was accomplished using a rabbit cDNA for aldolase A as a probe (2) to screen a human liver cDNA library (3) by colony hybridization techniques. The positive clones were confirmed as aldolase B by RNA blotting techniques (4) against liver RNA. The cDNA clones were subcloned into M13 vectors (5) and sequenced by the dideoxy termination method (6). The largest cDNA for human aldolase B was used to probe a human genomic library by plaque hybridization techniques (7). The positive clones were isolated and characterized by Southern blotting (8). DNA restriction fragments were subcloned into M13 and pUC vectors (9) and their sequence determined as before.

RESULTS. The cDNA clones and their relationship to the mRNA as well as the sequencing strategy is shown in Figure 1. The clones code for 80% of the mRNA. The amino acid and nucleotide homology of this human liver aldolase isozyme is highly conserved in comparison to rabbit muscle aldolase. The largest clone, pHL413, was used to probe the human genomic library in charon 4A. Two separate screenings of 8×10^5 plaques were done, each yielding a single clone corresponding to a partial segment of the aldolase B gene. The two clones, λH201 and λH313, were characterized and partially sequenced. The results are summarized in Figure 2. The clone λH201 contained the 3' most portion of the gene including the last exon coding for amino acid 333 to 363 and including all of the 3'-untranslated region. Further in the 5'-direction from

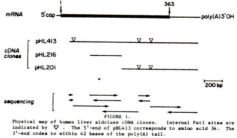

FIGURE 1.
Physical map of human liver aldolase cDNA clones. Internal PstI sites are indicated by ∇ . The 5'-end of pHL413 corresponds to amino acid 34. The 3'-end codes to within 42 bases of the poly(A) tail.

amino acid 333 there is a large intron of >3 kb. The clone λH313 contains at least two exons, one corresponding to amino acids 1 to 37, the other extending from amino acid 38. These two clones do not overlap as determined by their restriction digestion patterns and the sequences at their boundaries.

A canonical transcription initiation sequence is not seen in the upstream sequence at the position expected from the size of the mRNA. There is a sequence starting 10 bases upstream from the initiation methionine codon which correspond to an intron/exon junction. There may be an intron in the 5'-untranslated region of this gene. Studies are underway to sequence the mRNA by primer extension (2), as well as finish the isolation and sequencing of the remainder of the gene.

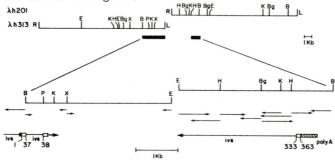

FIGURE 2.

Restriction map and sequence summary of two lambda clones coding for the human aldolase B gene. The restriction map of two clones are at the top and the regions which hybridize to the cDNA probe (███) expanded at the bottom. Arrows underneath depict regions and extent of sequence analysis, a schematic of the coding region is below that. Numbers refer to amino acid numbers, letters are: E, EcoRI; B, BamHI; Bg, BglI; H, HindIII; K, KpnI; P, PstI; X, XbaI; ivs, intervening sequence; L, left arm; R, right arm.

SUMMARY. The partial characterization of the human aldolase B gene has revealed a gene which is at least 7 kb in size, and contains at least 3 introns. When the complete structure and sequence of the gene is determined it will be used for comparison to the aldolase B genes from patients with hereditary fructose intolerance. Analysis of these mutations will help to understand the structure and catalytic properties of a mammalian enzyme as well as elements that affect the control of expression of this glycolytic, "housekeeping" gene. The studies will yield methods for simple diagnosis and detection of carriers for the disease.

REFERENCES. (1) Gitzelmann, R., Steinmann, B. and Van den Berghe, G. (1983) In "Metabolic Basis of Inherited Disease", pp. 118-140; (2) Tolan, D., Amsden, A., Putney, S., Urdea, M., and Penhoet, E. (1983) J. Biol. Chem., in press; (3) gift from R. Hollewell; (4) Thomas, P. (1980) Proc. Natl. Acad. Sci. USA 77, 5201; (5) Messing, J., Crea, R. and Seeburg, P. (1981) Nuc. Acids Res. 9, 309; (6) Sanger, F., Nicklen, S. and Coulsen, A. (1977) Proc. Natl. Acad. Sci. USA 74, 5463; (7) Maniatis, T., Hardison, R., Lacy, E., Laver, J., O'Connell, C., Quon, D., Sim, G., Efstratiadis, A. (1978) Cell 15, 687; (8) Southern, E. (1975) J. Mol. Biol. 98, 503; (9) Viera, J. and Messing, J. (1982) Gene 19, 259.

CHARGE HETEROGENEITY OF PROTEINS SYNTHESIZED IN CELL - FREE
PROTEIN SYNTHESIS AND E. COLI MINICELLS

K. Trinks[1], K. Beyreuther, P. Habermann[2]
Inst. f. Genetik, Univ. o. Cologne, Weyertal 141, D - 5000
Cologne 41

Radiolabled DNA directed protein synthesis in a Zubay type in
vitro system as well as in E. coli minicells exhibits an unexpected
ambiguity of the gene products. Highly expressed proteins that
look homomogenous upon SDS gel electrophoresis are separated into a
series of spots when analysed according to the method of O'Farrell
(1). Inactivation of one particular gene by a deletion or an
insertion event leads to the loss of only a single series of spots.
They are encoded by one single gene and are only distinguishable by
charge. This charge heterogeneity can not be explained by
secondary modification during protein extraction, because only
newly synthesized proteins are affected. These proteins can be
easily distinguished from host proteins that form homogenously
stained spots. A similar phenomenon was observed for de novo
synthesized proteins in E. coli and eukaryotic cells under
conditions of amino acid starvation (2). According to the
prediction of Parker et al. this is due to translational errors
that lead to codon specific replacements of histidine by glutamine
and of asparagine by lysine. The highest rate of misreading was
supposed to appear during translation of the asparagine specific
codon AAU (3). Radiolabeled microsequence analysis enabled us to
test this hypothesis more directly.

According to the DNA sequence data for E. coli
uridyltransferase (4) AAU encoded asparagine should be found in
position 5 of the protein sequence. Plasmids were constructed,
that contain the E. coli Gal - operon (pKS 100) and a mutated
operon that contains an IS1 - insertion in gal T (pKS 116).

Radiolabeled protein synthesis driven by pKS 100 gives rise to
three Gal - enzymes gal E, gal T and gal K of MR 39 Kd, 40Kd and
42Kd respectively (5). However in the presence of pKS 116 a stable
MR 28Kd chain termination polypeptide, is synthesized instead of
uridyltransferase. The in vitro synthesized chain termination
product is well separated from other synthesis products in SDS
gels. Electrophoretically pure protein was isolated and further
characterized. We confirmed the identity of the 28Kd polypeptide
as the N-terminal polypeptide of gal T by partial radiolabeled
sequence analysis. All Gal - operon encoded enzymes including the
28Kd chain termination polypeptide were heterogenous in charge.

1 Hoechst AG, Pflanzenschutzf. Biologie, D - 6230 Frankfurt 80, FRG
2 Dept. of Molec. Biol., Mass. Gen. Hospital, Boston, MA, 02114,USA

The release of $[^3H]$ - asparagine radioactivity in automated
Edman degradation clearly showed that asparagine is located at
position 5 of the MR 28Kd protein as expected from DNA sequence
information. When the 28Kd polypeptide is synthesized in presence
of $[^{14}C]$ - lysine however, a significant amount $[^{14}C]$ - activity is
detected in postion 5. For each analysis the full complement of
the 20 non-radioactive aminoacids was added. In our experiments
each third or fourth gal T chain termination peptide contained
lysine instead of asparagine at position 5. From these results we
conclude that the charge heterogeneity observed during our DNA
directed in vitro and minicell synthesis studies is in the majority
of cases based on frequent misreading of the asparagine specific
codon AAU.

Lit.: (1) O'Farrell, P.H.: J. Biol. Chem. 250, 4007 (1975); (2)
Parker, J. et al. Proc. Natl. Acad. Sci. 75, 1091 (1978); (3)
Parker, J. et al. Molec. gen. Genet. 180, 275 (1980); (4) Grindley,
N.D.F., et al. Proc. Natl. Acad. Sci. 77, 7176 (1980); (5) Trinks,
K. et al. Hoppe Seyler's Z.F. Phys. Chem. 360, 388 (1979)

Alu and KpnI Sequences are Found Adjacent to Alphoid DNA in the Human Genome.

P. W. Turk, G. J. Graham, T. J. Hall and M. R. Cummings
Department of Biological Sciences and Institute for the
Study of Developmental Disabilities, University of Illinois
Chicago, Illinois.

In the genomes of higher eucaryotes, DNA sequences are differentially represented. Some sequences are present in single copies and presumably code for particular gene products; others are present thousands or hundreds of thousands of times. Among the highly repetitive sequences present in primate genomes are tandem repeats that have varying degrees of homology to the alpha satellite sequence of the African green monkey (1). The alphoid family, concentrated at the centromeric regions of chromosomes (2), has a basic repeat length of 170 bp in the monkey genome. In humans, partial digestion of genomic DNA produces a ladder pattern of alphoid bands, confirming the tandem arrangement of these sequences. Upon complete digestion with EcoRI, two prominent fragments, one of 340 bp, and a dimer aproximately 680 bp in length are produced. The 340 bp repeat unit accounts for some 0.75% of the human genome. Among other highly repetitive sequences, families such as the short (500 bp) Alu family and the longer (up to 6.2 kb) KpnI family are interspersed with low copy number sequences (3,4). Although no functions have been ascribed to highly repetitive sequences, their molecular organization and arrangement have been intensively investigated.

In studies using a screening method which selects for chromosome 21-specific sequences from the human library (5), we have isolated a clone that contains alphoid sequences and adjacent or embedded KpnI and Alu sequences. Digestion of this clone (designated λH1) with EcoRI generates six fragments. One of these, approximately 680 bp long, has been subcloned into pACYC184. This subclone has a restriction pattern similar to that of the consensus human (6) alphoid sequence (Fig. 1) and also shows strong homology when hybridized to a human alphoid sequence. Digests of human genomic DNA hybridized with the subclone or an alphoid sequence produce similar (7) band patterns (Fig. 2).

Hybridization of EcoRI fragments of λH1 with the 1.2 kb and 1.8 kb KpnI repeats indicates that a single fragment approximately 7.8 kb in length is homologous to both probes (Fig. 3). Since there is no homology between λH1 and other elements of the 6.2 kb KpnI repeat, it indicates that portions of the long KpnI repeat occur independently in the human genome. The 7.8 kb fragment also contains sequences homologous to the Alu family (data not shown). When the 680 bp alphoid subclone is used as a probe, the results indicate that no alphoid sequences are interspersed with the KpnI or Alu sequences (Fig.3). Similar relationships between tandem alphoid sequences, KpnI and Alu families have been reported in the AGM

(8,9). These results suggest that the divergence in alphoid sequences between monkey and humans occurs independently of the relationship with other repetitive sequences in the genome.

Recently, a short KpnI sequence with flanking direct repeats has been found embedded in monkey alphoid DNA (9). Examination of the nucleotide sequences which flank the KpnI region in λH1 will determine whether longer KpnI elements in or near alphoid sequences have flanking repeats associated with transposable elements.

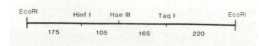

Fig. 1 Restriction map of the 680 bp subclone from λH1.

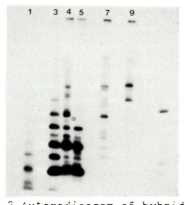

Fig. 2 Autoradiogram of hybridization of nick-translated 680 bp subclone from λH1 to Southern blots of human genomic DNA digested with various endonucleases: (1)MboII; (3)HaeIII; (4)EcoRI; (5)HinfI; (7)HindIII; (9)BamH1.

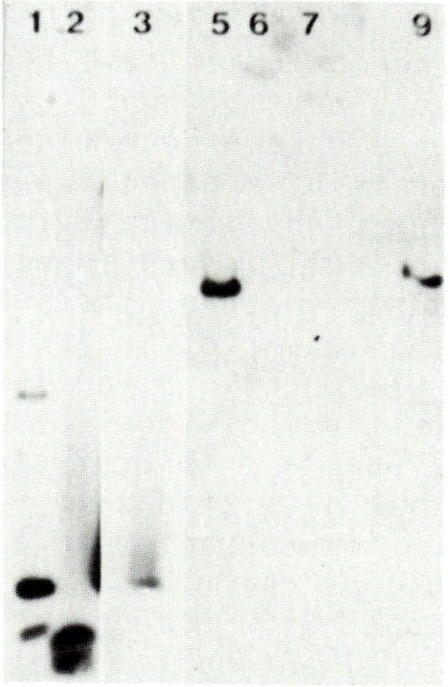

Fig. 3 Autoradiogram of Southern blots of λH1 digested with EcoRI (lanes 1,5,9), alphoid DNA digested with EcoRI (lane 2), and the 680 bp subclone from λH1 (lane 3): lanes 1,2 and 3 were probed with the 680 bp subclone DNA from λH1; lane 5 with a KpnI 1.8 kb clone; lane 9 with a KpnI 1.2 kb clone.

REFERENCES (1). Singer, 1982. Int Rev Cytol 76: 67; (2). Manuelidis, 1978. Chromosoma 66: 23; (3). Manuelidis and Wu, 1978. Nature 276: 92; (4). Duncan, et al, 1979. Proc Nat Acad Sci 76: 5095; (5). Graham, et al, 1984. Am J Hum Genet (in press); (6). Wu and Manuelidis, 1980. J Mol Biol 142: 363; (7). Darling, et al, 1982. J Mol Biol 154: 51; (8). Grimaldi and Singer, 1982. Proc Nat Acad Sci 79: 1497; (9). Thayer and Singer, 1983. Mol and Cell Biol 3: 967.

Acknowledgements: We would like to thank Jeff Doering for providing us with the alphoid clone used in the hybridization experiments, and Tom Maniatis for the human library. We also thank S. McCutcheon and D. Baro for quotidian discussions.

262

PRODUCTION AND CHARACTERIZATION OF MONOCLONAL ANTIBODIES THAT DISCRIMINATE AMONG INDIVIDUAL S100 POLYPEPTIDES

Linda J. Van Eldik

Dept. of Pharmacology and Howard Hughes Medical Institute
Vanderbilt University, Nashville, TN   37232

INTRODUCTION. The term S100 refers to a heterogeneous fraction of low molecular weight, acidic, calcium binding proteins (for review, see 1). The S100 fraction is a mixture of polypeptides, only some of which have been isolated and characterized. The amino acid sequences of two S100 proteins from bovine brain, S100α and S100β, have been determined. The physiological functions of the S100 proteins are not known. Although assay of immunoreactive S100 has been used clinically to screen tumors of neural origin, as an index of cell injury in various disorders, and as an index of malignancy, most of the antisera used in previous studies react with more than one protein in the S100 fraction. Even the currently available monoclonal antibodies against S100 (2-4) do not appear to measure the individual S100α and S100β components. In order to unequivocally interpret studies on the localization of S100 and its potential alterations in various disease states, and on the validity of S100 immunoreactivity as a diagnostic tool for tumor diagnosis, it would be useful to have antibodies that discriminate among the individual S100 components. We report here the production of monoclonal antibodies that appear to be specific for S100β.

MATERIALS AND METHODS. Protein Purification - S100 proteins were purified from bovine brain and from human brain fractions essentially as described (5). The individual S100 polypeptides were homogeneous by several criteria, including amino acid composition and limited amino acid sequence analysis.

Production of Monoclonal Antibodies - Purified bovine brain S100β was used as the immunogen. Mouse myeloma cells (X63-Ag8.6.5.3) were fused with spleen cells from immunized Balb/C mice by following standard procedures (6). Hybridomas were cloned by limiting dilution or by soft agar until stable clones were achieved.

ELISA - Antibody production was monitored by using an enzyme-linked immunosorbent assay (ELISA) and the Vectastain ABC kit for detection of mouse IgG (Vector Laboratories). Antibody reactivity was quantitated with a Multiskan MC plate reader (Flow Laboratories).

RESULTS. Two clones have been produced that secrete antibodies which appear to be specific for S100β. Both monoclonal antibodies are of the IgG$_1$ κ isotype. The antibodies were produced against bovine S100β, but cross-react with human S100β. Analysis of the reactivity of tissue culture supernatants from one of the two clones is shown in Fig. 1. Although not shown, the reactivity of the other antibody is similar. The antibodies react well with human S100β,

with half-maximal binding occurring at a supernatant dilution of
approximately 1:20. The antibodies also react with bovine, chicken,
and rat S100β, with half-maximal binding to bovine S100β occurring
at a supernatant dilution of approximately 1:1000. In contrast,
there is little or no reactivity with S100α (Fig. 1). The
antibodies show no reactivity with other calcium modulated proteins
such as calmodulin or troponin C.

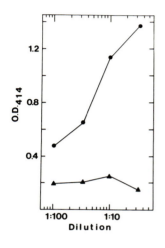

Figure 1. Reactivity of monoclonal
antibody supernatant in ELISA.
Various dilutions of supernatant
were incubated with a fixed
concentration (5 μg/ml) of human
S100β (●) or S100α (▲) that
had been absorbed to a microplate.
The ordinate shows the absorbance
at 414 nm.

DISCUSSION. This is the first
demonstration of monoclonal
antibodies against S100 that are
specific for an individual S100
polypeptide. Current studies are
directed toward establishing
immunocytochemical procedures for
analysis of S100 localization and distribution. The availability
of these antibodies will allow a more unambiguous interpretation of
the properties and potential functions of S100 proteins and may
provide new insight into the mechanisms of disease states,
differentiation, and tumorigenesis.

REFERENCES. (1) Van Eldik, L.J., Zendegui, J.G., Marshak, D.R.
and Watterson, D.M. (1982) Intl. Rev. Cytology 77, 1-61.
(2) Haan, E.A., Boss, B.D. and Cowan, W.M. (1982) Proc. Natl. Acad.
   Sci. USA 79, 7585-7589.
(3) Murakami, H., Masui, H., Sato, G.H., Sueoka, N., Chow, T.P. and
   Kano-Sueoka, T. (1982) Proc. Natl. Acad. Sci. USA 79, 1158-1162.
(4) Gillespie, G.Y. and Golden, P. (1983) Fed. Proc. 42, 2025.
(5) Marshak, D.R., Watterson, D.M. and Van Eldik, L.J. (1981) Proc.
   Natl. Acad. Sci. USA 78, 6793-6797.
(6) Galfre, G. and Milstein, C. (1981) Methods in Enzymol. 73, 3-46.

BIOCHEMICAL AND GENETIC STUDIES ON CELLS PRODUCING ABNORMAL IgM.   Luz M.
Vazquez, M. Patricia Beckmann, Marc J. Shulman*, and William J. Grimes, Department
of Biochemistry, University of Arizona, Tucson, AZ 85721, USA and *Department of
Medical Biophysics, University of Toronto, Toronto, Ontario, Canada M4X 1K9.

INTRODUCTION. The mouse immunoglobulin M (IgM) has been extensively studied at
both the DNA and protein level. We have selected this system as a model to study
glycoprotein biosynthesis and processing. The IgM heavy chain (μ) has five
homology domains: one variable (V), and four constant (C); followed by a "C"
terminal segment.   μ contains five glycosylation sites.   The carbohydrate
structures at each glycosylation site have been determined. The structures of the
carbohydrates show a gradient of processing with the NH_2-terminal having more
complex, and the COOH-terminal more simple, oligosaccharides.   Initial
glycosylation is a co-translational event. Final oligosaccharide processing
occurs in the Golgi apparatus. The observed complexity of the carbohydrate
structures on IgM and other glycoproteins indicates the requirement for a unique
system for their biosynthesis. Mutations that alter the μ chain can provide
information about regulation of the final glycosylation patterns on the protein.
    We present gene mapping and glycoprotein characterization of mutant cell lines
which secrete abnormal heavy chains.   The delineation of their structural
differences at the carbohydrate and protein levels is reported.

RESULTS. Biosynthetically labeled μ chains from mutant and wild type cells were
analyzed on SDS-PAGE under reducing conditions. Mutants 21 and 38 synthesize heavy
chains with slower than normal mobility. Mutant 562 presents a faster mobility
when compared to normal PC 700. The increase in molecular weight in 21 and 38 has
been shown to be due to hyperglycosylation (1). The 562 mutant chain is missing
portions of the constant domain. In further attempts to define the differences in
glycosylation of the μ chains, intracellular heavy chains from PC 700, 21, 38 and
562 were compared. Immunoprecipitated ^{35}S-methionine μ from all cell lines except
562, presented identical mobilities and endoglycosidase sensitivities in SDS-PAGE.
Treating the secreted IgM with endoglycosidase H shows that the hyperglycosylated
product has processed all the glycosylation sites to complex oligosaccharides. The
mutation appears to lead to an increase in carbohydrate processing. Studies of the
deletion mutants allow us to see how a change in the protein leads to alterations
in carbohydrate processing.

    To examine the gene structures of mutant cell lines, cellular DNA was digested
with restriction endonucleases and analyzed by Southern blots.   Hybridization
analysis of Eco RI digests using a Cμ probe gave the same molecular weight fragment
of 9.9 kb as expected for wild type cells. Bam HI restriction enzyme cleaves Cμ
into two fragments. Thus to assess changes at the 3' end of the molecule, cellular
DNA was treated with Bam HI. The presence of a 12.5 kb fragment on all cells
confirmed the conservation of the gene's 3' end.

DISCUSSION. Table 1 summarizes the mutant characteristics. The approach taken
is at both gene product and gene mapping level. Mutants 21 and 38 secrete
hyperglycosylated μ chains. Analysis of intracellular heavy chains shows that
these are normally glycosylated. This indicates that the increase in molecular
weight in the secreted form is not due to an extra glycosylation site, but rather
to a change in the carbohydrate processing.   Mutants which present
hyperglycosylated μ chains fail to secrete pentamers. It is not known whether
hyperglycosylation itself blocks pentamer formation. Mutant 562 produces a μ chain
with lower than normal molecular weight. This appears to be due to loss of one or
more constant domains (Figure 1). As with other mutants, 562 μ chain is released
as monomers and dimers, but some pentamer is also synthesized. Experiments are in
progress to examine the oligosaccharide structures at each glycosylation site.
Genetic mapping analysis indicates that none of these mutants have a major gene
change. However, Southern blots may not detect a point mutation. IgM deletions
may be the product of the introduction of a stop codon caused by a single base
change. Hyperglycosylation may be caused by a change in the cellular glycosylation
system.

SUMMARY. We have studied hybridoma cell lines which secrete altered IgM heavy chains. The analysis includes both genetic mapping and glycoprotein characterization. Recombinant DNA techniques were used to determine gene rearrangements. Comparison of mutant cells with wild type restriction enzyme mapping and Southern blots, indicate that the C_μ gene does not have a major gene change. While their intracellular forms present normal glycosylation, secreted μ chains from 21 and 38 mutant cells are retarded in their migration on SDS-PAGE. This difference is due to hyperglycosylation. Mutant 562 secretes a smaller than normal μ chain. A portion of C_μ is missing in this chain. Contrary to wild type cells, mutants produce IgM mainly as monomers and dimers. 562 secretes some pentamers as well.

REFERENCE. Shulman,M. et al., Mol.Cell.Biol. 2, 1033-1043, 1982.

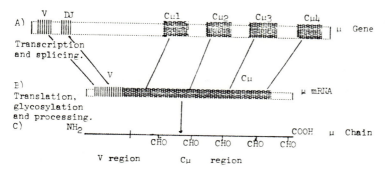

Figure 1. Schematic drawing of μ heavy chain. A) In the gene, the variable region (V) is formed by 3 gene segments V, D, and J interrupted by non-coding sequences (introns). The constant region (C μ) lies about 8 kb from the J segment. B) In the RNA, Cμ coding gene sequences (Cμ1 to Cμ4) are separated by introns. The transcriptional unit is a copy of the gene as shown, but the non-coding sequences are removed by splicing events which lead to a continuous coding sequence in the μ mRNA. C) On the protein, μ chain has 5 glycosylation sites. Each site has a specific set of oligosaccharide structures. There is a gradient of carbohydrate processing from the NH$_2$-terminal end to the COOH-terminus.

TABLE 1. SUMMARY OF MUTANT CHARACTERISTICS

Cell line	M.W. intra cellular	Chain extra	IgM secreted form	Cμ gene mapping
PC700 (wild type)	Normal	Normal	Pentamer	Normal
21 mutant	Normal	Hyperglycosylated	Dimer and Monomer	Normal
38 mutant	Normal	Hyperglycosylated	Dimer and Monomer	Normal
562 mutant	Deletion	Deletion	Pentamer, Dimer and Monomer	Normal

STUDIES OF THE HUMAN TRANSFERRIN GENE, Funmei Yang, J.B. Lum, John R. McGill, Charleen M. Moore, Peter H. van Bragt, W. David Baldwin and Barbara H. Bowman, Department of Anatomy - Division of Genetics, The University of Texas Health Science Center at San Antonio, San Antonio, Texas 78284.

Transferrin, the major iron binding protein in vertebrate serum, transports iron absorbed from the diet to the bone marrow and to all proliferating cells in the body (1). There is a family of transferrin-like proteins that bind iron. Lactoferrin is present in mammalian secretions, including milk (2). Ovotransferrin is synthesized in the chicken oviduct and appears to be controlled by the same gene as chicken serum transferrin (3). Melanoma antigen p97 is a membrane protein present on all human malignant melanoma cells (4). Two oncogenes found in chicken lymphoma DNA and in Burkitt's lymphoma DNA encode transforming proteins with strong homologies to the amino terminal sequence of human serum transferrin (5,6). Transferrin, ovotransferrin and lactotransferrin each have amino and carboxyl domains which share approximately 40% identity in their sequences. Structural evidence suggests that the transferrin-like proteins are products of gene duplications which occurred in vertebrates. The original gene is thought to have arisen in a pro-chordate ancestor. The ancient gene was probably the size of one domain or one-half the size of the present iron binding proteins. Antigen p97 and the transferrin receptor gene have been mapped to human chromosome 3 (8,9).

The goal of the study described here was to initiate study of the expression of the transferrin-like proteins by identifying, characterizing and mapping the human transferrin gene.

Recombinant plasmids containing human complementary DNA encoding transferrin (Tf) have been isolated by screening an adult human liver library with a synthesized oligonucleotide (7). One cDNA clone contained the coding for the entire transferrin sequence. A 19 amino acid leader sequence was deduced and found to be 56% homologous to the leader sequence of chicken ovotransferrin. The N and C domains of transferrin are homologous but reflect independent evolution in that 50% of codons specifying identical amino acid residues in the two domains differ in at least one nucleotide base. The duplicated gene product from this ancient intragenic amplification contrasts with that of a recent duplication, the $Hp\alpha^2$ gene, which arose in human populations and reflects a diversity of 3.6% in codons for the same amino acids in homologous domains.

Genomic clones from a human liver library have now been isolated that contain 27 and 11 kb inserts. The gene organization is being studied by the method of heteroduplex mapping. Introns from the transferrin gene are being studied by restriction endonuclease analysis of DNA fragments.

The *Tf* gene appears to map on chromosome 3 (7) which also carries genes encoding the melanoma antigen p97 and the transferrin receptor, presenting the possibility that not only the transferrin-like protein family but also their respective receptors may have a common evolutionary origin (1).

REFERENCES

1. Williams, J. 1982. *Trends Biochem. Sci.* 7, 394-397.
2. Metz-Boutique, M.H., Mazurier, J., Jollés, J., Spik, G., Montrevil, J. and Jollés, P. 1981. *Biochim. Biophys. Acta* 670, 243-254.
3. Cochet, M., Perrin, F., Gannon, F., Krust, A., Chambon, P., McKnight, G.S., Lee, D.C., Mayo, K.E. and Palmiter, R.D. 1979. *Nucleic Acids Res.* 6, 2435-2452.
4. Brown, J.P., Hewick, R.M., Hellström, K.E., Doolittle, R.F. and Dreyer, W.J. 1982. *Nature* 296, 171-173.
5. Goubin, G., Goldman, D.S., Luce, J., Neiman, P.E. and Cooper, G.M. 1983. *Nature* 302, 114-119.
6. Diamond, A., Cooper, G.M., Ritz, J. and Lane, M.A. 1983. *Nature* 305, 112-116.
7. Yang, F., Lum, J.B., McGill, J.R., Moore, C.M., van Bragt, P.H. and Baldwin, W.D. and Bowman, B.H. (submitted).
8. Enns, C.A., Suomaloinen, H.A., Gebhardt, J.E., Schroder, J. and Sussman, H.H. 1982. *Proc. Natl. Acad. Sci.* 79, 3241-3245.
9. Plowman, G.D., Brown, J.P., Enns, C.A., Schroder, J., Nikinmaa, B., Sussman, H.H., Hellström, K.E., Hellström, I. 1983. *Nature* 303, 70-71.

NONRADIOACTIVE COLONY HYBRIDIZATION.

Huey-Lang Yang and Norman Kelker.

Enzo Biochem, Inc., 325 Hudson Street, New York, NY 10013

Procedures for nonradioactive colony hybridization have been developed. Bacterial colonies, either imprinted or grown on a membrane matrix, were lysed and hybridized. Hybridization/ detection procedures (Langer et al., 1981) were employed using biotinylated DNA probes labeled by terminal transferase catalyzed addition of 2'-deoxyuridine 5'-triphosphate 5-allylamine biotin (Bio-11-dUTP). Detection was based on the binding of a protein complex (formed from streptavidin, a biotin binding protein, and biotinylated horseradish peroxidase) to hybridized, biotinylated DNA. Subsequent addition of the appropriate substrates yielded a colored precipitate. Using Col El::Tn3 DNA as a probe for amp^r (ampicillin resistance), amp^r and amp^s strains of Escherichia coli and Neisseria gonorrhoea were differentiated. Amp^r strains could be easily resolved from amp^s strains even when present as sectored colonies on crowded plates. As few as 10^7 amp^r E. coli cells (not treated for plasmid amplification) could be detected employing only one hour of hybridization. This method thus provides speed, safety, sensitivity and high resolution for genetic characterization of bacteria.

Langer, P.R., A. Waldrop and D. Ward (1981) Proc. Natl. Acad. Sci., U.S.A., 68, 6633.

MOLECULAR CLONING OF MAMMALIAN ADENOSINE DEAMINASE GENE SEQUENCES THROUGH GENE AMPLIFICATION

C.Y. Yeung*, D.E. Ingolia*, M.R. Al-Ubaidi*, A.G. Hook*, D.A. Wright[+], E.G. Frayne* and R.E. Kellems*

*Dept. of Biochemistry, Baylor College of Medicine and [+]Dept. of Genetics, M.D. Anderson Hospital and Tumor Institute, Houston, TX 77030

INTRODUCTION. Both genetic (1) and pharmacological (2) evidence has established that adenosine deaminase (ADA) deficiency invariably leads to severe depletion of both T and B lymphocytes in humans. In order to study the genetic defects associated with this form of genetic disorder, it is essential to isolate mammalian ADA cDNA sequences. We demonstrate here the successful isolation of both mouse and human ADA gene sequences. Mouse ADA sequences were isolated through the genetic enrichment of the ADA gene via gene amplification.

MATERIALS AND METHODS. The isolation of a mouse cell line, B-1/25, which overproduces ADA by ~3200-fold over parental Cl-1D cells has been previously described (3). A cDNA library complementary to total poly(A$^+$) RNA derived from the B-1/25 cells was constructed. The initial screening of both Northern blots and the cDNA library was accomplished using prehybridized single-stranded ^{32}P-labeled cDNA synthesized using B-1/25 poly(A$^+$) RNA as template. Non-amplified ^{32}P-labeled cDNA probe sequences were removed by prehybridization with a 2500-fold mass excess of parental (Cl-1D) derived RNA.

RESULTS. RNA blot analysis. Poly(A$^+$) RNA derived from both B-1/25 and Cl-1D cells was analyzed by blot analysis following electrophoresis in an agarose gel. The blot was probed with the prehybridized ^{32}P-labeled cDNA described above. The result (Fig. 1A) showed that three poly(A$^+$) RNA species (with sizes of 1.5, 1.7 and 5.2 kb, respectively) were overproduced in the B-1/25 cells. One cDNA clone, pADA600, derived from the B-1/25 cDNA library was identified using the prehybridized ^{32}P-labeled cDNA probe and was found to contain amplified gene sequences. This clone was radio-labeled and used to probe a RNA blot similar to the one used in Fig. 1A. The result (Fig. 1B) showed that the pADA600 clone hybridized to the same three mRNA species identified in Fig. 1A and is thus a likely ADA cDNA candidate.

Verification of pADA600 as an ADA cDNA clone. In order to prove that pADA600 contained mouse ADA gene sequences, the plasmid DNA was immobilized on nitrocellulose filters and used to hybridization-select homologous mRNA in the B-1/25 mRNA population. The hybridization-selected mRNA was translated by microinjection into Xenopus oocytes, and the translation products were identified by starch gel electrophoresis followed by histochemical staining for ADA activity. Plasmid pADA600 was found to hybridize with mouse ADA mRNA while a non-crosshybridizing control clone p5-72 did not. This established that pADA600 contained mouse ADA gene sequences.

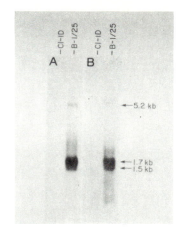

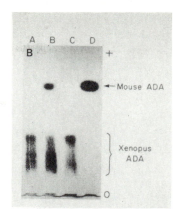

Fig. 1. (A) Northern blot of Cl-1D and B-1/25 poly(A⁺) RNA was analyzed using pre-hybridized ^{32}P-labeled cDNA as probe. (B) A similar blot analyzed using ^{32}P-labeled pADA600 as probe.

Fig. 2. ADA zymogram analysis of Xenopus oocyte translation products. Lane C contains uninjected oocyte lysate. Lane D contains mouse cell homogenate as a mouse ADA standard. Lanes B and A display oocyte translation products of mRNA "hybridization-selected" using plasmids pADA600 and p5-72, respectively.

Isolation of other mouse and human ADA cDNA clones. Clone pADA600 was used to identify 22 other mouse ADA clones. One of these clones (pCAM7-100) was found to contain an insert of ~1.8 kb and may contain the entire coding region of the mouse ADA mRNA. The longer (>1 kb) mouse ADA clones were found by Northern and Southern analysis to crosshybridize with human ADA gene sequences. By using one of these mouse ADA cDNA clones as a probe, 11 probable human ADA cDNA clones have been isolated from a human liver cDNA library.

DISCUSSION. The ease with which both mouse and human ADA cDNA was cloned here clearly shows genetic enrichment via gene amplification to be a powerful approach to cloning genes coding for relatively low-abundance mRNA species. The cloned ADA gene sequences reported here should soon lead to a clear understanding and possible cure (through gene replacement therapy) of genetic ADA deficiency in man.

References. (1) Giblett, E.R. et al. (1972) Lancet ii, 1067-1069; (2) Smyth, J.F. et al. (1978) Cancer Chemother. Pharmacol. 1, 49-51; (3) Yeung, C.Y. et al. (1983) J. Biol. Chem. 258, 8338-8345

Author Index

(invited speakers' names are in **bold**)

Aaronson, S.A. (145)
Adlakha, R. (224)
Al-Ubaidi, M.R. (270)
Annab, L. (254)
Arrand, J. (126)
Atherton, S.S. (128)

Baldwin, W.D. (266)
Banerji, J. (48)
Banks, A. (130)
Bardin, C.W. (190)
Barker, D. (86)
Baro, D.J. (132)
Barret, K. (180)
Barrett, J.C. (254)
Barths, J. (192)
Beckett, M.L. (236)
Beckmann, P. (264)
Beecroft, L.J. (134)
Bernstein, A. (222)
Beyreuther, K. (258)
Birnster, R.L. (52)
Birshtein, B.K. (22)
Blaxter, M. (94)
Bleskan, J. (152)
Blin, N. (192)
Bloom, A.L. (216)
Boggs, B.A. (136)
Boshart, M. (48)
Bower, J.R. (138)
Bowman, B.H. (266)
Boyd, D. (180)
Bradshaw, H. (154)
Brakel, C. (219)
Bresser, J. (108)
Breyel, E. (202)
Brizzard, B.L. (210)
Brousseau, R. (240)
Brown, M.S. (104)
Brownlee, G.G. (216)
Burt, D.W. (134)

Caillol, D. (67)
Campbell, A.E. (236)
Carr, B.I. (32)
Carradonna, S. (154)
Case, S.T. (138)
Caskey, C.T. (90)

Chaganti, R.S.K. (182)
Chan, R. (226)
Cherbas, L. (230)
Cherbas, P. (230)
Chinault, A.C. (90)
Chiu, I. (141)
Cho-Chung, Y.S. (142)
Chung, D.W. (100)
Clark, J.C. (160)
Cohen, D. (144)
Coleman, M.S. (208)
Cooper, G.M. (3)
Crampton, J. (180)
Crawford, B.D. (238)
Cummings, M.R. (132, 260)
Cutroneo, K.R. (243)

Damotte, M. (67)
Daniels, G.R. (146)
Dausset, J. (144)
Davidson, A.A. (148)
Davidson, J.N. (148)
Davie, E.W. (100)
Davies, B.L. (216)
Davies, K. (94)
Davis, L.M. (150)
Davis, R.E. (152)
Deak, S. (156)
Degen, S.J.F. (100)
Deininger, P.L. (146, 154)
Delovitch, T.L. (67)
de Villiers, J. (48)
Dickson, L.A. (156)
Dickson, R.C. (208)
Dilella, A.G. (188, 198)
Dinh, Y.T. (158)
Drayna, D. (86)
Drobetsky, E. (126)
Drysdale, J. (180)
Duband, J.L. (250)
Dubreuil, J. (67)
Dush, M.K. (160)

Eckhardt, L. (22)
Edenberg, H.J. (162)
Eng, C.E.L. (244)
Erlich, H.A. (164)